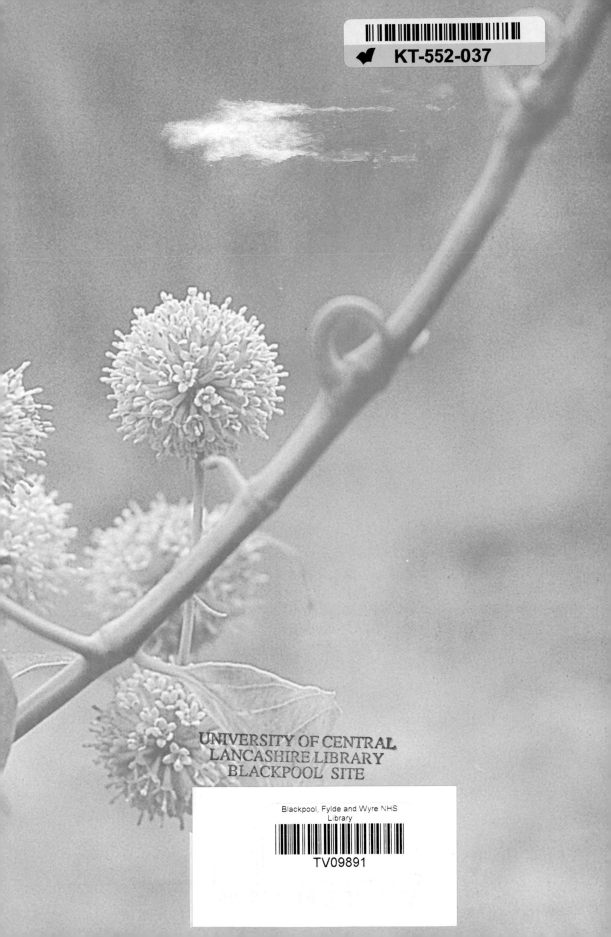

Vol. 1

International

Collation

of

Traditional

and

Folk Medicine

NORTHEAST
ASIA

Part I

International Collation of Folk and Traditional Medicine

Vol. 1　　　　　　A project of UNESCO　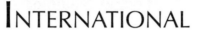

INTERNATIONAL

COLLATION

OF

TRADITIONAL

AND

FOLK MEDICINE

Editor-in-Chief

Takeatsu Kimura
Daiichi College of Pharmaceutical Sciences

Editors

Paul P. H. But
The Chinese University of Hong Kong

Ji-Xian Guo
Shanghai Medical University

Chung Ki Sung
Chonnam National University

NORTHEAST ASIA

Part I

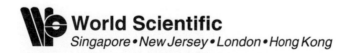 **World Scientific**
Singapore • New Jersey • London • Hong Kong

Published by

World Scientific Publishing Co Pte Ltd
P O Box 128, Farrer Road, Singapore 912805
USA office: Suite 1B, 1060 Main Street, River Edge, NJ 07661
UK office: 57 Shelton Street, Covent Garden, London WC2H 9HE

Library of Congress Cataloging-in-Publication Data
Northeast Asia / editors, Takeatsu Kimura . . . [et al.].
        p.   cm. -- (International collation of traditional and folk medicine ; vol. 1)
     "A project under the aegis of UNESCO."
     Includes bibliographical references and index.
     ISBN 981022589X
     1. Materia medica, Vegetable -- East Asia.   2. Medicinal plants -- East Asia.
3. Traditional medicine -- East Asia.   I. Kimura, Takeatsu.   II. UNESCO.
III. Series.
     [DNLM: 1. Medicine, Herbal.   2. Plants, Medicinal -- chemistry.
3. Plant Extracts -- therapeutic use.   4. Drug Design.
5. International Cooperation.   WB 925 N874 1996]
RS180.E18N67   1996
615'.321'095--dc20   96-4659
DNLM/DLC   CIP
for Library of Congress

British Library Cataloguing-in-Publication Data
A catalogue record for this book is available from the British Library.

Front cover: Cornus officinalis (p. 108).
Shan-zhu-yu (C), San-tsue-yue (H), San-shu-yu (J), San-su-yu (K).

Back cover: Uncaria rhynchophylla (p. 134).
Gou-teng (C), Ngou-teng (H), Kagikazura (J).

Printed in Singapore.

FOREWORD

The plant floras in China, Hong Kong, Japan, and Korea — located nearly in the same temperature zone — share much similarity with the result that traditional folk medical experiences in this region are comparable in nature. Nonetheless, since folk medical experience in different countries have been developed rather independently each with a long history, both similarities and differences coexist in traditional folk medical knowledge from different countries.

Folk medical knowledge may be regarded as clinical experience obtained naturally. However, part of the experience might be mythical reflecting regional differences in culture. The task of separating fact from myth and isolating placebo-effects from objective bioactivity in folk and traditional medicines is a difficult one. We believe that when folk medical experiences derived from the same plant are collated comparatively the real medical effects associated with plant bioactivity will emerge. From this perspective, an international collation of folk medical knowledge should help in establishing objective and reliable medical experience.

The search for bioactive components from plants as a source of lead compounds in drug development, is a major endeavor in phytochemical research. This book is aimed at assisting phytochemists to identify the plant species which most likely contain bioactive components of interest and which may warrant further investigation.

The folk medical knowledge of each entry in the book includes the botanical and local names of the drug, special processing involved, method used for administration, apparent folk medical efficacy in each country, contra-indications and side effects. Also included is the information concerning modern scientific data relating to the associated chemistry and pharmacology as well as references to the available literature.

The first volume covers the outcome generated by the "international collaborating project" propelled by the Regional Network for the Chemistry of Natural Products in Southeast Asia, operated by the United Nations Educational, Scientific and Cultural Organization (UNESCO). The Ministry of Education, Republic of Korea has kindly provided financial support for this ongoing project. On behalf of the Managing Board, I am most grateful to Professor T. Kimura, the *Editor-in-Chief* of volume I, and other members of the editorial board who undertook the painstaking job of making a literature survey, as well as writing and editing this volume. My sincere gratitude is also extended to the UNESCO Office, Jakarta (ROSTSEA) and the Korean National Commission for UNESCO for their valuable help in the planning and organizing this project.

Byung Hoon Han, Prof., Ph.D.
Chairman, Managing Board

v

CONTENTS

xii

EXPLANATIONS AND ABBREVIATIONS

Plant Name
Two hundred important medicinal plants are presented in this volume. The sequence of the plant families follows the classification and arrangement of plant families of Engler's system[1] and the sequence of the individual species in a family follows the alphabetical order of their scientific names. Synonyms are shown as (=). Each representative vernacular name is shown in Roman script followed by an abbreviation of a country/region name.[2] Chinese characters of the herb and plant names are shown in the "Chinese Character Index." Related plants are shown in similar manner.

Part
Pharmacopoeias which adopt a particular herb are shown in abbreviations.[3] Local drug names are the standard or representative vernacular names for that particular herb.

Processing
Procedures for processing the crude drug.

Method of Administration
Routes of administration and preparation methods.

Folk Medicinal Use
Names of diseases or symptoms treated with the herb, followed by an abbreviation of the country which uses the herb for that purpose.

Contra-indications and Side Effects
Warnings for conditions to be avoided in the application of a particular herb and adverse reactions that may be induced by the herb.

---

[1] H. Melchior, E. Werdermann: "A. Engler's Syllabus der Pflanzenfamilien" 12 Aufl., 1 band (1954), 2 band (1964), Gerbrüder Borntraeger, Berlin.

[2] C: China, H: Hong Kong, J: Japan, K: Korea.

[3] CP: Zhong-hua Ren-min Gong-he-guo Yao-dian (Pharmacopoeia of the People's Republic of China) **1990**, Beijing, China.
JP: Dai 12 Kaisei Nihon Yakkyokuho (The Pharmacopoeia of Japan, 12th ed) **1991**, Tokyo, Japan.
KR: Je Yook Gae-Jung Daihan Yak Jeun (The Korea Pharmacopoeia, Sixth Revision), Seoul, Korea.

Scientific Research

Chemical components and pharmacology reported before 1993 are summarized.

Literature

Format of the literature citation is as follows: First author, *journal title or book title* (in italics), **year** (boldface), volume, and first page.

1. *Digenea simplex* C. Agardh   (Rhodomelaceae)

Hai–ren–cao (C), Makuri, Kaininso (J), Hae–In–Cho (K)

Whole plant (JP, KP)
Local Drug Name: Zhe–gu–cai (C); Makuri, Kai–nin–so (J); Hae–In–Cho (K).
Processing: Air dry.
Administration: Oral (decoction: C, J, K).
Folk Medicinal Uses:
        1) Parasitic diseases (ascaris) (C, J, K).
Side Effects: Temporary abdominal pain, diarrhea, nausea, vomitting, xanthopsia or tinnitis.

Scientific Researches:
  Chemistry
    1) Amino acid: α–kainic acid, α–allokainic acid [1].
  Pharmacology
    1) Anthelmintic (α–kainic acid) [2,3].

Literatures:
[1] Murakami, S. et al.:*Yakugaku Zasshi* **1953,** 73, 1026, 1055; **1955**, 75, 866, 869; Miyazaki, M. et al.:
   ibid. **1955**, 75, 693; Ueno, Y. et al.:*ibid.* **1955**, 75, 807; Morimoto, H.:*ibid.* **1955**, 75, 901.
[2] Aoki, D.: *Keio Igaku* **1936**, 16, 1255.
[3] Tamura, S.: *Yakugaku Zasshi* **1955**, 75, 283.

[T. Kimura]

2. *Coriolus versicolor* Quel.   (Polyporaceae)

Yun–zhi (C), Won–gee (H), Kawaratake (J), Un–ji–beo–seot (K)

Fruiting body
Local Drug Name: Yun–zhi (C), Won–gee (H); Kawara–take (J); Un–ji (K).
Processing: Dry under the sun (J, K).
Method of Administration: Oral (decoction: H, J, K).
Folk Medicinal Uses:
        1) Gastric cancer (J, K).
        2) Heart disorder (J, K).
        3) Pyrexia (J).
        4) Leukopenia in radio– & chemotherapy (H).
        5) Heptidis (C).
Scientific Researches:
  Chemistry
    1) Glycoproteins: PSK (krestin) [1, 8].
    2) Glucopeptides: PSP [3, 12, 15, 17].
    3) Polysaccharides: coriolan [2,7].
  Pharmacology
    1) Antitumor activity (PSK) [1, 4, 12, 17].
    2) Immunostimulant action (PSK) [3, 12, 15, 17].
    3) Competitive effect against immunosuppressive factor [5].
    4) Stimulation of macrophage function [6].
    5) Antimutagenic action [7].
    6) Inhibition of HIV infection (in vitro) [8].

7) Inhibition of reverse transcriptase (in vitro) [9].
8) Prevention of acute radiation injury [10].
9) Angiogenesis inhibition [11].
10) Stimulation of human peripheral blood polymorphonuclear cell iodination (PSK) [13].
11) Anti–injurious effects (PSK) [16].

Literatures:
[1] Muto, S. et al.:*Proc. Int. Congr. Chemother., 13th,* **1983,** 17, 287/37.
[2] Takahashi, H. et al.:*Jpn. Kokai Tokkyo Koho,* 79 59,398, 12 May **1979.**
[3] Seo, S. et al.:*Agent Actions* **1979,** 9, 344.
[4] Ito, H. et al.:*Japanese J. Pharmacol.* **1979,** 29, 953.
[5] Matsunaga, K. et al.:*Gan to Kagaku Ryoho* **1980,** 7, 496.
[6] Saito, H. et al.:*Igaku to Seibutsugaku* **1984,** 108, 193.
[7] Hang, B. et al.:*Nanjing Yaoxueyuan Xuebao* **1986,** 17, 305.
[8] Tochikura, T. et al.:*Biochem. Biophys. Res. Commun.* **1987,** 148, 726.
[9] Hirose, K. et al.: *Biochem. Biophys. Res. Commun.* **1987,** 149, 562.
[10] Patchen, M. et al.: *Comments Toxicol.* **1988,** 2, 217.
[11] Kanoh, T. et al.:*Eur. Pat. Appl. EP* 353,861, 07, Feb. **1990.**
[12] Yang, Q.: *Faming Zhuanli Shenqing Gongkai Shuomingshu* CN 1,034,957, 23, Aug. **1989.**
[13] Sakagami, H. et al.:*Anticancer Res.* **1990,** 10, 697.
[14] Ren, H. et al.:*Ziran Zazhi* **1990,** 13, 255.
[15] Li, X. et al.:*Zhongguo Yaoli Xuebao* **1990,** 11, 542.
[16] Wu, G. et al.:*Zhongguo Yaoke Daxue Xuebao* **1991,** 22, 301.
[17] Yang, Q. Y. et al.:*EOS–Riv. Immunol. Immunofarmacol.* **1992,** 12, 29.

[C.K. Sung]

3   *Ganoderma lucidum* **(Leyss. ex Fr.) Karst.**   (Polyporaceae)

Ling–zhi(C), Ling–gee (H), Mannentake (J), Young–ji–beo–seot (K)

Fruiting body
Local Drug Name: Ling–zhi (C), Ling–gee (H), Rei–shi (J), Young–ji (K).
Processing: Dry in the shade (C, H), dry under the sun (J, K).
Method of Administration: Oral (water extract: C, H, J, K),(powder: C).
Folk Medicinal Uses:

        1) Hepatitis (J, K).
        2) Cough (C, H).
        3) Insomnia (C, H, J).
        4) Neurasthenia (C, H).
        5) Indigestion (C, H).
        6) Asthma (C, H).
        7) Tumor (J, K).
        8) Weakness (J, K).
        9) Debility (H).
        10) Climacterium disorder (J).
        11) Dyspepsia (C, J).

Scientific Researches:
Chemistry
  1) Triterpenes: Ganoderic acid A, B [1], C[5], D, E [7], G, I [8], T, V, W, X, Y, Z [2, 3], F, H [10],
             lucidenic acid A, B, C [5], D, E [7], F [10], lucidone A, B [7], ganolucidic acid A, B [8],

ganoderenic acid A, B, C, D, E, F, G [14], ganoderal A, ganoderol A, B [15].
2) Polysaccharides: Ganoderan A, B4 [11], C, D [16], ganoderan I [13].
3) Inorganics: Ca, Mg, Na, Mn, Fe, Zn, Ge [6].
4) Nucleosides: adenosine [9].
5) Proteins: LZ–81 [7].
6) Steroids: Ergosta–7,22–dien–3–yl–linoleate [18].
Pharmacology
1) Antitumor activity [12, 19].
2) Immunostimulating activity [17, 19].
3) Inhibition of platelet aggregation (adenosine) [9, 20].
4) Cytotoxic activity against hepatoma cell (ganoderic acid U–Z) [2, 3, 18].
5) Inhibitionof angiotensin converting enzyme (ganoderal A) [15].

Literatures:

[1] Kubota, T. et al.:*Helv. Chim. Acta* **1982,** 65, 611.
[2] Toth, J. O. et al.: *Tetrahedron Lett.* **1983,** 24, 1081.
[3] Toth, J. L. et al.:*J. Chem. Res.,* **1983,** 299.
[4] Wang, C. et al.:*Linchan Huaxue Yu Gongye,* **1984,** 4(3), 42.
[5] Nishitoba, T. et al.:*Argic. Biol. Chem.* **1985,** 49(6), 1793.
[6] Shin, H. W. et al.:*Han'guk Kyunhakhoechi,* **1985,** 13(1), 53.
[7] Nishitoba, T. et al.:*Agric. Biol. Chem.* **1985,** 49(5), 1547.
[8] Kikuchi, T. et al.:*Chem. Pharm. Bull.* **1985,** 33(6), 2628.
[9] Shimizu, A. et al.:*Chem. Pharm. Bull.* **1985,** 33(7), 3012.
[10] Nishitoba, T. et al.:*Agric. Biol. Chem.* **1984,** 48(11), 2905.
[11] Hikino, H. et al.:*Planta Med.,* **1985**(4), 339.
[12] Mizuno, T. et al.:*Nippon Nogei Kagku Kaishi,* **1985,** 59(11), 1143.
[13] Misaki, A. et al.:*Japan Kokai Tokkyo Koho* JP 60,188,402, 25 Sep. **1985.**
[14] Komoda, Y. et al.:*Chem. Pharm. Bull.* **1985,** 33(11), 4829.
[15] Morigiwa, A. et al.:*Chem. Pharm. Bull.* **1986,** 34(7), 3025.
[16] Tomoda, M. et al.:*Phytochemistry* **1986,** 25(12), 2817.
[17] Kino, K. et al.:*J. Biol. Chem.* **1989,** 264(1), 472–8.
[18] Lin, C. N. et al.:*J. Nat. Prod.* **1991,** 54(4), 998.
[19] Lee, K. H. et al.: *PCT Int. Appl.* WO 92 10,202, 25 Jun. **1992.**
[20] Kawagishi, H. et al.:*Phytochemistry* **1993,** 32(2), 239–41(1993)

[C.K. Sung]

4.   *Polyporus umbellatus* Fries   (Polyporaceae)

Zhu–ling (C), Tsue–ling (H), Choreimaitake (J), Jeo–Ryung (K)

Sclerotium   (CP, JP, KP)
Local drug name: Zhu–ling (C), Tsue–ling (H), Cho–rei (J), Jeo–Ryung (K).
Processing: Air dry.
Administration: Oral (decoction: C, H, J, K).
Folk Medicinal Uses:
1) Edema (C, H, J, K).
2) Urethritis (J).
3) Oliguria or dysuria (C, H, J).
4) Diarrhea (C, H, J).
5) Excessive leukorrhea (C, H).
6) Beriberi (H).

Side Effects: Dehydration on over dosis.

Scientific Researches:
Chemistry:
  1) Steroids: Ergosterol and its derivatives [1].
  2) Fatty acids: α–hydroxyteracosanoic acid [2].
  3) Polysaccharides [3].
Pharmacology:
  1) Platelet coagulation (ergosterol derivertive) [1].
  2) Diuretic (water extract) [4–7].
  3) Antitumor (polysaccharides) [8].

Literatures:
[1] Lu, W. et al.:*Chem. Pharm. Bull.* **1985**, 33, 5083.
[2] Yosioka, I. et al.:*Yakugaku Zasshi* **1964,** 84, 742.
[3] Miyazaki, T. et al.:*Carbohydrate Res.* **1979**, 69, 165; Y. Ueno, et al.:*ibid.* **1982**, 101, 160.
[4] Tsurumi, S. et al.:*Gifu Ikadaigaku Kiyo***1963**, 11, 129; Haginiwa, T. et al.:*Shoyakugaku Zasshi* **1963**, 17, 6.
[5] Yamaguchi, I.:*Chosen Igakkai Zasshi***1928**, 86, 173.
[6] Wang, R. et al.:*Yaoxue Xuebao* **1964**, 11, 815.
[7] Aburada, M.:*Hinyo Kiyo* **1981**, 27, 677.
[8] Miyazaki, T. et al.:*Carbohydr. Res.* **1978**, 65, 235.

[T. Kimura]

5.   ***Poria cocos* Wolf** (= *Pachyma hoelen* Rumph.)   (Polyporaceae)

Fu–ling (C), Fuk–ling (H), Matsuhodo (J), Bok–Ryung (K)

Sclerotium   (CP, JP, KP)
Local Drug Name: Fu–ling (C), Fuk–ling (H), Buku–ryo (J), Bok–Ryung (K)
Processing: Steam briefly after soften in water, separate the skin immediately and cut into pieces then dry
           (C). Air dry after removing skin (J).
Method of Administration: Oral (decoction: C, H, J, K).
Folk Medicinal Uses:
              1) Edema (C, H, J, K).
              2) Urinary tract diseases (C, H, J).
              3) Dysuria (H).
              4) Anxiety neurosis (C, J, K).
              5) Pain (J).
              6) Weakness (C, J, K).
              7) Diarrhea (C, H, J, K).
              8) Sputum (H).
              9) Spermatorrhea (H).
              10) Hiccup (H).
              11) Infantile epilepsy (H).

Scientific Researches:
Chemistry
  1) Polysaccharides: pachyman [1].
  2) Triterpenoids: eburicoic acid, pachymic acid [2].
  3) Steroids: ergosterol [1].

Pharmacology
  1) Diuretic (water extract) [3,4].
  2) Antiulcer effect (water extract) [5,6].
  3) Blood sugar depression (water and ethanol extract) [7].

Literatures:

[1] Narui, T. et al.: *Carbohydr. Res.* **1980**, 87, 161; Kanayama, H. et al.:*Yakugaku Zasshi* **1986,** 106, 199, 206.
[2] Shibata, S. et al.: *Chem. Pharm. Bull.* **1958**, 6, 608; Kanematsu, A. et al.:*Yakugaku Zasshi* **1970**, 90, 475; Natori, S.:*Gendai Toyo Igaku* **1986**, 7, 66.
[3] Yamaguchi, I.: *Chosen Igakkaishi,* **1928,** No.86, 173; Haginiwa, T. et al.:*Shoyakugaku Zasshi* **1963**, 17, 6; Tsurumi, S. et al.:*Gifu Univ. Med. Kiyo* **1963**, 129; Uchizumi, S. et al.:*Jap. J. Oriental Med.* **1953**, 3(2)–4(1), 1.
[4] Tanaka, S. et al.: *Yakugaku Zasshi* **1984**, 104, 601.
[5] Tomisawa, S.:*Jap. J. Oriental Med.* **1962**, 13, 5.
[6] Yamasaki, M. et al.:*Shoyakugaku Zasshi* **1981**, 35, 96.
[7] Min, H.: *Nippon Yakubutsugaku Zasshi* **1930**, 11, 22, 181.

[T. Kimura]

6.   *Blechum orientale* **L.**   (Blechnaceae)

Wu–mao–jue (C), Woo–mo–kuet (H), Hiryushida (J).

Rhizome
  Local Drug Name: Wu–mao–guan–zhong (C), Goon–jong (H).
  Processing: Dry under the sun (C).
  Method of Administration: Oral (decoction: C).
  Folk Medicinal Uses:
              1) Influenza (C, H).
              2) Parotitis (C, H).
              3) Artificial abortion (C).
              4) Postpartum hemorrhage (C).

Scientific Researches:
  Chemistry
    1) Organic acids: chlorogenic acid [1].
    2) Steroids: sterol [2].
  Pharmacology:
    1) Excitatory effect on uterus [3].

Literatures:

[1] Bolun, B.A.: *Phytochem.* **1968**, 7, 1825.
[2] Chiu. P.L. et al.: *Phytochem.* **1988**, 27(3), 819.
[3] Wang, Y.S. et al.: '*Zhongyao Yaoli Yu Yingyong*", **1983**, 728.

[J.X. Guo]

7.   ***Ginkgo biloba* L.** (Ginkgoaceae)

Yin–xing (C), Bak–gwo–sue (H), Icho (J), Eun–Haeng–Na–Mu (K)

Seed (CP)
Local Drug Name: Bai–guo (C), Bak–gwo (H), Haku–ka (J), Baek–Gwa (K).
Processing: Remove outer seed coat, and remove seed coat when use.
Method of Administration: Oral (decoction: C, H, J, K).
Folk Medicinal Uses:
           1) Asthma (C, J, K).
           2) Sputum and coughing (C, J, K).
           3) Leukorrhea (C, K).
           4) Spermatorrhea (C).
           5) Euresis, frequent urination (C).
Contraindications: Firm diseases.
Side Effects: Contact dermatitis by fleshy seed due to ginkgolic acid and bilobol; excessive ingestion
        resulted in food poisoning causing convulsions, loss of consciousness, and a death rate of
        25 percent due to an antipyridoxine substance (4-O-methyl pyridoxine), especially in
        individuals with lower body levels of pyrodoxine (vitamin B_6) on a poor substitute diet [1].

Leaf
Local Drug Name: Bai–guo–ye (C); Baek–Gwa–Yeop (K)
Processing: Dry under the sun.
Method of Administration: Oral (decoction: C).
Folk Medicinal Uses:
           1) Chest distention (C).
           2) Palpitation (C).
           3) Sputum and coughing (C, K).
           4) Leukorrhea (C).
           5) Diarrhea (C).
           6) Frostbite (topical, J).
Contraindications: Firm diseases.

Root
Local Drug Name: Bai–guo–gen (C), Baek–Gwa–Geun (K).
Method of Administration: Oral (decoction: C).
Folk Medicinal Uses:
           1) Leukorrhea (C).
           2) Spermatorrhea (C).
Contraindications: Cold disease.

Scientific Researches:
Chemistry
  1) Monoterpenes (from wood):p-cymene, thymol, α–, β–ionone, t–linalool oxide.
  2) Sesquiterpenes (from wood): bilobanone, α–bilobalide, elemol, eudesmol, dihydroatlantone.
  3) Diterpenes (from leaf and root bark): ginkgolides.
  4) Steroids (from leaf): β–sistosterol, β–sitosterol glucoside, stigmasterol.
  5) Flavonols: isorhamnetin, kaempferol, quercetin and their analogs [14].
  6) Flavones: luteolin, tricetin.
  7) Biflavones: amentoflavone, bilobetin, ginkgetin, isoginkgetin, 5'-methoxybilobetin, sciadopitysin [7,8].
  8) Tannins: catechins, prosanthocyanidins.
  9) Flavonol triglycosides: quercetin 3-O-[α–rhamnosyl–(1→2)–α–rhamnosyl(1→6)–β–glycoside,
        kaempferol 3-O-[α–rhamnosyl–(1→2)–α–rhamnosyl(1→6)–β–glycoside [4].

10) Flavonol glycosides: kaempferol 3–*O*–coumaryoyl glucorhamnoside, quercetin 3–*O*–coumaryoyl glucorrhamnoside [6], isorhamnetol–3–*O*–rutinoside, kaempferol–3–*O*–rutinoside, syringetin–3–*O*–rutinoside, kaempferol–3–*O*–α–(6'''–p–coumaroylglucosyl–β–1,4–rhamnoside, kaempferol 7–*O*–glucoside, quercetol–3–*O*–rutinoside, quercetol–3–*O*–rhamnoside, quercetol–3–*O*–glucoside, quercetol–3–*O*–α–(6'''–p–coumaroylglucosyl–β–1,4–rhamnoside [7,10,11,12,15].

11) Polysaccharides with a rhamnogalacturonan backbone and arabinogalactan side chains [5,9].

12) Acids: 6–hydroxykynurenic acid [7].

13) Nonacosan–10–ol, τ–tocopherol, acetates on epiculticular leaf wax [19].

14) Protein: legumin–like protein (seed) [21].

Pharmacology

1) Antibacterial effect (leaf extracts).

2) Antifungal effect (leaf extract).

3) Platelet–activating factor (ginkgolides).

4) Enhancing retention of learned behavior [3].

5) Antiradical properties (leaf) [4].

6) Bilobalide and ginkgolide A shorten sleeping time induced by hexobarbital [13].

7) Antiobesity uses [16].

8) Anti–oxidant effects of the extract (EGB 761) protects rat retina against lipid peroxidation [17].

9) Beneficial effects of the extract (EGB 761) on vestibular syndromes [18].

10) Beneficial effects of the extract (EGB 761) on cortical hemiplegia [20].

11) Benefical uses in enhancing hyperbaric O therapy [23, 24].

Literature

[1] Huh, H. et al.: *J. Herbs, Spices Aromatic Pl.* **1992**, 1, 91.

[2] Braquet, P.: "*Ginkgolides: Chemistry, Biology, Pharmacology and Chemical Perspectives* ", Vol. 1–2. H.R. Prous Science Pub., Barcellona, Spain, **1988–89**.

[3] Petkov, V.D. et al.: *Planta Med.* **1993**, 59, 106.

[4] Vanhaelen, M. et al.: *Planta Med.* **1989**, 55, 202.

[5] Kraus, J. et al.: *Planta Med.* **1989**, 55, 583.

[6] Lobstein, A. et al.: *Planta Med.* **1991**, 57, 430–3.

[7] Victoire, C. et al.: *Planta Med.* **1988**, 54, 245–7.

[8] Lobstein–Guth, A. et al.: *Planta Med.* **1988**, 54, 555–6.

[9] Kraus, J.: *Phytochem.* **1991**, 30, 3017–20.

[10] You, S. et al.: *J. Shenyang Coll. Pharm.* **1989**, 6, 284.

[11] Nasr, C. et al.: *Phytochem.* **1986**, 25, 770.

[12] Nasr, C. et al.: *Phytochem.* **1987**, 26, 2869.

[13] Wada, K., et al.: *Biol. Pharm. Bull.* **1993**, 16, 210.

[14] Zhuang X.P. et al.: *Zhongcaoyao* **1992**, 23, 122–4.

[15] Hasler, A. et al.: *Phytochem.* **1992**, 31, 1391–4.

[16] Soudant, E. et al.: *Fr. Demande FR* 2,669,537. **1992**.

[17] Droy–Lefaix, M.T. et al.: *Drugs Exp. Clin. Res.* **1991**, 17, 571.

[18] Yabe, T. et al.: *Pharmacol., Biochem. Behav.* **1992**, 42, 595.

[19] Guelz, P.G. et al.: *Z. Naturforsch., C: Biosci.* **1992**, 47, 516.

[20] Brailowsky, S. et al.: *Restor. Neurol. Neurosci.* **1991**, 3, 267.

[21] Haeger, K.P. et al.: *Phytochem.* **1992**, 31, 523.

[22] Huguet, F. et al.: *J. Pharm. Pharmacol.* **1992**, 44, 24–7.

[23] Schumann, K.: *Ger. Offen.* DE 4,023,788 **1992**.

[24] Schumann, K.: *Ger. Offen.* DE 4,023,789 **1992**.

[25] DeFeudis, F.V.: "*Ginkgo biloba extract (EGb 761), Pharmacological Activities and Clinical Applications.*" Elsevier, Paris, **1991**, 1–187.

[P.P.H. But]

8.
Biota orientalis (L.) Endl. (Cupressaceae)
(= *Thuja orintalis, Platycladis orientalis*)

Ce–bai (C), Bin–pak(H), Konotegashiwa (J), Cheuk–baek–na–mu (K)

Twig and leaf
Local Drug Name: Ce–bai–ye (C), Bin–pak–yip (H), Soku–haku–yo (J), Cheuk–baek–yeop (K).
Processing: Eliminate hard twigs and foreign matter, dry in the shade or carbonize by stir–frying (C, K).
Method of Administration: Oral (decoction: C, H, J, K). Topical (Powder, J).
Folk Medicinal Uses:
> 1) Hemorrhagic disease (C, H, J).
> 2) Chronic tracheitis (C).
> 3) Acute or chronic bacillary dysentery (C, H, K).
> 4) Rheumatalgia (H).
> 5) Hypertension (H).
> 6) Erysipelas (H).
> 7) Mumps (H).
> 8) Burnt (H).
> 9) Alopecia (J).
> 10) Hematemesis, epistaxis, hemoptysis (K).

Seed
Local Drug Name: Ce–bai–ren (C), Pak–gee–yan (H), Haku–shi–nin (J), Baek–ja–in (K).
Processing: Eliminate foreign matter and remaining testa (C, K).
Method of Administration: Oral (decoction: C, H, J, K).
Folk Medicinal Uses:
> 1) Neurasthenia, insomnia (C, H, J).
> 2) Constipation (C, H).
> 3) Spermatorrhea (H).
> 4) Palpitation (H).
> 5) Hair loss (H, J).
> 6) Stomatitis (J).
> 7) Weakness of the body (K).
> 8) Liver tonic (K).

Scientific Researches:
Chemistry
> Leaf: 1) Flavonoids: quercetin, myricetin [1], hinokiflavone, amentoflavone [2], kaempferide [3].
>   2) Essential oil: fenchone, thujene, thujone [4].
>   3) Tannins [4].
> Seed: 1) Fatty oils, saponins, volatile oils [5].

Pharmacology: (Leaf)
> Leaf: 1) Antitussive effect [4].
>   2) Expectorant effect [4].
>   3) Antiasthmatic effect [4].
>   4) Hemostyptic effect (flavonoids, tannins) [6].
>   5) Antibacterial effect [4].

Literatures:
[1] Natarajon, S. et al.:*Phytochem.* **1970**, 9, 575.
[2] Pelter, A. et al.:*ibid*, **1970**, 9, 1897.
[3] Takahashi, M. et al.:*Yakugaku Zasshi*, **1960**, 80, 1488.
[4] Wang, Y.S. et al.: "*Zhongyao Yaoli Yu Yingyong*", **1983,** 690.
[5] "*Zhongyao Zhi* ", **1984,** Vol.3, 479.
[6] Xu, Z.W. et al.:*Zhongyao Tongbao*, **1983**, 8, 30.
[J.X. Guo]

9. *Ephedra sinica* Stapf (Ephedraceae)

Cao–ma–huang (C), Ma–wong (H), Shinamao (J), Cho–ma–hwang (K)

Related plants: *Ephedra distachya* L.: Futamatamao (J), Ssang–su–ma–hwang (K);
E. equisetina Bunge: Kidachimao (J), Mok–jeok–ma–hwang (K);
E. intermedia Schrenk et C. A. Meyer: Jung–ma–hwang (K).

Herbaceous stem (CP, JP, KP)
Local Drug Name: Ma–huang (C), Ma–wong (H), Ma–o (J), Ma–hwang (K).
Processing: Remove the woody stems and roots, and cut into section (C). Dry under the sun (J).
Method of Administration: Oral (decoction: C, H, J, K).
Folk Medicinal Uses:
1) Asthma (C, H, J, K).
2) Cough (C, H, J, K).
3) Fever (C, H, J, K).
4) Common cold (C, H, J, K).
5) Edema (C, H, J, K).
6) Articular rheumatism (J, K).
7) Rheumatalgia (H).
Contraindications : Hypertension.
Side effects: Central nervous system stimulation.

Root (CP)
Local Drug Name: Ma–huang–gen (C), Ma–wong–gun (H), Ma–o–kon(J).
Method of Administration: Oral (decoction: C, H, J); Topical (powder: C).
Folk Medicinal Uses:
1) Polyhydrosis (H).
2) Spontaneous sweating, night sweating (C).

Scientific Researches:
Chemistry
1) Alkaloids: (–)–ephedrine, (+)–pseudoephedrine [1], ephedroxane [2],
pseudoephedroxane [3], (–)–norephedrine, (–)–*N*–methylephedrine, (+)–*N*–methylpseudoephedrine,
(+)–norpseudoephedrine [2].
2) Flavonoids [4].
3) Tannins [4].
4) Glycans: ephedran A, B, C, D, E [5].
Pharmacology
1) Antitussive (water extract, (–)–ephedrine) [6].
2) Promotion of bronchial secretion (water extract) [7].
3) Anti–inflammatory ((–)–ephedrine, (+)–pseudoephedrine) [1,8,9], (water extract) [10].
4) Adrenergic effect, central nervous stimulation: ((–)–ephedrine) [11,12].
5) Diuretic ((+)–pseudoephedrine) [13].
6) Antihyperglycemia (ephedrane A–E) [5].

Literatures:
[1] Hikino, H. et al.:*Chem. Pharm. Bull.* **1980**, 28, 2900.
[2] Konno, C. et al.:*Phytochem.* **1979**, 18, 697.
[3] Kasahara, Y. et al.:*Planta Med.* **1985**, 51, 325; Sugawara, M. et al.:*Ensho* **1986**, 6, 245.
[4] Kinjo, Y. et al.:*27th Ann. Meeting of Jap. Soc. Pharmacognosy, Abstr* **1980,** 53.
[5] Konno, C. et al.:*Planta Med.* **1985**, 51, 162.
[6] Miyagoshi, M. et al.:*Planta Med.* **1986**, 52, 275.
[7] Akiba, K. et al.:*Oyo Yakuri* **1981**, 22, 339.

[8] Cho, S.: *Shoyakugaku Zasshi* **1982,** 36, 78.

[9] Harada, H. et al.:*J. Pharm. Dyn.* **1981,** 4, 691.

[10] Kasahara, Y. et al.:*Shoyakugaku Zasshi* **1984,** 38, 159.

[11] Chen, K. K. et al.:*J. Pharmacol. Exptl. Therap.* **1925,** 24, 339; Rowe, L. W.:*J. Am. Pharm. Assoc.* **1927,** 16, 912.

[12] Astrup, A. et al.:*Metabolism* **1986,** 35, 260.

[13] Okanishi, T.: *Manshu Igaku Zasshi* **1930,** 13, 1.

[T. Kimura]

10.　　　　　*Myrica rubra* Sieb. et Zucc. (Myricaceae)

Yang–mei (C); Yeung–mui (H); Yamamomo (J); So–gwi–na–mu (K)

Fruit

Local Drug Name: Yang–mei (C); Yeung–mui (H); Yama–momo (J); Yang–mae (K).

Processing: Dry under the sun or use when fresh.

Method of Administration: Oral (fresh, prickled, tincture, ash, C,H,J).

Folk Medicinal Uses:
> 1) Thirst (C).
> 2) Anorexia (H).
> 3) Dysentery (C).
> 4) Stomach distention (H).
> 5) Sputum (J).
> 6) Berberi (J).

Contraindications: Avoid excessive ingestion; blood heat.

Root

Local Drug Name: Yang–mei–gen (C), Yeung–mui–gun (H), Yang–mae–geum (K).

Processing: Dry under the sun or use when fresh.

Method of Administration: Oral (decoction: C, H). Topical (decoction: C, H).

Folk Medicinal Uses:
> 1) Toothache (C, H).
> 2) Hematemesis, uterine hemorrhage (C, H).
> 3) Hemorrhoidal bleeding (C, H).
> 4) Traumatic injury; fractures (C, H).
> 5) Gastric and duodenal ulcer (C, H).
> 6) Enteritis, dysentery (C, H).
> 7) Pruritus (C).
> 8) Burns (C).

Stem bark

Local Drug Name: Yang–mei–shu–pi (C), Yeung–mui–sue–pay (H), Yo–bai–hi (J), Yang–mae–su–pi (K).

Method of Administration: Oral (decoction: C, H, J).

Folk Medicinal Uses:
> 1) Toothache (C, H, J).
> 2) Hematemesis, uterine hemorrhage (C, H).
> 3) Hemorrhoidal beleeding (C, H).
> 4) Traumatic injury; fractures (C, H, J).
> 5) Gastric and duodenal ulcer (C, H).
> 6) Enteritis, dysentery (C, H, J).

7) Eye diseases (C, H).
8) Diarrhea (J).
9) Abscess, boil, swelling (J).
10) Bruise (topical) (J).

Scientific Researches:
Chemistry
1) Taraxerol, taraxerone, myricadiol, sitosterol,α–amyrin, lupeol, myoinositol, vanillic acid [5–6].
2) Diarylheptanoids (bark) [1].
3) Saccharides, acids [3].
4) Glycosides: myricanol 5–O–α–D–glucopyranosyl–(1–6)–β–D–glucopyranoside, myricanol 5–O–β–D–glucopyranosyl–(1–3)–β–D–glucopyranoside, myricanol 5–O–α–D–(6'–O–galloyl)–glucopyranoside, myricanol 5–O–α–L–arabinofuranosyl–(1–6)–β–D–glucopyranoside [4, 5].
5) Triterpenoids: maslinic acid, alphitolic acid, arjunolic acid, myricolal, oleanolic acid, oleanolic acid acetate [5], 28–hydroxy–D–friedoolean–14–en–3–one [6].
Pharmacology
1) Hepatoprotective effect (methanol extract of bark) [2].

Literatures:
[1] Inoue, T. et al.:*Yakugaku Zasshi* **1984**, 104, 37.
[2] Ohta, S. et al.: *Yakugaku Zasshi* **1992**, 112, 244.
[3] Li, X. M.:*Zhonghua Yufang Yixue Zazhi* **1991**, 25, 371.
[4] Sakurai, N. et al.:*Phytochem.* **1991**, 30, 3077.
[5] Yaguchi, Y. et al.:*Chem. Pharm. Bull.* **1988**, 36, 1419.
[6] Sakurai, N. et al.:*Phytochem.* **1986**, 26, 217.

[P.P.H. But]

11.   *Salix babylonica* L.   (Salicaceae)

Chui–liu (C), Lau–sue (H), Shidareyanagi (J), Su–yang–beo–deul(K)

Related plants: *Salix subfragilis* Anders. (Tachiyanagi:J)

Bark or twig
Local Drug Name: Chui–liu (C), Ryu–haku–hi, Ryu–shi(J), Yu–baek–pi(K).
Processing: Grind into powder or bake dry and grind into fine powder, mix well with sesame oil (C). Dry under the sun (J, K).
Method of Administration: Oral (decoction: C, J, K); Topical (powder: C).
Folk Medicinal Uses:
1) Antipyretic (J, K).
2) Neuralgia (K).
3) Diuretic (K).
4) Astringent (K).
5) Frost bite (K).
6) Urticaria (K).
7) Peritonitis (K).
8) Pruritus or itching (K).
9) Metrorrhagia (K).
10) Toothache (J, K).

11

11) Common cold (J).
12) Enterobiasis (C).
13) Impetigo (C).

Scientific Researches:
Chemistry
1) Phenolic glycosides: salicin, benzyl ester of gentisic acid 2'-O-acetyl-D-glucoside [1], trichocarpin, an ester of terephthalic acid [1].
2) Catechols: pyrocatechol, diacetylpyrocatechol [2].
3) Flavonoids: kaempferol 7-O-glucoside, apigenin 7-O-galactoside, luteolin 4'-O-glucoside [1].
Pharmacology
1) Antipyretic.
2) Effect against vaginal Pseudomonas infection (diacetylpyrocatechol) [2].

Literatures:
[1] Khatoon, F. and Khabiruddin, M.: *Phytochem.* **1988,** 27(9), 3010.
[2] Wang, J. and Zhang, L.: *Yaoxue Tongbao* **1988,** 23(1), 15.

[C.K. Sung]

12.   *Morus alba* **Linn.**   (Moraceae)

Sang (C), Song (H), Kuwa, Maguwa (J), Bbong–na–mu (K)

Related plants: *Morus bombycis* Koidz.: Yamaguwa (J), San–bbong–na–mu (K).
                  M. multicaulis Perr.: Roso (J).

Root bark   (CP, JP, KP)
Local Drug Name: Sang–bai–pi (C), Song–bak–pay (H), So–haku–hi (J), Sang–baek–pi (K).
  Processing: 1) Remove the cork, soften briefly with water, cut into slivers and dry (C, J).
                2) Stir–fry the slivers with honey (C).
  Method of Administration: Oral (decoction: C, H, J, K).
  Folk Medicinal Uses:
                1) Cough (C, J, K).
                2) Phlegm (J).
                3) Anasarca with oliguria (C, H, J, K).
                4) Dysuria (J, K).
                5) Asthma (C).
                6) Constipation (K).

Leaf
  Local Drug Name: Sang–ye (C), Song–yip (H), So–yo (J), Sang–yeop (K) .
  Processing: Dry under the sun (J, K).
  Method of Administration: Oral (decoction or herb tea: H, J, K).
  Folk Medicinal Uses:
                1) Hypertension (J, K).
                2) Arteriosclerosis (J).
                3) Influenza (H).
                4) Cough (H).
                5) Sore eyes (H).
                6) Rheumatism (H).
                7) Edema (H).

8) Weakness (J, K).

Branch
Local Drug Name: Sang–zhi (C), Song–gee (H), So–shi (J).
Method of Administration: Oral (decoction: C, H).
Folk Medicinal Uses:
        1) Arthritis (H).
        2) Lumbago (H).

Fruit
Local Drug Name: Sang–shen (C), Song–sum (H), So–jin (J).
Method of Administration: Oral (decoction: H).
Folk Medicinal Uses:
        1) Chronic hepatitis (H).
        2) Anemia (H).
        3) Neurasthenia (H).

Scientific Researches:
Chemistry
  1) Triterpenoids: α–amyrin, β–amyrin, betulinic acid [1].
  2) Prenylflavones: morusin, cyclomorusin, kuwanon A–F, G (moracenin B, albanin F), H (moracenin A, albanin G), moracenin C, D [1].
  3) Cumarins: umbelliferone.
Pharmacology
  1) Blood sugar depression (water or ethanol extract [2], moran A [3]).
  2) Antihypertensive (90% ethanol extract, prenylflavones) [4].
  3) Vasodilator activity (90% ethanol extract) [4].
  4) Peripheral parasympathomimetic activity [4].
  5) Analgesic (butanol soluble fraction) [5].
  6) Antitussive (butanol soluble fraction) [5].
  7) Antiinflammatory (water extract) [5].
  8) Anti–tumor–promoter (phenolic compounds) [6].

Literatures:
[1] Nomura, T., et al.:*Chem. Pharm. Bull.* **1978**, 26, 1394, 1453; **1980**, 28, 2548; Idem:*Tetrahedron Lett.*, **1981**, 22, 2195; Idem:*Heterocycles* **1981**, 15, 1531; **1981**, 16, 983; **1983**, 20, 585; Oshima, Y. et al.: *Tetrahedron Lett.* **1980**, 21, 3381; Idem.:*Heterocycles* **1981**, 15, 1531; Kimura, Y. et al.: *Chem. Pharm. Bull.* **1986**, 34, 1223; Idem.:*J. Nat. Prod.* **1986**, 49, 639; Nomura, T. et al.:*Chem. Pharm. Bull.* **1983**, 31, 2936; **1984**, 32, 808, 1260; **1985**, 33, 1088, 3195, 4288;*Planta Medica* **1984**, 50, 127;*Phytochem.* **1985**, 24, 159;*Heterocycles* **1984**, 22, 1791, 2729;**1985**, 23, 819; **1986**, 24, 1251, 1381, 1807, 2603; Nikaido, T. et al.:*Chem. Pharm. Bull.* **1984**, 32, 4929.
[2] Konno, C.:*Ann. Meeting of Japanese Soc. Pharmacognosy, Abstract***1984,** 49; Hano, Y.:*ibid.*, **1984,** 59; Bin, H.:*Nippon Yakubutsugaku Zasshi***1930,** 11, 22, 181.
[3] Hikino, H. et al.:*Planta Med.* **1985**, 51, 159.
[4] Tanemura, I.:*Nippon Yakurigaku Zasshi***1960**, 56, 704.
[5] Yamatake, Y. et al.:*Japan. J. Pharmacol.* **1976**, 26, 461.
[6] Yoshizawa, S. et al.:*Phytother. Res.* **1989**, 3, 193.

[T. Kimura]

13. *Boehmeria nivea* (L.) Gaud. (Urticaceae)

Zhu–ma (C), Tzue–ma (H), Karamushi (J), Mo–si–pul (K)

Root, Rhizome and Leaf
Local Drug Name: Zhu–ma (C), Tzue–ma (H), Cho–ma (J), Jeo–ma–geun (Root, K), Jeo–ma–yeop
(Leaf, K).
Processing: Dry under the sun (C, J, K).
Method of Administration: Oral (decoction: C, H, J, K).
Folk Medicinal Uses:
1) Urinary tract infection (C, H, J, K).
2) Hemorrhagic disease (C, H, J, K).
3) Threatened abortion (C, H, J, K).
4) Colds, fever (H).
5) Measles (H).
6) Hemorrhoid (H).
7) Traumatic injury (H).
8) Ulcers (H).
9) Boils (H).
10) Snake bite (H).

Scientific Researches:
Chemistry
1) Organic acids: chlorogenic acid [1].
2) Flavonois: rhoifolin [2].
3) Phenols: protocatechuic acid [3].
4) Alkaloids [4].
Pharmacology
1) Hemostyptic effect [3].
2) Antibacterial effect [4].
3) Miscarriage prevention [5].

Literatures:
[1] Wehmer, C.: *"Die Pflanzenstoffe"* Vol.2, **1929**, 254.
[2] Nakaoki, T. et al.: *Yakugaku Zasshi* **1957**, 77, 112.
[3] Nanjing College of Pharmacy: *"Zhongcaoyao Xue"* Vol. 2, **1976**, 125.
[4] Sheng, Z.M. et al.: *Zhongguo Shouyi Zazhi,* **1984**, 10(5), 38.
[5] Chen, G.S.: *Jiangxi Zhongyiyao* **1988**, 19(6), 33.

[J.X. Guo]

14. *Polygonum tinctorium* Ait. (= *Persicaria tinctoria* H. Gross) (Polygonaceae)

Liao–lan (C), Ai, Tadeai (J), Jjok (K)

Leaf (CP)
Local Drug Name: Liao–da–qing–ye (C), Ran–yo (J), Dae–cheong–yeop (K).
Processing: Dry under the sun (C, J, K).
Method of Administration: Appropriate quantity of the fresh leaves to be pounded into paste and
applied topically (C).
Folk Medicinal Uses:
1) Fever and eruptions in epidemic diseases (C, J, K).

2) Cough and asthma due to heat in the lung (C, J).

3) Inflammation of the throat, mumps, erysipelas, carbuncle (C, J, K).

4) Hemorrhoid (J).

5) Insect bite (J).

6) Bleeding (J).

7) Tonsillitis (J).

Scientific Researches:

Chemistry

1) Glucosides: indican [1].

Pharmacology

1) Augmented leucocyte phagocytosis [1].

2) Anti-inflammatory effect [1].

3) Antipyretic effect [1].

Literature:

[1] Nanjing College of Pharmacy: "*Zhongcaoyao Xue*" Vol. 2, **1976**, 366.

[J.X. Guo]

15.   *Polygonum aviculare* L.   (Polygonaceae)

Bian-xu (C), Bin-chuk (H), Michiyagi (J), Ma-di-pul (K)

Related plant: *Polygonum aviculare* L. var. *vegetum*

Herb (CP)

Local Drug Name: Bian-xu(C), Bin-chuk (H), Hen-chiku (J), Pyun-chuk (K).

Processing: Cut into sections and dry (C). Dry under the sun (J, K).

Method of Administration: Oral(decoction: C, H, J, K), external(decoction: C).

Folk Medicinal Uses:

           1) Dysuria (C, H, J, K).

           2) Edema (H, J, K).

           3) Jaundice (H, J, K).

           4) Ascariasis (H, J, K).

           5) Hemorrhoid (H, C).

           6) Leukorrhea (H, C).

           7) Febrile diseases (H, C).

           8) Catarrhal enteritis (J).

           9) Vomiting (K).

           10) Diarrhea (K).

           11) Eczema (C).

           12) Vulval itching with morbid leukorrhea (C).

Scientific Researches:

Chemistry

1) Flavonoids: avicularin, quercetin, quercitrin [1], vitexin, isovitexin, luteolin, rhamnetin-3-O-
β-D-galactopyranoside, quercetin-3-O-β-D-galactopyranoside [2, 3].

2) Coumarins: umbelliferone, scopoletin [1].

3) Tannins: rhatannin [4], gallotannin.

4) Fatty acids [5].

5) Phenols: ferulic, sinapic, vanillic, syringic, p-coumaric, gallic acid, etc.

Pharmacology
1) Cholesterol lowering effect.
2) Angiotensin–converting enz. inhibiting action (tannins) [4].
3) Platelet aggregation inhibiting action (flavonoids) [2].
4) Allelopathic effect (Na salts of fatty acids).

Literatures:
[1] Khvorost, P. P.:*Khim. Prir. Soedin,* **1980**, 840.
[2] Panosyan, A. G. et al.:*Khim. Farm. Zh.* **1986,** 20, 190.
[3] Zhang, Z. et al.:*Yaoxue Xuebao* **1983,** 18, 468.
[4] Inokuchi, J. et al.:*Chem. Pharm. Bull.* **1985,** 33(1), 264.
[5] Alsaadawi, I. S. et al.:*J. Chem. Ecol.* **1983,** 9(6), 761.

[C.K. Sung]

16. 　　　　　*Polygonum multiflorum* Thunb.　　(Polygonaceae)
　　　　　　　　　(= *Pleuropterus multiflorus* Turcz.)

He–shou–wu (C), Ho–sau–woo (H), Tsuru–dokudami (J), Ha–su–o (K)

Root (CP)
Local Drug Name: He–shou–wu (C), Ho–sau–woo(H), Ka–shu–u (J), Ha–su–o (K).
Processing:　　　1) Eliminate foreign matter, wash, macerate, soften thoroughly, cut into thick slices or pieces, and dry (C, H, J, K).
　　　　　　　　2) Stew with balck bean juice, steam alone or steam after mixed with black bean juice, dry to semidryness, then cut into slices and dry (C, H).
Method of Administration: Oral (decoction: C, H, J, K).
Folk Medicinal Uses:
　　　　　　　1) Lymphadenitis, carbuncles, urticaria with itching (C, J).
　　　　　　　2) Constipation (C, H, J, K).
　　　　　　　3) Hyperlipemia (C, H, J).
　　　　　　　4) Backache (H).
　　　　　　　5) Knee pain, lumbago (H).
　　　　　　　6) Premature greying of hair (H).
　　　　　　　7) Hypercholesterolemia (H).
　　　　　　　8) Coronary heart disease (H).
　　　　　　　9) Neurasthenia, insomnia (H).
　　　　　　　10) Tuberculous adenopathy (H).
　　　　　　　11) Chronic enteritis (J).
　　　　　　　12) Weakness of the body (K).
Contraindications: Loose stool (C).
Side Effects: Alimentary tract reaction.

Vine
Local drug name: Yair– gwau–teng (H).
Processing: Dry under the sun.
Folk Medicinal Uses:
　　　　　　　1) Insomnia (H).
　　　　　　　2) Carbuncle (H).

Scientific Researches:
Chemistry

1) Anthraquinones: emodin, chrysophanol, monomethylether, rhein, chrysophanol anthrone [1].

2) Lipids: lethin [2].

3) Stilbenes: rhapontin [1], 2,3,5,4'–tetrahydroxystilbene–2–*O*–β–D–glucoside [3], 2,3,5,4'–tetrahydroxy–
stilbene–2–*O*–D–glucofuranoside–2"–*O*–monogalloyl ester, 2,3,5,4'–tetrahydroxystilbene–2–*O*–
D–glucopyranoside–3"–*O*–monogalloyl ester [4].

4) Phenolic glycosides: polygoacetophenoside [5].

Pharmacology

1) Retarding heart rate [6].

2) Alleviating atheroscleorsis [7].

3) Increasing cold–resistant ability [6].

4) Antibacterial effect [6].

5) Senility–resistant effect [8].

6) Liver–protective effect (stilbene) [9].

Literatures:

[1] Tsukida, K.: *Yakugaku Zasshi* **1954**, 74, 230.

[2] "*Zhongyao Zhi*", Vol. 1, **1979**, 487.

[3] Hata, K.: *Yakugaku Zasshi* **1975**, 95, 211.

[4] Nonaka, G. et al.: *Phytochem.* **1982**, 21, 429.

[5] Yoshizaki, M. et al.: *Planta Med.* **1987**, 53, 273.

[6] Wang, Y.S. et al.: "*Zhongyao Yaoli Yu Yingyong*", **1983,** 533.

[7] Wang, W. et al.: *Zhongxiyi Jiehe Zazhi* **1984**, 4, 748.

[8] Yao, M.C. et al.: *Yaoxue Tongbao* **1984**, 19, 28.

[9] Kimuta, Y. et al.: *Planta Med.* **1983**, 49, 51.

[J.X. Guo]

17.   *Polygonum orientale* L. (Polygonaceae)
                           (= *Persicaria pilosa* Kitagawa)

Hong–liao (C), Oketade (J), Teol–yeo–ggwi (K)

Herb

Local Drug Name: Shui–hong–cao (C), Sui–ko–so (J), Hong–cho (K).

Processing: Dry under the sun (C, J).

Method of Administration: Oral (decoction: C, J).

Folk Medicinal Uses:

1) Rheumatic arthritis (C).

2) Dysentery (C, J).

3) Rheumatic edema (C, J).

4) Colic (J).

5) Urethritis (J).

Fruit (CP)

Local Drug Name: Shui–hong–hua–zi (C).

Processing: Eliminate foreign matter (C).

Method of Administration: Oral (decoction: C); Topical (plaster: C).

Folk Medicinal Uses:

1) Mass in the abdomen (C).

2) Goitre with pain (C).

3) Epigastric pain (C).

4) Distension due to indigestion (C).

Scientific Researches:
Chemistry
  1) Flavonoids: vitexin, isovitexin, orientin, isoorientin, luteolin–7–glucoside [1].
          3,3',5,6,7,8–hexa–methoxy–4',5'–methylenedioxyflavone, 5–hydroxy–3,3',6,7,8–
          pentamethoxy–4',5'–methylene–dioxy–flavone, 3'–hydroxy–3,4',5,5',6,7,8–
          heptamethoxyflavone, 3,3',5,8–tetramethoxy–4',5',6,7–bis(methylenedioxy)
          flavone, 3'–hydroxy–3,4',5,5',8–pentamethoxyflavone, 3',5–dihydroxy–3,4',5',8–
          tetramethoxy–6,7–methylenedioxyflavone [2], taxifolin (fruit) [3].
  2) Quinones: plastoquinone–9 [1].
  3) Steroids: β–sitosterol [2].
Pharmacology
  1) Dilate coronary artery [4].
  2) Anoxiatolerant effect [4].
  3) Bronchiectasts effect [4].
  4) Antitumor effect (vitexin) [1].
  5) Antibacterial effect (fruit) [5].
  6) Diuretic (fruit) [6].

Literatures:

[1] Nanjing College of Pharmacy: *"Zhongcaoyao Xue"* Vol. 2, **1976,** 163.
[2] Kuroyanagi, M.:*Chem. Pharm. Bull.***1982,** 30, 1163.
[3] Zhang, Z. J. et al.:*Zhongcaoyao* **1990,** 21, 7.
[4] Wang, G.Q. et al.:*Fujian Yixue Zazhi* **1984,** 6, 28.
[5] Nanjing College of Pharmacy:*Yaoxue Xuebao* **1966,** 13, 93.
[6] Chen, F.L.:*Zhongyi Zazhi,* **1979,** 27.

[J.X. Guo]

18.   *Rheum palmatum* Linn.   (Polygonaceae)

Zhang–ye–da–huang (C), Die–wong (H), Momijiba–daio (J), Gae–jang–gun–pul (K).

Related plants: *Rheum tanguticum* Maxim.; *R. officinarum* Baillon, Yak–dae–hwang (K),
          R. coreanum Nakai, Jang–gum–pul (K)

Rhizome   (CP, JP, KP)
Local Drug Name: Da–huang (C), Die–wong (H), Dai–o (J), Dae–hwang (K).
  Processing: 1) Remove skin then dry under the sun (J, K).
          2) Cut into slices or pieces and dry in the air (C, J).
          3) Stir–fry with wine to dryness (C).
          4) Stew or steam with wine until dark (C).
          5) Carbonize by stir–frying until the outer surface is charred and the inner surface turns to
              darkbrown (C).
Method of Administration: 1) Oral (decoction or powder: C, H, J, K). 2) Topical (C).
Folk Medicinal Uses:
          1) Constipation (C, H, J, K).
          2) Gastrointestinal disorder (C, H, J, K).
          3) Hypertension (J).
          4) Dysentery (H).
          5) Hematuria (H).
          6) Heat in the blood; Hemoptysis (C, H), Epistaxis (C, H), eye inflammation, swelling of
              the throat (C, H).

7) Appendicitis with abdorminal pain (C, J).
8) Hemorrhage from the upper gastrointestinal tract (C).
9) Amenorrhea due to blood stasis (C).
10) Edema (H).
11) Dysuria (H).
12) Boils, sores and abscess (C).
13) Traumatic injuries (C).
14) External use for scalds and burns (C, H).

Scientific researches:
Chemistry
1) Bis-anthrone glucosides: sennoside A, B, C, D, E, F [1, 2, 3,].
2) Anthrone glycosides: rheinoside A, B, C, D [4].
3) Anthraquinones: rhein aloe-emodin, emodin, physcion, chrysophanol [1, 3, 5, 6] and their glycosides [1, 3, 6, 7].
4) Stilbene glycosides [8, 9].
5) Naphthalene glycosides [10].
6) Chromones [11].
7) Phenylbutanone glycosides [8, 12].
8) Tannins: rhatannin and relative compounds [6, 9, 13].
Pharmacology
1) Purgative (water extract, ethanol extract [14], sennoside A~F [5], and rheinoside A~D [2, 3, 4]).
2) Antibacterial (water extract [15]. Rhein and emodin [16, 17, 18]).
3) Antiviral (water extract) [19].
4) Choresterol-lowering (water extract) [20].
5) Blood urea nitrogen lowering (rhatannin) [21, 22, 23].

Literatures:

[1] Zwaving, J. H.: *Planta Medica* **1965**, 13, 474; Idem: *J. Chromatogr.* **1968**, 35, 562.
[2] Miyamoto, M. et al.: *Yakugaku Zasshi* **1967**, 87, 1040; H. Oshio et al.: *Chem. Pharm. Bull.* **1974**, 22, 823; **1978**, 26, 2458.
[3] Oshio, H.: *Shoyakugaku Zasshi* **1978**, 32, 19.
[4] Yamagishi, T. et al.: *Chem. Pharm. Bull.* **1987**, 35, 3132.
[5] Matsuoka, T.: *Shoyakugaku Zasshi* **1961**, 15, 113.
[6] Schnelle, F. et al.: *Planta Medica* **1966**, 14, 194.
[7] Hörhammer, L. et al.: *Chem. Ber.* **1964**, 97, 1662; **1965**, 98, 2859; Okabe, H. et al.: *Chem. Pharm. Bull.* **1973**, 21, 1254.
[8] Murakami,T. et al.: *Yakugaku Zasshi* **1973**, 93, 733.
[9] Nonaka, G. et al.: *Chem. Pharm. Bull.* **1977**, 25, 2300; **1984**, 32, 3501; *Phytochem.* **1983**, 22, 1659.
[10] Tsuboi, M. et al.: *Chem. Pharm. Bull.* **1977**, 25, 2708.
[11] Kashiwada, Y. et al.: *Chem. Pharm. Bull.* **1984**, 32, 3493.
[12] Nonaka, G. et al.: *Chem. Pharm. Bull.* **1981**, 29, 2862; **1983**, 31, 1652.
[13] Kashiwada, Y. et al.: *Chem. Pharm. Bull.*, **1986**, 34, 3208, 4083.
[14] Fujimura, H. et al.: *Nippon Yakurigaku Zasshi* **1969**, 65, 81.
[15] Gaw, H. Z., Wang, H. P.: *Science* **1949**, 110, 11.
[16] Inagaki, I.: *Ann. Rep. Nagoya City Univ.*, **1967**, 15, 27.
[17] Chen, L. et al.: *Yaoxue Xuebao* **1964**, 11, 258; Fuzellier, M. C. et al.: *Ann. Pharm. Fr.* **1981**, 39, 313.
[18] Cyong, J.-C. et al.: *J. Ethnopharmacol.* **19**, 279 (1987).
[19] May, G. et al.: *Arzneim.-Forsch.* **1978**, 28, 1.
[20] Aonuma, S. et al.: *Yakugaku Zasshi* **1957**, 77, 1303.
[21] Nagasawa, T. et al.: *Yakugaku Zasshi* **1979**, 99, 71; Ibid.: *Chem. Pharm. Bull.* **1980**, 28, 1736.
[22] Shibutani, S.: *Yakugaku Zasshi* **1980**, 100, 434.
[23] Ohura, H. et al.: *Igaku no Ayumi* **1983**, 126, 837; Shibutani, S. et al.: *Chem. Pharm. Bull.* **1983**, 31,

2378; Nagasawa, T. et al.:*ibid.* **1985,** 33, 715, 4494.

[T. Kimura]

19.   *Phytolacca esculenta* **Van Houtt.**(= *P. acinosa* Roxb.) (Phytolaccaceae)

Shang–lu (C), Sheung–luk (H), Yamagobo (J), Ja–ri–gong (K)

Related plant: Phytolacca americana L.: Chui–liu–shang–lu (C)

Root (CP)
  Local Drug Name: Shang–lu (C), Sho–riku (J), Sang–ryuk (K).
  Processing: 1) Radix Phytoloccae: cut into slices or pieces, and dry (C).
            2) Radix Phytoloccae (processed with vinegar): add vinegar to Radix Phytoloccae and mix
            thoroughly in a closed vessel until they are infused completely. Place them in a pot and roast
            to dryness, take out and cool. Use 30kg of vinegar per 100kg of Radix Phytoloccae. (C).
            3) Cut and dry under the sun (J, K).
  Method of Administration: Oral (decoction: C, H, J, K), topical (paste of fresh root or powder of the dry root:
            C).
  Folk Medicinal Uses:
            1) Edema (H, J, K).
            2) Beri–beri (J, K).
            3) Tinea pedis (K).
            4) Heart exitability (K).
            5) Gastric disease (K).
            6) Furunculosis (H).
            7) Lumbago (K).
            8) Arteriosclerosis (J).
            9) Anascaria with oliguria and constipation (C).
            10) External use for carbuncles and sores (C).
            11) Ascites (H).
            12) Oliguria (H).
            13) Cervical erosion (H).
            14) Leukorrhea (H).
            15) Pyodermas (H).
  Contraindications: Pregnancy(C)

Scientific Researches:
  Chemistry
    1) Saponins: phytolaccoside B, D, E, G, 3–O–β–D–glucopyranosyl–jaligonic acid [1], esculentoside [2],
            jaligonic acid [3], esculentoside J [6].
    2) Steroids: stigmasterol, α –spinasterol [4].
    3) Organic acids: γ –aminobutyric acid [5].
  Pharmacology
    1) Antiinflammatory action (saponins) [1].
    2) Hypotensive action (γ –aminobutyric acid, histamine) [5].

Literatures:
  [1] Yi, Y. H.: *Chin. Trad. Herb Drugs* **1984,** 15, 55.
  [2] Wang, Z. L. and Yi, Y. H.:*Yaoxue Xuebao* **1984,** 19, 825.
  [3] Woo, W. S.: *Yakhak Hoeji* **1971,** 15(3–4), 99.
  [4] Woo, W. S.: *Yakhak Hoeji* **1973,** 17(3), 152.

[5] Funayama, S.:*J. Nat. Prod.* **1979,** 42(6), 672.
[6] Yi, Y. and Dai, F.:*Planta Med.* **1991,** 57(2), 162.

[C.K. Sung]

20.   *Stellaria media* **(L.) Cyr.** (Caryophyllaceae)

Fan–lu (C), Fan–lau (H), Hakobe, Kohakobe (J), Byeol–ggot (K).

Herb
  Local Drug Name: Fan–lu (C), Fan–lau (H), Han–ro (J), Beon–ru (K).
  Processing: Dry under the sun (C).
  Method of Administration: Oral (decoction: C, H).
  Folk Medicinal Uses:
          1) Enteritis (C, H, J).
          2) Dysentery (C, H).
          3) Hepatitis (C, H).
          4) Appendicitis (H),
          5) Hemorrhoids (H).
          6) Anal fissure (H).
          7) Urinary tract infection (H).
          8) Toothache (H, J).
          9) Endometritis (H).
          10) Pyodermas, mastitis, traumatic injury (H).
          11) Lactation deficiency (J).
          12) Bruise, swelling (J).
          13) Edema (J).
          14) Gingivitis, alveolar pyorrhea (J).

Scientific Researches:
  Chemistry
    1) Flavonoids: 7,2"–di–O–β–glucopyranosyl isovitexin, 7–O–β–galatopyranosyl–2"–O–β–glucopyrano-
            syl isobitexin [1].
    2) Saponins: gypsogenin glycoside [2].
    3) Phenolic acid: vanillic acid, p–hydroxyvenzoic acid, ferulic acid, caffeic acid, chlorogenic acid [3].
    4) Coumarins [4].
  Pharmacology
    1) Antioxidative effect (orientin, isoorientin) [5].

Literatures:
[1] Budzianowski, J. et al.:*Planta Med.* **1991,** 57, 290.
[2] Hodisan, V. et al.:*Farmacia (Bucharest)* **1989,** 37, 105.
[3] Kitanov, G.:*Pharmazie* **1992,** 47, 470.
[4] Khromatogr:*Metody Farm.* **1977,** 172.
[5] Budzianowski, J. et al.:*Pol. J. Pharmacol. Pharm.* **1991,** 43, 395.

[J.X. Guo]

21.   *Achyranthes aspera* L.   (Amaranthaceae)

Tu–niu–xi (C), Do–kou–cho (H), Indo–inokozuchi (J)

Root
Local Drug Name: Dao–kou–cao (C), To–ngau–chut (H).
Processing: Herb: Dry under the sun (C). Root: Use in fresh (C).
Method of Administration: Oral (decoction: C, H).
Folk Medicinal Uses:

1) Fever due to common cold (C, H).
2) Headache due to summer–heat (C).
3) Malaria (C, H).
4) Dysentery (C, H).
5) Urethral calculus (C, H).
6) Chronic nephritis (C, H).
7) Tonsillitis, mumps (H).
8) Rheumatoid arthritis (H).
9) Traumatic injury (H).
10) Nephritic edema (H).
11) Dysmenorrhea (H).
12) Amenorrhea (H).

Scientific Researches:
Chemistry
1) Saponins: asperasaponin A, B [1].
2) Alkaloids: achyanthin [2].
3) Aliphalic ketones: 36,47–dihydroxyhentacontan–4–one [3].
4) Steroids: ecdysterone [4].
Pharmacology
1) Protein assimilation (ecdysterone) [5].
2) Raising blood pressure, stimulating respiration (alkaloids) [6].
3) Antispasmodic effect on intestine (alkaloids) [6].
4) Antiduretic effect (alkaloids) [6].
5) Contraceptive and absortifacient effect [7, 8].
6) Antifungal effect (volatile oil) [9].

Literatures:
[1] Hariharan, V. et al.:*Phytochem.* **1970**, 9, 409.
[2] Ratra, P. S.:*Curr. Treuds Life Sci.* **1979**, 4, 81.
[3] Mista, T. N. et al.:*Phytochem.* **1991**, 30, 2076.
[4] Banerji, A. et al.:*ibid*, **1971,** 10, 2225.
[5] Otaka, T. et al.: *Chem. Pharm. Bull.* **1968**, 16, 2426; **1969**, 17, 1352, 1883.
[6] Kapoor, V. K. et al.:*Ind. J. Pharm.* **1967**, 29, 285.
[7] Wadhwa, V. et al.:*Planta Med.*, **1986**, 231.
[8] Pakrashi, A. et al.:*Ind. J. Exp. Biol.* **1977**, 15, 856.
[9] Misra, T. N. et al.:*Phytochem.* **1992**, 31, 1811.

[J.X. Guo]

22. *Achyranthes bidentata* Blume (Amaranthaceae)

Niu–xi (C), Ngau–sut (H), Okinawa–inokozuchi (J), Dang–u–Seul (K)

Related plant: *Achyranthes bidentata* Blume var. *tomentosa* Hara: Hinata–inokozuchi (J)
A. bidentata Blume var. *japonica*: Inokozuchi (J), Soe–Mu–Reup (K)
Cyathula officinalis Kuan, *C. capitata* Moquin

Root (CP, JP, KP)
Local Drug Name: Niu–xi (C), Ngau–sut (H), Go–shitsu (J), U–seul (K).
Processing: 1) Remove the rhyzomes and cut into sections (C).
2) Fumigate with sulfur then dry under the sun (C, K).
3) Stir–fry with wine(C).
Method of Administration: Oral (decoction or powder: C, J).
Folk Medicinal Uses:
1) Pain (C, J).
2) Edema (J, K)
3) Lumbago (C, J).
4) Gynecologic backache, menstrual disorder (C, H, J).
5) Pain on calculus (J).
6) Rheumatism (H, J, K).
7) Dizziness due to hyperactivity of the liver (C).
8) Hematuria (H).
9) Traumatic injury (H).
10) Furunculosis (H).
11) Ouadriplegia (H).
Contraindications: Metrorrhagia in pregnancy.

Scientific Researches:
Chemistry
1) Saponins: oleanolic acid glycoside.
2) Phytoecdysons: ecdysterone inokosterone [1].
Pharmacology
1) Diureic activity was not observed (decoction) [2].
2) Antiallergic (water extract) [3].
3) Antitumor on Ehrlich's ascites carcinoma (water or methanol extract) [4].

Literatures:
[1] Takemoto, T. et al.: *Yakugaku Zasshi* **1967,** 7, 1521; **1968,** 88, 1293; **1971,** 91, 916.
[2] Haginiwa, T. et al.: *Shoyakugaku Zasshi* **1963,** 17, 6.
[3] Koda, A. et al.: *Nippon Yakurigaku Zasshi* **1970,** 66, 366.
[4] Kosuge, T. et al.: *Yakugaku Zasshi* **1985,** 105, 791.

[T. Kimura]

23. *Celosia argentea* L. (Amaranthaceae)

Qing–xiang (C), Ching–sheung (H), Nogeito (J), Gae–maen–deu–ra–mi (K)

Seed (CP)
Local Drug Name: Qing–xiang–zi (C), Ching–sheung–gee (H), Sei–sho–shi (J), Cheong–sang–ja (K).
Processing: Dry under the sun.

Method of Administration: Oral (decoction: C, H, J, K).
Folk Medicinal Uses:
> 1) Conjunctivitis, keratitis (H, J, K).
> 2) Chronic uveitis (H, J).
> 3) Hypertension (H, J).
> 4) Pruritus (C, J).
> 5) Hemorrhinia (C).
> 6) Liver fire (C).

Contraindications: Glaucoma.

Flower
Local Drug Name: Qing–xiang–hua (C), Sei–sho–ka (J), Cheong–sang–hwa (K).
Processing: Eliminate foreign matter, wash clean, and dry under the sun.
Method of Administration: Oral (decoction: C, J). Topical (decoction: C).
Folk Medicinal Uses:
> 1) Hematuria (C).
> 2) Conjunctivitis (C).
> 3) Leucorrhea (C).
> 4) Menoxenia (C).
> 5) Hematorrhea (C).
> 6) Hematemesis (J).
> 7) Menorrhagia (J).
> 8) Epistaxis (J).

Whole plant
Local Drug Name: Qing–xiang (C), Ching–sheung (H), Sei–sho (J), Cheong–sang (K).
Method of Administration: Oral (decoction: C, H, J). Topical (juice: J).
Folk Medicinal Uses:
> 1) Dysentery (H).
> 2) Urinary tract infection (H).
> 3) Pruritus (C, J).
> 4) Rheumatalgia (C).
> 5) Hemorrhoid (J).
> 6) Skin parasites (J).
> 7) Traumatic injury (J).

Scientific Researches:
Chemistry
1) β–sitosterol, cholesteryl palmitate, 3,5–dihydroxy–benzaldehyde, 4–hydroxybenzoic acid, 3,4–dihydroxybenzoic acid, n–butyl–β –D–fructoside, and sucrose [1].

Literature:
[1] Fu, H.Z. et al.:*Zhongcaoyao* **1992**, 23, 344.

[P.P.H. But]

24.   *Celosia cristata* L.   (Amaranthaceae)

Ji–guan–hua (C), Gait–kwun–fa (H), Keito (J), Maen–deu–ra–mi (K)

Flower (CP)
Local Drug Name: Ji–guan–hua (C), Gait–kwun–fa (H), Kei–kan–ka (J), Gye–gwan–hwa (K).
Processing: (a) Eliminate foreign matter and remains of stems, cut into sections, and dry under the sun.

(b) Carbonize by stir-frying the sections until they become charred black.

Method of Administration: Oral (decoction: C, H, J, K).

Folk Medicinal Uses:

      1) Hemorrhinia, hemoptysis, hematemesis, hemorrhoidal bleeding, hematuria (C, H, J, K).

      2) Functional uterine bleeding (C, H, J).

      3) Dysentery (C, H, J, K).

      4) Leukorrhea (C, H).

      5) Urinary tract infection (H).

Contraindications: Patient weak in qi.

Seed

Local Drug Name: Ji-guan-zi (C), Kei-kan-shi (J), Gye-gwan-ja (K).

Processing: Remove from flowers, dry under the sun.

Method of Administration: Oral (decoction: C, J).

Folk Medicinal Uses:

      1) Hemorrhoidal bleeding, hematuria (C, J).

      2) Dysentery (C).

      3) Leukorrhea (C).

      4) Conjunctivitis (J).

Leaf and stem

Local Drug Name: Ji-guan-miao (C).

Method of Administration: Oral and topical (decoction: C, J).

Folk Medicinal Uses:

      1) Dysentery (C, J).

      2) Urticaria (C, J).

      3) Hematemesis, hemorrhinia, uterine bleeding (C, J).

      4) Centipede bite (C).

Scientific Researches:

Chemistry

  1) Kaempferitrin, amaranthin.

  2) Lauric acid, myristic acid, palmitic acid, stearic acid, oleic acid, linoleic acid, linolenic acid, hexadecadienoic acid, tricosanoic acid, lignoceric acid, cerotic acid, 1,1'-[3-(2-cyclopentylethylidene)-1,5-pentanediyl]-bis-cyclopentane [1-2].

  3) Amino acids: α-aminobutyric acid [2].

Literatures:

[1] Raie, M. Y. et al.:*Pak. J. Sci. Ind. Res.* **1987**, 30, 372.

[2] Nam, H. K. et al.:*Han'guk Yongyang Siklyong Hakhoechi* **1988**, 17, 172.

[P.P.H. But]

25.   *Magnolia denudata* Desr. (= *M. heptapeta* Dandy) (Magnoliaceae)

Yu-lan (C), Hakumokuren (J), Baek-mok-ryeon (K)

Related Plants: *M. praecocissima* Koidz (= *M. kobus* DC.): Kobushi (J),
                        M. salicifolia Maxim.: Tamushiba (J).

Flower   (CP, JP, KP)

Local Drug Name: Xin-yi (C), Sun-yi (H), Shin-i (J), Sin-i (K).

Processing: Collect before blooming and dry in the shade (C, J, K).
Method of Administration: Oral or appropriate quantity for external use (decoction: C, H, J, K).
Folk Medicinal Uses:

      1) Headache and nasal obstruction in colds (C, H, J, K).

      2) Sinusitis with purulent discharge (C, H, J).

      3) Toothache (J).

Contraindications: in pregnacy (C).
Side Effects: Stimulant effect on mucous membrane.

Scientific Researches:
Chemistry
  1) Volatile oil: 1,8–cineole, eugenol [1].
  2) Flavonoids: rutin [2].
Pharmacology
  1) Local astringency, local stimulation, and local anesthetic effect [3].
  2) Antihypertensive effect (water or alcohol extract) [3].
  3) Excitatory effect on ulterus [3].
  4) Antimicrobial effect [3].

Literatures:

[1] Xue, Z.L. et al.: *Zhongguo Zhongyao Zazhi* **1989**, 14, 38.
[2] Sato. M. et al.: *Phytochem.* **1992**, 31, 3413.
[3] Wang, Y.S. et al.: *"Zhongyao Yaoli Yu Yingyong"* **1983,** 540.

[J.X. Guo]

26.   *Magnolia obovata* **Thunb.**   (Magnoliaceae)

Honoki (J), Wang–Hu–Bak–Mu (K)

Related plants: *Magnolia officinalis* Rehd. et Wils.: Hou–po (C), Dang–hu–bak–na–mu (K)
                   M. officinalis Rehd. et Wils. *var. biloba* Rehd. et Wils.: Ao–ye–hou–po (C)

Bark   (JP, KP)
Local Drug Name: Wa–ko–boku (J), Hu–bak (K).
  Processing: Dry under the sun (J, K).
Method of Administration: Oral (decoction or powder: J, K).
  Folk Medicinal Uses:

      1) Gastrointestinal disorder (J, K).

      2) Pain (J, K).

      3) Convulsive diseases (J)

Scientific Researches:
Chemistry
  1) Monoterpenes: α–, β–pinene, camphene, limonene, bornyl acetate [1].
  2) Sesquiterpenes: β–eudesmol, α–eudesmol, γ–eudesmol, caryophyllene, caryophyllene epoxide, cryptomeridiol, eudesobovatol A, B [1].
  3) Phenylpropanoids: magnolol, honokiol [1], magnoloside A, B, C [2].
  4) Alkaloids: magnocurarine, magnoflorine, anonaine, michelarbine, liriodenine, salicifoline [3].
Pharmacology
  1) Gastric contract stimulation, intestine movement depression (water extract) [4].
  2) Muscle relaxation and antispasmodic activity (water [5] and ether extract [6], and

magnocurarine [7]).

3) Central nervous system depressing and anlgesic (ether extract [6], magnolol and honokiol [8]).

4) Spinnal reflex depressing (ether extract [6], magnolol and honokiol [8]).

5) Antiulcer and antimicrobial (magnolol and honokiol) [9,10].

Literatures:

[1] Fujita, M., et al.:*Yakugaku Zasshi* **1973**, 93, 415, 422, 429; Fukuyama, Y. et al.:*Tetrahedron Lett.* **1989**, 30, 5907.

[2] Hasegawa, T. et al. :*Chem. Lett.* **1988,** 163; Idem.: *Chem. Pharm. Bull.* **1988**, 36, 1245.

[3] Tomita, M. et al.:*Yakugaku Zasshi* **1951**, 71, 1069; Ito, I. et al.:*Yakugaku Zasshi* **1966**, 86, 124.

[4] Hosono, S. et al.:*Jap. J. Oriental Med.* **1953**, 3, 16.

[5] Sugaya, A. et al.:*Planta Med.* **1983**, 47, 59.

[6] Watanabe, K. et al.:*Chem. Pharm. Bull.* **1973**, 21, 1700.

[7] Ogiu, K., et al.:*Nippon Yakurigaku Zasshi* **1955**, 51, 209.

[8] Watanabe, K., et al.:*Japan. J. Pharmacol.* **1975**, 25, 605; Watanabe, K. et al.: Planta Med.**1983**, 49, 103; Watanabe, H.:*J. Pharm. Dyn.* **1983**, 6, 184.

[9] Yamahara, J., et al.:*Wakan Iyaku Gakkaishi* **1987**, 4, 100.

[10] Watanabe, K., et al.:*Nippon Yakurigaku Zasshi* **1979**, 75, 60.

[T. Kimura]

27.   *Schisandra chinensis* Baillon   (Schisandraceae)

Wu–wei–zi (C), Ng–may–gee (H), Chosen–gomishi (J), O–mi–ja (K)

Related plants: *Kadsura japonica* Dunal: Sanekazura (J)
                      Schisandra sphenanthera Rehd et Wils.

Fruit   (CP, JP, KP)

Local Drug Name: Wu–wei–zi (C), Ng–may–gee (H), Go–mi–shi (J), O–mi–ja (K).

Processing: 1) Dry under the sun. Break into pieces before use (C, J, K).

                  2) Steam with vinegar until the drug becomes black in colour (C).

Method of Administration: Oral (decoction or powder: C, H, J, K).

Folk Medicinal Uses:

              1) Cough (C, H, J. K).

              2) Phlegm (H, J).

              3) Weakness (C, J, K).

              4) Nocturnal emission, spermatorrhea (C, H).

              5) Enuresis, frequent urination (C).

              6) Protracted diarrhea (C), dysentery (H).

              7) Spontaneous sweating, night sweating (C, H).

              8) Wheezing (H).

              9) Jaundice (H).

              10) Impairment of body fluid with thirst, shortness of breath and feeble pulse (C).

              11) Diabetes caused by internal heat (C).

              12) Palpitation and insomnia (C).

Scientific Researches:

Chemistry

  1) Lignans: schizandrin [1], deoxyschizandrin, gomisin A, B, C, D, E, F [2].

  2) Sesquiterpenes: (+)–ylangene, sesquicarene [3].

Pharmacology

1) Central nervous system depression (petroleum ether extract [4, 5], gomisin A [6] and schizandrin [7]).
2) Hepatotoxic substance activity depression (γ–schizandrin) [7, 8].
3) Antitussive (gomisin A) [6].
4) Antiallergic (50% methanol extract) [6, 9].
5) Antiinflammatory (gomisin A) [6].

Literatures:

[1] Kochetkov, N. K., et al.:*J. Gen. Chem.(U.S.S.R.)* **1961**, 31, 3218; *Tetrahedron Letters* **1968**, 2483.
[2] Taguchi, H. et al. :*Chem. Pharm. Bull.* **1975**, 23, 3296; Ikeya, Y. et al.:*Tetrahedron Letters* **1976**, 1359; Taguchi, H. et al.:*Chem. Pharm. Bull.* **1977**, 25, 364; Ikeya, Y. et al.:*ibid.* **1978**, 26, 328, 682, 3257; **1979**, 27, 1383, 1395, 1576, 1583, 2536, 2695 (1979);**1980**, 28, 2422; **1981**, 29, 2893; **1982**, 30, 132, 3202, 3207;**1985**, 33, 3599; **1988**, 36, 3974; Taguchi, H.:*Gendai Toyo Igaku* **1985**, 6, 65.
[3] Hirose, H. et al.:*Tetrahedron Letters* **1968**, 1251, 2483.
[4] Volicer, L. et al.:*Arch. Int. Pharmacodyn.* **1966**, 163, 249.
[5] Niu, X. Y. et al.:*Zhonghua Yixue Zazhi* **1975**, 55, 348.
[6] Maeda S. et al.:*Yakugaku Zasshi* **1981**, 101, 1030; Takeda, S. et al.:*Oyo Yakuri* **1987**, 33, 229; Nagai, H., et al.:*Wakan Iyaku Gakkaishi* **1990**, 7, 46.
[7] Bao, T. T. et al.:*Yaoxue Xuebao* **1979**, 14, 1 (1979); Liu, G. T. et al.:*ibid.* **1980**, 15, 206; Maeda, S. et al.:*Yakugaku Zasshi* **1982**, 102, 579; Maeda, S., et al.:*Japan J. Pharmacol.* **1985**, 38, 347; Takeda, S. et al.:*Nippon Yakurigaku Zasshi* **1985**, 85, 193; **1986**, 87, 169; **1986**, 88, 321; **1987**, 90, 51; **1988**, 91, 237; Hikino, H. et al.:*Planta Med.* **1984**, 50, 213; Kiso, Y., et al.:*ibid.* **1985**, 51, 331; Mizoguchi, Y. et al.:*Kanzo* **1986**, 27, 538; Ohkura, Y., et al.:*Japan. J. Pharmacol.* **1987**, 44, 179; **1990**, 52, 331; Mizoguchi, Y. et al.:*Wakan Iyaku Gakkaishi* **1989**, 6, 135; Nagai, H. et al.:*Planta Med.* **1989**, 55, 13.
[8] Bao, T. T. et al.:*Zhonghua Yixue Zazhi* **1974**, 54, 275; Bao, T. T. et al.:*ibid.* **1975**, 55, 498.
[9] Koda, A. et al.:*Nippon Yakurigaku Zasshi* **1982**, 80, 31.

[T. Kimura]

28. *Cinnamomum cassia* **(Presl.) Blume**   (Lauraceae)

Rou–gui (C), Yuk–gwai (H), Kei (J), Gye–pi–na–mu (K)

Related plants: *Cinnamomum okinawaense* Hatsushima (= *C. sieboldii* Meisn.): Nikkei (J), *C. burmanii* Blume, *C. iners* Blume.

Bark (CP, JP, KP)
Local Drug Name: Rou–gui (C), Yuk–gwai (H), Kei–hi (J), Gye–pi (K).
Processing: Dry in the shade (C, J).
Method of Administration: Oral (decoction or powder: C, H, J, K).
Folk Medicinal Uses:
    1) Stomachic (C, H, J, K).
    2) Common cold (H, J, K).
    3) Fever and pain (J, K).
    4) Headache (C, H, J, K).
    5) Cough and wheezing (H).
    6) Diarrea due to cold (H, C).
    7) Rheumatism, rheumatalgia (H, C).
    8) Dysmenorrhea (H).
    9) Traumatic bleeding (C).
    10) Hypertension (H).

11) Frost–bite (H).
Contraindications: Pregnancy.

Twig
Local Drug Name: Gui–zhi (C), Gwai–gee (H), Kei–shi (J).
Processing: Dry in the shade.
Method of Administration: Oral (decoction: C, H, J, K).
Folk Medicinal Uses:
     1) Common cold (C, H, J, K).
     2) Amenorrhea (H).
     3) Rheumatism (H).
     4) Phlegm (H).

Scientific Researches:
Chemistry
 1) Phenyl propanoids: cinnamaldehyde, cinnamyl acetate, phenylpropyl acetate, cinnamic
    acid, salicylaldehyde [1].
 2) Diterpenoids: cinnzeylanine, cinnzeylanol, cinncassiol A, B, C_1, C_2, C_3, D_1, D_2, D_3, D_4, E and their
    glycosides [2].
 3) Tannins: (–)-epicatechin, procyanidin B–2, B–5, C–1, cinnamtannin I [3, 4].
 4) Glycosides: cassioside, cinnamoside [3].
 5) Polysaccharide: arabinoxylan [5].
Pharmacology
 1) Antipyretic (water extract [6], 70% methanol extract and cinnamaldehyde [7]).
 2) Antiallergic (water extract) [8, 9].
 3) Antiulcer (decoction, 3–(2–hydoxyphenyl)–propanoic acid, cassioside and cinnamoside) [10].
 4) Antitumor (water extract) [11].
 5) Anticoagulant (70% methanol extract and cinnamaldehyde) [12, 13].
 6) Bowel movement stimulation (essential oil) [14].

Literatures:
[1] Heide, R.:*J. Agr. Food. Chem.* **1992,** 20, 747; Lockwood, G. B.:*Planta Med.* **1979,** 36, 380;
 Kakinuma, K. et al.:*Agric. Biol. Chem.* **1984,** 48, 1905; Tsai, S. Y. et al.:*J. of Nat. Prod.* **1984,** 47,
 536; Sagara, Y. et al.:*J. Chromatogr.* **1987,** 409, 365.
[2] Nohara, T. et al.:*Chem. Pharm. Bull.* **1980,** 28, 1432, 1969, 2682; **1981,** 29, 2451, 2686; *Tetrahedron*
 Lett. **1980,** 2647; *Yakugaku Zasshi* **1981,** 101, 1052 (1981);*Phytochem.* **1982,** 21, 2130; **1985,** 24,
 1849.
[3] Nohara, T. et al.:*Phytochem.* **1983,** 22, 215.
[4] Morimoto, S. et al.:*Chem. Pharm. Bull.* **1985,** 33, 2281; **1986,** 34, 633, 643.
[5] Kanari, M. et al.:*Chem. Pharm. Bull.* **1989,** 37, 3191.
[6] Noguchi, M.:*Shoyakugaku Zasshi* **1967,** 21, 17.
[7] Harada, M. et al.:*Yakugaku Zasshi* **1972,** 92, 135.
[8] Koda, A. et al.:*Nippon Yakurigaku Zasshi* **1970,** 66, 366.
[9] Nagai, H. et al.:*Japan. J. Pharmacol.* **1982,** 32, 813, 823.
[10] Akira, T. et al.:*Planta Med.* **1986,** 52, 440; Tanaka, S. et al.:*ibid.* **1989,** 55, 245.
[11] Haranaka, R. et al.:*Wakan Iyaku Gakkaishi* **1987,** 4, 49.
[12] Matsuda, H. et al.:*Chem. Pharm. Bull.* **1987,** 35, 1275.
[13] Takenaga, M. et al.:*J. Pharmacobio–Dyn.* **1987,** 10, 201.
[14] Sone, Y. et al.:*Tohoku J. Exptl. Med.* **1937,** 30, 540.

                  [T. Kimura]

29.   *Aconitum carmichaeli* **Debx.**   (Ranunculaceae)

Wu–tou (C), Woo–Tau (H), Kara–torikabuto (J), Ba–ggot (K)

Related plants: *Aconitum japonicum* Thunb.: Yama–torikabuto (J).,
                    A. kusnezofii Reichb., *A. koreanum*: Baek–bu–ja (K)

Root   (CP, KP)
Local Drug Name: Chuanwu, Fu–zi (C), Foo–gee (H), Bushi, Uzu (J), Bu–Ja (K).
Processing: 1) Dry under the sun (Caowutou (C), So–uzu (J)).
                  2) Macerate in water until there is no dry core, and boil in water for 4–6 hours, or steam
                     for 6–8 hours (H, C).
                  3) Steam in high pressure (1 kg/cm^2, 120°) for 30–40 min. (Kako bushi: J), (K).
Method of Administration: Oral (decoction or powder of processed drug) (C, H, J, K).
Folk Medicinal Uses:
                  1) Chill in legs and arms (C, J, K).
                  2) Collapse (H, J).
                  3) Articular pain (C, J, K).
                  4) Epigastric pain (C).
                  5) Abdominal colic due to cold (C).
                  6) Anesthesis (C).
                  7) Rheumatism (H, J).
                  8) Hemiplegia (H).
                  9) Edema (H).
                  10) Infantile epilepsy (H).
Contraindications: Excessive and heat syndrome. Pregnancy.
Side Effects: Very potent and quick acting poison, causing arrhythmia and lowering of blood pressure, if
              not processed to degradate diester type alkaloids like aconitine [6–8].

Scientific Researches:
Chemistry
   1) Alkaloids: aconitine, mesaconitine, jesaconitine, hypaconotine, benzoyl aconine, benzoyl mesaconine,
      aconine [1], hygenamine, coryneine [2].
   2) Degradation of toxic alkaloids [5].
Pharmacology
   1) Analgesic (mesaconitine, aconitine) [3].
   2) Atrioventricular transmission disturbance (aconitine) [4].
   3) Cardiac (higenamine, coryneine) [2].

Literatures:
[1] Okamoto, T.: *Kagaku to Kogyo* **1961,** 14, 792; Ochiai, E.: *Jap. J. Oriental Med.* **1968,** 19, 51.
[2] Kosuge, T. et al.: *Chem. Pharm. Bull.*, **24**, 176 (1976); Idem.: *Yakugaku Zasshi* **1978,** 98, 1370; Konno,
    C. et al.: *Planta Medica* **1979,** 35, 150.
[3] Hikino, H. et al.: *Yakugaku Zasshi* **1979,** 99, 252; Idem.: *J. Pharm. Dyn.* **1979,** 2, 78.
[4] Imai, H.: *Tokyo Igakkai Zasshi* **1949,** 7, 40.
[5] Hikino, H. et al.: *Yakugaku Zasshi* **1956,** 97, 359; Goto, M.: *Nippon Yakurigaku Zasshi* **1956,** 52, 496,
    511.
[6] Tai, Y. T. et al.: *PACE*, **1992,** 15, 831.
[7] Tai, Y. T. et al.: *Lancet* **1992,** 340, 1254.
[8] But, P. P. H. et al: *Vet. Hum. Toxicol.* **1994,** 35, in press.

[T. Kimura]

30.   *Cimicifuga dahurica* Maxim.   (Ranunculaceae)

Bei–sheng–ma (C), Sing–ma (H), Shoma (J), Nun–bit–seung–Ma (K)

Related plants: *Cimicifuga simplex* Wormsk.: Sarashina–shoma (J), Chot–dae–seung–Ma (K)
                        C. heracleifolia Komarov, *C. foetida* Linn.

Rhizome   (JP, CP, KP)
  Local Drug Name: Sheng–ma (C), Sing–ma (H), Sho–ma (J), Seung–Ma.
  Processing: 1) Dry under the sun (J).
                     2) Cut into thick slices and dry (C).
  Method of Administration: Oral (decoction: C, H, J, K).
  Folk Medicinal Uses:
                  1) Fever (J, K).
                  2) Headache (C, H, J, K).
                  3) Pharyngitis, tonsillitis (C, H, J).
                  4) Food poisoning (J).
                  5) Hemorrhoidal diseases (H, J).
                  6) Ulcers in the mouth (C).
                  7) Measles with inadequate eruption and other eruptive febrile diseases (C).
                  8) Prolapse of the rectum and uterus (C, H).
                  9) Dysentery (H).
                  10) Leukorrhea (H).
                  11) Erythema (H).
    Contraindications: Erupted measles.

Scientific Researches:
  Chemistry
    1) Triterpenoids: Cimigenol, cimigenol–3–xyloside, dahurinol, acetylshengmanol xyloside [1].
    2) Chromones: Visamminol, visnagin, cimifugin, (Z)–3–(3'–methyl–2'–butenylidene)–2–indolinone
            I , II [2, 3, 4].
  Pharmacology
    1) Antipyretic (ether extract, butanol soluble fraction) [5].
    2) Analgesic (ether extract, buthanol soluble fraction) [5].
    3) Antiinflammatory (ether extract, butanol soluble, water soluble) [5].
    4) Reduction of experimental periproctitis (butanol soluble, water soluble) [5].
    5) Antispasmodic (methanol extract, visamminol, visnagin) [6, 7].
    6) Central nervous system depression (methanol extract, cimifugin) [8].
    7) Others [9].

Literatures:
  [1] Takemoto, T. et al.: *Yakugaku Zasshi* **1970**, 90, 68; Sakurai, N. et al.: *ibid.*: **1972**, 92, 724; Kusano,
     G. et al.: *Chem. Pharm. Bull.* **1977**, 25, 3182; Sakurai, N.: *Chem. Pharm. Bull.* **1981**, 29, 955; Kimura,
     O. et al.: *Yakugaku Zasshi* **1983**, 103, 293.
  [2] Ito, M. et al.: *Chem. Pharm. Bull.* **1976**, 24, 580.
  [3] Inoue, T. et al.: *Shoyakugaku Zasshi* **1970**, 24, 76.
  [4] Baba, K. et al.: *Chem. Pharm. Bull.* **1981**, 29, 2182.
  [5] Shibata, M. et al.: *Yakugaku Zasshi* **1975**, 95, 539; Idem.: *ibid.* **1977**, 97, 911.
  [6] Shibata, M. et al.: *Yakugaku Zasshi* **1980**, 100, 1143.
  [7] Ito, M. et al.: *Chem. Pharm. Bull.* **1976**, 24, 580.
  [8] Kondo, Y. et al.: *Chem. Pharm. Bull.* **1972**, 20, 1940.
  [9] Hemmi, H. et al.: *J. Pharm. Dyn.* **1979**, 2, 339; Idem.: *ibid.* **1980**, 3, 636, 643; Yamahara, J. et al.:
     Shoyakugaku Zasshi **1985**, 39, 80.   [T. Kimura]

31.   *Coptis chinensis* Franch   (Ranunculaceae)

Huang–lian (C), Wong–lin (H).

Related plants: *Coptis omeiensis* C. Y. Cheng, *C. deltoidea* C. Y. Cheng, *C. teeta* Wallich,
                        C. japonica Makino *var. japonica* Satake; Kikuba–oren (J), Hwang–ryun (K),
                        C. japonica Makino *var. dissecta* Nakai; Seriba–oren (J)

Rhizome   (CP, JP, KP)
Local Drug Name: Huang–lian (C), Wong–lin (H), O–ren (J), Hwang–ryun (K).
Processing: 1) Cut off and burn the roots, then dry under the sun (C, J).
                      2) Soften, cut into slices and dry in air (C).
                      3) Stir–fry with ginger juice or wine to dryness (C).
                      4) Mix with the decoction of Evodia fruits and stir–fry to dryness (C).
Method of Administration: 1) Oral (decoction or eye solution: C, H, J, K). 2) Topical (C).
Folk Medicinal Uses:
            1) Dyspepsia and anorexia (C, J, K).
            2) Diarrhea (C, H, J, K).
            3) Food intoxication (C, J).
            4) Fever (C, H, J).
            5) Bleeding (C, J, K).
            6) Eye edema (C, J, K).
            7) Tuberculosis (H).
            8) Boils (H).
            9) Sore throat (H).
            10) Eczema and skin diseases with exudation (C, H, J).
            11) Burns (H).
            12) Whooping cough (H).
            13) Ascariasis (H).
            14) Attack of damp–heat manifested by stuffiness and fullness sensation in the abdomen,
                or causing acute dysentery of jaundice (C).
            15) Fidgetness and insomnia due to exuberant fire (C).
            16) Spitting of blood and epistaxis caused by heat in the blood (C).
            17) Acid regurgitation (C).
            18) Toothache (C).
            19) Diabetes (C).
            20) Carbuncles and sores (C).
            21) Purulent discharge from the ear (C).

Scientific Researches:
Chemistry
  1) Alkaloids: Berberine, palmatine, jateorrhizine [1], coptisine, worenine [2], magnoflorine [3].
  2) Phenylpropanoids: Ferulic acid [4].
Pharmacology
  1) Gastric secretion increasing (water extract, decoction) [5].
  2) Pancreas protease precursor activation (water extract) [6].
  3) Gastric movement (water extract) [7].
  4) Antispasmodic (35% ethanol extract) [8].
  5) Antiulcer (water extract) [9].
  6) Antiinflammatory (methanol extarct, berberine) [10, 16].
  7) Antibacterial (50% ethanol extract, berberine, coptisine) [11, 13].
  8) Antihypertensive (berberine) [12, 14].
  9) Antipyretic (berberine) [15].

10) Choleretic (berberine) [17].
11) Blood sugar lowering (berberine) [18].
12) Blood choresterol lowering (berberine) [19].
13) Anti–tumor–promoter (berberine) [20].
14) Central nervous system depressing (berberine) [21].
15) Hepatotonic (35% ethanol extract) [22].
16) Acetylcholine supressing (berberine) [23].

Literatures:
[1] Tani, C. et al.:*Yakugaku Zasshi* **1957**, 77, 805.
[2] Kitazato, Z.:*Yakugaku Zasshi* **1927**, 47, 315.
[3] Tomita, M. et al.:*Yakugaku Zasshi* **1956**, 76, 1425.
[4] Ito, H. et al.:*Yakugaku Zasshi* **1954**, 74, 812; Yahara, S. et al.:*Chem. Pharm. Bull.* **1985**, 33, 527.
[5] Sato, I.:*Kyotofuritsu Ikadaigaku Zasshi***1936**, 16, 443; Ikuta, M.:*Osaka Igakkai Zasshi* **1940**, 39, 2072;
 1941, 40, 711, 727.
[6] Uchiyama, T. et al.:*Wakan Iyaku Gakkaishi***1989**, 6, 201.
[7] Suga, S.: *Osaka Igakkai Zasshi***1942**, 41, 649.
[8] Haginiwa, T. et al.: *Yakugaku Zasshi* **1962**, 82, 726.
[9] Takase, H. et al.:*Japan. J. Pharmacol.* **1989**, 49, 301.
[10] Otsuka, K. et al.:*Yakugaku Zasshi* **1981**, 101, 883.
[11] Chang, N. C.:*Proc. Soc. Exptl. Biol. Med.***1948**, 69, 141; Yamahara, J. et al.:*Shoyakugaku Zasshi*,
 1972, 26, 84; Sawada, T. et al.:*Shoyakugaku Zasshi* **1971**, 25, 74.
[12] Aonuma, S. et al.:*Yakugaku Zasshi* **1957**, 77, 1303.
[13] Ukita, T. et al.: *Penishirin* **1949**, 2, 534; Amin, A. H. et al.:*Canad. J. Microbiol.* **1969, 15**, 1067; Sun,
 D. et al.:*Antimicrob. Agents Chemother.***1988**, 32, 1274, 1370; Higaki, S. et al. :*Wakan Iyaku*
 Gakkaishi **1987,** 4, 458; Lahiri, S. C. et al.:*J. Indian Med. Assoc.* **1967**, 48, 1; Dutta, N. K. et al.:
 Br. J. Pharmacol. **1972**, 44, 153; Sabir, M. et al.:*Indian J. Med. Res.* **1977**, 65, 305.
[14] Suzuki, S.:*Tohoku J. Exptl. Med.* **1939**, 36, 134.
[15] Sabir, M. et al.:*Indian J. Physiol. Phamacol.* **1978**, 22, 9.
[16] Fujimura, H. et al.:*Yakugaku Zasshi* **1970**, 90, 782.
[17] Oshiba, S. et al.:*Nihon Univ. J. Med.* **1974**, 16, 69.
[18] Chen, Q. M. et al.:*Yaoxue Xuebao* **1986**, 21, 401; **1987**, 22, 161.
[19] Vad, B. G. et al.:*Indian J. Pharm.* **1971**, 33, 23.
[20] Nishino, H. et al.:*Onchology* **1986,** 43, 131.
[21] Shanbhag, S. M. et al.:*Japan. J. Pharmacol.* **1970,** 20, 482.
[22] Yang, L. L. et al.:*Wakan Iyaku Gakkaishi***1990**, 7, 28.
[23] Uchizumi, S. et al.:*Nippon Yakurigaku Zasshi***1957**, 53, 63; Shimamoto, T. et al.:*ibid.* **1957**, 53, 75.

[T. Kimura]

32.   *Nandina domestica***Thunb.**   (Berberidaceae)

Nan–tian–zhu (C), Nam–tin–chuk (H), Nanten (J), Nam–cheon (K)

Fruit
 Local Drug Name: Tian–zhu–zi (C), Tin–chuk–gee (H), Nan–ten–jitsu (J), Nam–cheon–juk–ja (K).
 Processing: Dry under the sun (C, J, K).
 Method of Administration: Oral (decoction: C, H, J, K).
 Folk Medicinal Uses:
                1) Cough (C, H, J, K).
                2) Asthma (C, H, J, K).
                3) Wheezing (H).

Contraindications: Cough caused by wind and cold (C).

Stem, Leaf and Root
Local Drug Name: Nan– tian–zhu (C), Nan–tin–chuk–gun (H), Nan–ten–chiku (J), Nam–chen–juk (K).
Processing: Dry under the sun (C, J, K).
Method of Administration: Oral (decoction: C, H, K).
Folk Medicinal Uses:
 (Stem and leaf)1) Diarrhea (C).
　　　　　　　2) Hernia (C).
　　　　　　　3) Scald (C).
　　　　　　　4) Rheumatic arthritis (H).
　　　　　　　5) Juandice (H).
　　　　　　　6) Acute gastroenteritis (H).
　　　　　　　7) Beriberi (K).
　　　　　　　8) Anxiety (K).
 (Leaf)　　　　1) Hemorrhage (C).
　　　　　　　2) Cough (C, H, J).
　　　　　　　3) Conjunctivitis for eye wash (H).
　　　　　　　4) Excoriation (J)
 (Root)　　　　1) Rheumatalgia (C,H).
　　　　　　　2) Ascites due to cirrhosis (C).
　　　　　　　3) Cervical lymph tuberculosis (C).
　　　　　　　4) Jaundice (H).
　　　　　　　5) Acute gastroenteritis (H).
　　　　　　　6) Urinary tract infection (H).
　　　　　　　7) Sciatica (H).

Scientific Researches:
 Chemistry
　1) Alkoloids: pseudocolumbamine [1], domesticine, nantenine, berberine, jatrorrhizine, nandazuine, protopine, menisperrine, magnoflorine [2], isoboldine [3], isocorydine [4], sinoacutine [5], nornantenine, hydroxynatenine, dehydronatenine, nuciferine, dehydroisoboldine [6], 1,2–dimethoxy–9,10–methylene–dioxy–7–oxodibenzo–quinoline, 4,5–dioxo–dehydronantenine [7].
　2) Flavonoids: amentoflavone, nantenoside A, B [8].
　3) Lignans: (–)–episyringaresinol [9].
　4) Cyanohydrins: nandinin [10].
　5) Cyanoyenic glycosides: p–glucosyloxymandelonitrile [11].
 Pharmacology:
　1) Antihypertensive effect (nantenine) [12].
　2) Excitatory effect on central nervous system (nantenine) [13].
　3) Bacteriostatic effect [14].
　4) Serotonergic receptor anttagonist (nantenine) [15].

Literatures:
[1] Moriyasu, M. et al.: *Shoyakugaku Zasshi* **1992**, 46, 143.
[2] Tomita,M. et al.: *Yakugaku Zasshi* **1961**, 81, 1090.
[3] Chikamatsu, et al.: *Nippon Kagakukashi* **1961**, 82, 1708.
[4] Kunitomo, J. et al.: *Yakugaku Zasshi* **1972**, 92, 207.
[5] Kunitomo, J. et al.: *ibid*, **1974**, 94, 97.
[6] Kunitomo, J. et al.: *ibid*, **1974**, 94, 1149.
[7] Kunitomo, J. et al.: *Shoyakugaku Zasshi* **1979**, 33, 84.
[8] Morita, N. et al.: *Chem. Pharm. Bull.* **1974**, 22, 2750.
[9] Kunitomo, J. et al.: *Yakugaku Zasshi* **1975**, 95, 445.

[10] Olechno, J. D. et al.:*Phytochem.* **1984**, 23, 178.

[11] Abrol, Y. P. et al.:*Phytochem.* **1966**, 5, 1021.

[12] *Japan Pat.* Jp 58. 183, 617 [83, 183, 617], 26 Oct. 1983, Appl. 82 1 66, 719, 21 Apr. 1982, 5pp.

[13] Ikomi, F. et al.:*Yakugaku Kenkyu* **1954**, 26, 507.

[14] Nanjing College of Pharmacy: *"Zhongcapyao Xue"* Vol. 2, **1976**, 281.

[15] Shoji, N. et al.:*J. Pharm. Sci.* **1984**, 73, 568.

[J.X. Guo]

33.   *Akebia quinata* **Decaisne**   (Lardizabalaceae)

Mu–tong (C), Muk–tung (H), Akebi (J), Eu–reum–deong–gul (K).

Related plants: *Akebia trifoliata* Koidz.: Mitsuba–akebi (J), *A. pentaphylla* Makino: Goyo–akebi (J),
                 A. trifoliata Koidz. *var. austoralis* (Diels) Rehder: Bai–mu–tong (C),
                 A. quinata Decne. *var. polyphylla* Nakai: Pal–son–eu–reum (K)

Stem   (JP, KP)

Local Drug Name: Mu–tong (C), Muk–tung (H), Moku–tsu (J), Mok–tong (K).

Processing: Dry under the sun (J, K).

Method of Administration: Oral (decoction: C, H, J, K).

Folk Medicinal Uses:

        1) Edema (H, J, K).

        2) Nephritis (J, K).

        3) Dysuria (H, K).

        4) Gonorrhea (J, K).

        5) Sore throat (H).

        6) Amenorrhea (H).

        7) Neuralgia (K).

Fruit (CP)

Local Drug Name: Yu–zhi–zi (C), Hachi–gatsu–satsu (J).

Processing: Wash clean, dry under the sun. Break to pieces before use (C).

Method of Administration: Oral (decoction: C).

Folk Medicinal Uses:

        1) Epigastric and hypochondriac distension and pain (C).

        2) Amenorrhea, dysmenorrhea (C).

        3) Oliguria (C).

        4) Snake and insect bite (C).

Scientific Researches:

Chemistry

  1) Saponins: Akeboside St [1].

  2) Inorganic compounds: Potassium salts.

Pharmacology

  1) Diuretic (water extract, 50% methanol extract) [2, 4].

  2) Prevention against stress ulcer (50% methanol extract, saponin) [3].

  3) Congestive edema inhibition (50% methenol extarct) [4].

  4) Inhibition of serum cholesterol and lipid ascending (50% methanol extract) [5].

  5) Antiinflammatory and gastric secretion decreasing (oleanolic acid glycoside) [6].

Literatures:

[1] Higuchi, R. et al.: *Chem. Pharm. Bull.* **1976**, 24, 1021.

[2] Yamaguchi, I.: *Chosen Igakkai Zasshi* **1928**, No.86, 173; Haginiwa, T. et al.: *Shoyakugaku Zasshi* **1963**, 17, 6; Tsurumi, S. et al.: *Gifu Daigaku Igakubu Kiyo* **1963**, 11, 129.

[3] Yamahara, J. et al.: *Yakugaku Zasshi* **1975**, 95, 1179.

[4] Yamahara, J. et al.: *Chem. Pharm. Bull.* **1979**, 27, 1464.

[5] Onishi, E. et al.: *Chem. Pharm. Bull.* **1984**, 32, 646.

[6] Takezaki, T. et al.: *90th Ann. Meeting of Jap. Pharm. Soc., Abstr.* **1970**.

[T. Kimura]

34.　　　　　　　*Menispermum dauricum* DC.　　(Menispermaceae)

Bian–fu–ge (C), Pin–fuk–got (H), Komorikazura (J), Sae–mo–rae–deong–gul (K)

Rhizome (CP)

Local Drug Name: Bei–dou–gen, bian–fu–ge–gen (C), Pin–fuk–got (H), Hen–puku–kak–kon (J), San–du–geun (K).

Processing: Cut into thick sections and dry under the sun (C, H, J, K).

Method of Administration: Oral (decoction: C, H, J, K).

Folk Medicinal Uses:

   1) Cancer (C, K).

   2) Gastric cancer (K).

   3) Lumbago (C, J).

   4) Rheumatism (J).

   5) Swelling (J).

   6) Edema (J).

   7) Laryngitis (J).

   8) Stomach ache (J).

   9) Scrofula (C).

   10) Sore throat (C).

   11) Colitis (C).

   12) Dysentery (C).

   13) Rheumatic arthralgia (C).

Scientific Researches:

Chemistry

 1) Alkaloids: dauricine [1, 2, 19], dauricinoline [3], dauricoline [4], daulisoline [5], daurisoline [6], menisperine [7], sinomenine [8], stepharine, stepholidine [9], bianfugecine, bianfugedine, bianfugenine [10, 11, 12], menisporphine [13], acutumidine, acutumine [14].

 2) Nitrile glucoside: menisdaurin [17].

Pharmacology

 1) Hypotensive action (dauricine) [15, 18].

 2) Antiarrhythmic action (dauricine) [16].

Literatures:

[1] Kondo, H. and Narita, S.: *J. Pharm. Soc. Japan* **1927**, (542), 279.

[2] Tomita, M. et al.: *Yakugaku Zasshi* **1964**, 84, 1030; Sun Y. Q. et al.: *J. Shenyang Coll. Pharm.* **1984**, 1, 223.

[3] Tomita, M. et al.: *Yakugaku Zasshi* **1970**, 90, 1182.

[4] Tomita, M. et al.: *Yakugaku Zasshi* **1970**, 90, 1178.

[5] Tomita, M. et al.: *Yakugaku Zasshi* **1965**, 85, 456.

[6] Zheng, X. W.: *Kexue Tongbao* **1979**, 24, 285.

[7] Tomita, M. et al.:*Pharm. Bull. Jpn.* **1955,** 3, 100.

[8] Ilinskaya, T. N.:*Dokl. Akad. Nauk. SSSR***1956,** 108, 1081.

[9] Okamoto, Y. et al.:*Yakugaku Zasshi* **1971,** 91, 684.

[10] Hou, C. Y. et al.:*Acta Pharm. Sin.* **1985,** 20, 112.

[11] Hou, C. Y. et al.:*Acta Pharm. Sin.* **1984,** 19, 471.

[12] Takani, M. et al.: *Chem. Pharm. Bull.* **1983,** 31, 3091.

[13] Kumitomo, J. et al.:*Tetrahedron* **1983,** 39, 3261.

[14] Tomita, M. et al.: *Chem. Pharm. Bull.* **1971,** 19, 770.

[15] Chen, S. H. et al.:*Acta Pharmacol. Sin.* **1982,** 3, 178.

[16] Li, G. R. et al.:*Acta Acad. Med. Wuhan***1983,** 12, 280.

[17] Takahashi, K. et al.:*Chem. Pharm. Bull.* **1978,** 26(6), 1677.

[18] Pan, X.: *Faming Zhuanli Shenqing Gongkai Shuomingshu*CN 1,047,861, 19 Dec.**1990.**

[C.K. Sung]

35.   *Sinomenium acutum* Rehder et Wilson   (Menispermaceae)

Qing–teng (C), Ching–fung–teng (H), Otsuzurafuji (J), Bong–gi (K).

Stem (CP), **Stem and Rhizome** (JP, KP)
Local Drug Name: Qing–feng–teng (C), Ching–fung–teng (H), Bo–i (J), Bong–gi (K).
Processing: Dry under the sun.
Method of Administration: Oral (decoction: C, H, J, K).
Folk Medicinal Uses:
        1) Pain (C, J, K).
        2) Edema (H, J, K).
        3) Neuralgia (J, K).
        4) Articular pain (J, K).
        5) Myalgia (J).
        6) Rheumatism (C, H, J, K).
        7) Paralysis (C).
        8) Itching (C).

Scientific Researches
Chemistry
  1) Alkaloids: Sinomenine, disinomenine, sinactine, tuduranine, acutumine, magnoflorine, isosinomenine
        [1].
Pharmacology
  1) Central nervous system depressing (sinomenine) [2].
  2) Analgesic (sinomenine) [3].
  3) Antiinflammatory (sinomenine) [4].
  4) Antiallergic (decoction) [5].
  5) Congestive edema inhibition (50% methanol extract) [6].
  6) Others [7].

Literatures:
[1] Kunitomo, J.:*Gendai Toyo Igaku* **1986,** 7, 54.

[2] Feng, J. Y. et al.:*Yaoxue Xuebao* **1965,** 12, 81.

[3] Sanuki, K.:*Japan. J. Pharmacol.* **1957,** 6, 69; Ono, H.:*Nippon Yakurigaku Zasshi***1958,** 54, 407; **1959,**
    55, 109, 126.

[4] Irino, S.:*Acta Med. Okayama* **1958,** 12, 93, 112.

[5] Koda A. et al.:*Nippon Yakurigaku Zasshi***1970,** 66, 366; **1973,** 69, 88.

[6] Yamahara, J., et al.:*Chem. Pharm. Bull.* **1979,** 27, 1464.

[7] Yamashita, T.:*Jap. J. Oriental Med.* **1959,** 10, 81; Haginiwa, T. et al.:*Shoyakugaku Zasshi* **1963,** 17, 6; Wang, N. Q. et al.:*Yaoxue Xuebao,* **1965,** 12, 86; Yamazaki, H. et al.:*Arerugi* **1954,** 2, 239; Mayeda, H.:*Japan. J. Pharmacol.* **1953,** 3, 62; Nishiyama, R.:*Okayama Igakkai Zasshi* **1959,** 71, 93, 107, 115; Saikawa, H.:*Arerugi* **1965,** 14, 312; Li, Z. X. et al.:*Yaoxue Xuebao* **1987,** 22, 561.

[T. Kimura]

36.   *Stephania cepharantha* Hayata   (Menispermaceae)

Tou–hua–qiang–jin–teng (C), Tamazaki–tsuzurafuji (J).

Root

Local Drug Name: Jin–xian–diao–wu–gui (C), Haku–yaku–shi(J).

Processing: Dry under the sun.

Method of Administration: Oral (decoction: C, J).

Folk Medicinal Uses:

     1) Whooping cough (J).

     2) Diabetes mellitus (J).

     3) Hyperacidity (J).

     4) Gastric ulcer (J).

     5) Areatic alopecia (J).

     6) Internal hemorrhage (C).

     7) Gastroenteritis, bacillary dysentery, appendicitis (C).

     8) Innominate swelling pain (J).

     9) Pain due to pathogenic wind–dampness, nephritic edema (C).

Scientific Researches:

Chemistry

     1) Alkaloids: Cepharanthine, isotetrandrine, cycleanine, berbamine, homoaromoline, cephalamine, cepharanoline, trilobine, tetrandrine [1].

Pharmacology

     1) Antimicrobial against human tuberclosis and leprosy (cepharanthine) [2].

     2) Antihypertensive (cepharanthine) [2].

     3) Antiinflammatory (isotetrandrine) [2].

     4) Antipyretic analgesic (isotetrandrine) [2].

     5) Leucopenia recovery (cepharanthine) [2].

Literatres:

[1] Tomita, M. et al.:*Yakugaku Zasshi* **1967,** 87, 1203; **1969,** 89, 1678.

[2] Harborne, J. B. et al.: *"Phytochemical Dictionary",* 201 (1993), Taylor & Francis, London.

[T. Kimura]

37.   *Nuphar pumilum* **(Timm.) DC.**   (Nymphaeaceae)

Ping–peng–cao (C), Nemuro–kohone (J), Wae–gae–yeon–ggot (K)

Related plant: *Nuphar japonicum* DC.: Kohone (J), Gae–yeon–ggot (K)

Rhizome (JP)
 Local Drug Name: Ping–peng–cao (C), Sen–kotsu (J), Pyung–bong–cho–geum (K)
 Processing: Dry under the sun (C, J, K).
 Method of Administration: Oral (decoction or powder: C, J, K).
 Folk Medicinal Uses:
>   1) Antipyretic, analgesic (C, J).
>   2) Anti–inflammatory (C, J).
>   3) Weakness (K).
>   4) Antitussive, hemostatic amenorrhea due to blood stasis (C).

Scientific Researches:
 Chemistry
  1) Alkaloids: Nupharidine, nupharamine, deoxynupharidine [1].
  2) Tannin [1].
 Pharmacology
  1) Congestive hydropsy depression (50% methanol extract) [2].
  2) Diuretic (50% methanol extract) [2].

Literatures:
 [1] Nishizawa M. et al.:*Chem. Pharm. Bull.* **1982**, 30, 1094; **1987**, 35, 3127; **1989**, 37, 1735.
 [2] Yamahara J. et al.:*Chem. Pharm. Bull.* **1979**, 27, 1464.

[T. Kimura]

38.   *Houttuynia cordata* Thunb.   (Saururaceae)

Ji–cai (C), Yue–sang–cho (H), Dokudami (J), Yak–mo–mil (K)

Herb (aerial part with flowers, CP, JP)
 Local Drug Name: Yu–xing–cao (C), Yue–sang–cho (H), Ju–yaku (J), Eo–seong–cho (K).
 Processing: Dry under the sun (C, J, K).
 Method of Administration: 1) Oral (decoction or herb tea: C, H, J, K). 2) Topical (C).
 Folk Medicinal Uses:
>   1) Chronic constipation (J).
>   2) Edema (H, J).
>   3) Suppuration (J, K).
>   4) Poisoning (J, K).
>   5) Lung abscess with purulent expectoration (C), pulmonary empyema (H).
>   6) Heat in the lung with cough and dyspnea (C).
>   7) Acute dysentery (C), enteritis, dysentery (H).
>   8) Acute urinary infection (C).
>   9) Carbuncles and sores (C).
>   10) Mastitis (H).
>   11) Cellulitis (H).
>   12) Tympanitis (H).
>   13) Urethritis, nephritis (H).

Leaf (fresh)
 Processing: Fresh leaf or leaf juice.
 Method of Administration: Topical.
 Folk Medicinal Uses:
>   1) Empyema (J).

2) Tympanitis (J).

3) Eczema, water eczema (J).

4) Traumatic injury (J, K).

5) Urticaria (H).

Scientific Researches:

Chemistry

1) Flavonoids: Quercitrin [1], isoquercitrin [2] and their glycosides [3].

2) Fatty aldehydes: decanoylacetaldehyde, laurylaldehyde, methyl nonylketone (fresh plant).

3) Benzamide: *cis*– and *trans*–*N*–(4–hydroxystyryl)–benzamide [4].

Pharmacology

1) Various edema depressing (Water extract) [5].

2) Antiinflammatory (Water extract, ethanol extract) [5].

3) Antivirus and vitamin P like activity (quercitrin) [6,7].

4) Platelet coaguration depressing: (*N*–(4–hydroxystyryl)–benzamides) [8].

5) Antifungal and antimicrovial: (decanoylacetaldehyde, laurylaldehyde, methylnonylketone) [9].

Literature

[1] Nakamura H. et al.: *Yakugaku Zasshi* **1936**, 56, 441.

[2] Kimura Y. et al.: *Yakugaku Zasshi* **1953**, 73, 196.

[3] Takagi S.: *Shoyakugaku Zasshi* **1978**, 32, 123.

[4] Nishiya H. et al.: *Chem. Pharm. Bull.* **1988**, 36, 1902.

[5] Suzuki Y.: *Oyo Yakuri* **1985**, 30, 403.

[6] Wacker A. et al.: *Arzneim. Forsch.* **1978**, 28, 347; Mucsi, I. et al.: *Experientia* **1985**, 41, 930.

[7] Ozawa H. et al.: *Yakugaku Zasshi* **1951**, 71, 1173.

[8] Nishiya H. et al.: *Chem. Pharm. Bull.* **1988**, 36, 1902.

[9] Kosuge T.: *Yakugaku Zasshi* **1952**, 72, 1227; **1953**, 73, 435.

[T. Kimura]

39.   *Chloranthus serratus* **(Thunb.) Roem. et Schult.**   (Chloranthaceae)

Ji–ji(C), Kup–gay (H), Futarishizuka (J), Ggot–dae (K)

Root or Herb

Local Drug Name: Ji–ji (C), Kup–gay (H), Kyu–ki (J), Geup–gi (K).

Processing: Dry under the sun or use in fresh (C).

Method of Administration: Topical (paste of fresh root, or wash of herb:), or oral (decoction: C, H).

Folk Medicinal Uses:

         1) Traumatic injury, or innominate inflammatory swelling (C, H).

         2) Scald (C, H).

         3) Anemia (C).

         4) Lumbago (H).

         5) Boils (H).

         6) Pyodermas (H).

         7) Tinea capitis (H).

         8) Snake bites (H).

Side Effects: Fast pulse, nausea, vomit, miosis, cardio palmus, coma.

Scientific Researches:

Chemistry

1) Sesquiterpene: neoacolamone, 7α–hydroxyneoacolamone, acoragermacrone, acolamone, zederone [1],

(−)–dihydropyrocurzerenone [2], schizukanolides E and F [3], shizukaols B, C, D [4].
2) Amide compounds: *N*–β–phenethyl–3–(3,4–methylene–dioxyphenyl)–propenamide, *N*–β–phenethyl–3–(3,4–dimethoxyphenyl)–propenamide [5].

Pharmacology
1) Bacteriostatic effect [6].

Literatures:
[1] Kawabata, J. et al.:*Agric. Biol. Chem.* **1985**, 49, 1479.
[2] Takemoto, T. et al.:*Chem. Pharm. Bull.* **1976**, 14, 531.
[3] Kawabata, J. et al.:*Agric. Biol. Chem.* **1989**, 53, 203.
[4] Kawabata, J. et al., *Phytochem.* **1992**, 31, 1293.
[5] Tokemoto, T. et al., *Chem. Pharm. Bull.* **1975**, 23, 1161.
[6] Nanjing College of Pharmacy: *"Zhongcaoyao Xue"*, **1976**, Vol.2, 98.

[J.X. Guo]

40.   *Sarcandra glabra* **(Thunb.) Nakai** (Chloranthaceae)

Cao–shan–hu (C), Gou–jit–cha (H), Senryo (J), Juk–jeol–cho (K)

Herb
Local Drug Name: Jiu–jie–cha (C), Gou–jit–cha (H), Kyu–setsu–cha (J), Gu–jeol–da (K).
Processing: Dry in the shade or use in fresh (C).
Method of Administration: Oral (decoction:) or topical (paste of fresh plant or powder mixed with spirits: C, H).
Folk Medicinal Uses:
1) Pneumonia, cholecystitis, appendicitis, acute gastroen teritis (C, H).
2) Traumatic fracture (C, H).
3) Rheumatic arthritis, lumbago (C, H).
4) Cancer of pancreas, stomach, nectum, liver, and esophagus (H).
5) Epidemic influenza, encephalitis B (H).
6) Pneumonitis (H).
7) Dysentery (H).
8) Appendicitis (H).
9) Furunculosis (H).

Scientific Researches:
Chemistry
1) Organic acids: fumaric acid, succinic acid [1].
2) Terpenes: (−)–istanbulin [2].
3) Coumarins: isofraxidin [3].
4) Others: flavonoids [4], lignans [5].
Pharmacology
1) Bacteriostatic effect [6].
2) Antitumor effect (flavonoids [7], isofraxidin [4]).
3) Catagmatic effect [8].
4) Antimycotic effect (volatile oils) [9].

Literatures:
[1] Wang, A. Q. et al.:*Zhongcaoyao Tongxun* **1979**, 10, 8.
[2] Wang, A. Q. et al.:*Yaoxue Xuebao* **1988**, 23, 64.
[3] Wang, A. Q. et al.:*Zhongcaoyao* **1983**, 14, 37.

[4] Liu, C. C. et al.:*Beijingdaxue Xuebao, Zira Kexue Ban***1981,** (2), 94.
[5] Shio, T. et al.:*Wood Res.* **1981,** 67, 43.
[6] Nanjing College of Pharmacy:*"Zhongcaoyao Xue"***1976,** Vol. 2, 99.
[7] Cai, X. L. et al.:*Pharm. Industry,* **1981,** 26.
[8] Shi, G. D. et al.:*Zhonghua Waike Zazhi***1985,** 23, 389.
[9] Li, S. L. et al.:*Zhongcaoyao* **1991,** 22, 435.

[J.X. Guo]

41. *Aristolochia debilis* Sieb. et Zucc. (Aristolochiaceae)

Ma–dou–ling (C), Ma–dou–ling (H), Umanosuzukusa (J)

Relative plants:*Aristolochia contorta Bunge.* Bei–ma–dou–ling (C), Jui–bang–ul (K).

Fruit (CP)
Local Drug Name: Ma–dou–ling (C), Ma–dou–ling (H), Ba–to–rei (J), Ma–du–ryung (K).
Processing:　　1) Sift, and rub the fruits into pieces (C, H, J, K).
　　　　　　　　2) Dilute the refined honey with a quantity of water, then add it to clean drug and mix well
　　　　　　　　　in a closed vessel untill they are infused thoroughly. Roast them in a pot with gentle heat
　　　　　　　　　until not sticky to fingers (C).
Method of Administration: Oral (decoction: C, H, J, K).
Folk Medicinal Uses:
　　　　　　　　1) Cough (H, J, K).
　　　　　　　　2) Sputum (H, J, K).
　　　　　　　　3) Chronic bronchitis (J).
　　　　　　　　4) Hemoptysis (H).
　　　　　　　　5) Loss of voice (H).
　　　　　　　　6) Hemorrhoid (H).
　　　　　　　　7) Asthma, cough and bloody sputum due to heat in the lung (C).
　　　　　　　　8) Bleeding, swollen and painful hemorrhoids due to heat in the large intestine (C).

Herb (CP)
Local Drug Name: Tian–xian–teng (C).
Processing: Eliminate foreign matter, cut into sections.
Method of Administration: Oral (decoction: C).
Folk Medicinal Uses:
　　　　　　　　1) Pricking pain in the epigastrium (C).
　　　　　　　　2) Arthralgia (C).
　　　　　　　　3) Edema of pregnancy (C).

Root
Local Drug Name: Qin–mu–xiang (C), Sei–mok–ko (J).
Processing: Dry under the sun (K).
Method of Administration: Oral (decoction) (J).
Folk Medicinal Uses:
　　　　　　　　1) Hypertension (J).
　　　　　　　　2) Rheumatism (J).
　　　　　　　　3) Bruise (J).
　　　　　　　　4) Sore throat (J).
Contraindications: in diarrhea by cold.
Side Effects: Nausea, vomitting.

Scientific Researches:

Chemistry

1) Nitro compounds: aristolochic acid A, C, debilic acid [1, 2, 3, 4], 9–hydroxyaristolochic acid I,
9–methoxyaristolochic acid [5], aristolochic acid II, IV, IVa, aristolochic acid methy ester [6].

2) Alkaloids: magnoflorine, cyclanoline [9], tetrandrine [10], allantoin [2].

3) Sesquiterpenes: aristolone [11, 12], 9–aristolene, 1(10)–aristolene, debilone [13], 3–oxoishwarene,
1(10)–aristolen–9–one [14].

Pharmacology

1) Antimicrobial activity (aristolochic acids) [15].

2) Antitumor activity (aristolochic acids).

3) Hypotensive activity (magnoflorine) [7, 8].

4) Immunostimulating activity (aristolochic acid A).

Literatures:

[1] Tseng, K. F. et al.:*Yaoxue Xuebao* **1958,** 6, 174.

[2] Tseng, K. F. et al.:*Yaoxue Xuebao* **1958,** 6, 33.

[3] Ku, Y. T. et al.:*Kexue Tongbao* **1957,** 761.

[4] Zhang, X. Q. et al.:*Yaowu Fenxi Zazhi* **1982,** 2, 72.

[5] Chen Z. L. et al.:*Huaxue Xuebao* **1981,** 39, 237.

[6] Huang B. S. et al.:*Zhongcaoyao* **1985,** 16, 482.

[7] Tomita, M. et al.:*Yakugaku Zasshi* **1957,** 77, 812.

[8] Chang, C. C. et al.:*Yaoxue Xuebao* **1964,** 11, 42.

[9] Tomita, J. et al.:*Yakugaku Zasshi* **1962,** 82, 1673.

[10] R cher, G. et al.:*Planta Med.* **1985,** 51, 183.

[11] Furukawa, S. and Soma, N.:*Yakugaku Zasshi* **1961,** 81, 559.

[12] Furukawa, S. and Soma, N.:*Yakugaku Zasshi* **1961,** 81, 565.

[13] Krepinsky, J. et al.:*Collect. Czech. Chem. Commun.* **1970,** 35, 745.

[14] Nishida, R. et al.:*Agric. Biol. Chem.* **1973,** 37, 341.

[15] Zhang, X. et al.:*Yaoxue Tongbao* **1981,** 16(9), 57.

[16] Ahmed Farag, I. S. et al.:*Cryst. Res. Technol.* **1988,** 23(6), 729.

[C.K. Sung]

42. *Asiasarum heterotropoides* F. Maekawa var. *mandshuricum* F. Maekawa
(*Asarum heterotropoides* F. Schum. var. *mandshuricum* F. Maekawa (Aristolochiaceae)

Liao–xi–xin (C), Sai–sun (H), Keirin–saishin (J), Jok–do–ri–pul (K)

Related plant: *Asiasarum sieboldii* F. Maekawa (=*Asarum sieboldii Miq.*): Hua–xi–xin (C), Sai–sun (H),
Usuba–saishin (J), Min–jok–do–ri–pul (K).

Whole herb (CP), **Rhizome** and **Root** (JP, KP).

Local Drug Name: Xi–xin (C), Sai–sun (H), Sai–shin (J), Se–sin (K).

Processing: Dry under the shade (C, J, K).

Method of Administration: Oral (decoction: C, H, J, K).

Folk Medicinal Uses:

1) Fever and headache (C, H, J, K).

2) Cough (C, H, J, K).

3) Common cold (C, J, K).

4) Edema (J).

5) Ulcer in the mouth (C).

6) Toothache (C, H).

7) Rheumatic arthritis (C, H).

8) Phlegm (H).

Scientific Researches:

Chemistry

1) Essential oil: methyleugenol, asaryl ketone, pinene, eucarvone, safrol, cineol, l–asarinin, limonene, 2,4,5–trimethoxy–1–allylbenzene, n–pentadecane, elemicin, 3,4,5–trimethoxytoluene, 2,3,5–trimethoxy–toluene, (±)–car–3–en–2–on–5–ol, (±)–epoxycaran–2–on–3–ol [1].

2) Acidamides: peritolin, 2 *E,4E,8Z,10E–N*–isobutyl–2,4,8,10–dodecatetraen–amide and 2 *E,4E,8Z,10Z–N*–isobutyl–2,4,8,10–dodecatetraenamide [2].

3) Alkaloids: hygenamine [3].

Pharmacology

1) Antihistamic (extracts) [3, 4, 5].

2) Antiallergic (acetone extract, elemicin) [6].

3) Cardiac (ethanol extract) [7].

4) Antipyretic analgesic and anti–inflammatory (essential oil) [8].

Literatures:

[1] Nagasawa M.: *Yakugaku Zasshi* **1961**, 81, 129; Saiki Y. et al.: *ibid.* **1967**, 87, 1524; Endo J. et al.: *ibid.* **1978**, 98, 789.

[2] Yasuda, I. et al.: *Chem. Pharm. Bull.* **1981**, 29, 564.

[3] Kosuge, et al.: *Chem. Pharm. Bull.* **1978**, 26, 2284.

[4] Koda, A. et al.: *Nippon Yakurigaku Zasshi* **1982**, 80, 31.

[5] Koda, A. et al.: *Nippon Yakurigaku Zasshi* **1970**, 66, 366; Itokawa, H. et al.: *Shoyakugaku Zasshi* **1983**, 37, 223.

[6] Yamahara, J. et al.: *Wankan Iyaku Gakkaishi* **1986**, 3, 153.

[7] Chen, Z. Z. et al.: *Yaoxue Xuebao* **1981,** 16, 721.

[8] Qu, S. Y. et al.: *Yaoxue Xuebao* **1982**, 17, 12.

[T. Kimura]

43.   *Paeonia lactiflora* **Pallas** (= *P. albiflora* Pall.) (Paeoniaceae)

Shao–yao (C), Bak–churk (H), Shakuyaku (J), Cham–Jak–Yak (K)

Root   (CP, JP, KP)

Local Drug Name: Bai–shao, Chi–shao (C), Bak–churk (H), Shaku–yaku (J), Jak–Yak (K).

Processing: 1) Steam short time then dry in air (J, K).

2) Stir–fry (C). Stir–fry with wine (C).

Method of Administration: Oral (decoction or powder: C, H, J, K).

Folk Medicinal Uses:

1) Pain (C, J, K).

2) Convulsion (C, J).

3) Women's disease, irregular menses, leukorrhea (C, H, J, K).

4) Blood circulation disorder (C, J, K).

5) Headache and dizziness (C).

6) Spontaneous sweating and night sweating (C, H).

7) Maculation in epidemic diseases (C).

8) Abdominal pain (H).

9) Inflammation of the eye (C).

10) Traumatic injuries (C).

11) Boils and sores (C).

Scientific Researches:

Chemistry

　1) Monoterpenoid glycoside: paeoniflorin, paeoniflorigenone, paeonilactone [1, 2, 3, 4].

　2) Tannins: gallo-tannins [5].

Pharmacology

　1) Antiinflammatory (paeoniflorin) [6].

　2) Sedative (paeoniflorin) [6].

　3) Analgesic (paeoniflorin) [6].

　4) Antiulcer (paeoniflorin) [6].

　5) Vasodilator (paeoniflorin) [6].

　6) Coaguration depressing (paeoniflorin [6]), benzoyl paeoniflorin [7].

　7) Blood urea nitrogen lowering (tannins) [8].

Literatures:

[1] Shibata, S. et al.: *Chem. Pharm. Bull.* **1963**, 11, 372, 379; Aimi, N. et al.:*Tetrahedron* **1969**, 25, 1825; Kaneda, M., et al.:*Tetrahedron* **1972**, 28, 4309.

[2] Shimizu, M. et al.:*Chem. Pharm. Bull.* **1983**, 31, 577.

[3] Hayashi, T. et al.: *Tetrahedron Letters* **1985**, 26, 3699.

[4] Lang, et al.:*Planta Med.* **1984**, 501.

[5] Nishizawa, M. et al.:*Chem. Pharm. Bull.* **1983**, 31, 2593.

[6] Takagi K. et al.:*Yakugaku Zasshi* **1969**, 89, 879, 887, 893.

[7] Ishida, H. et al.:*Chem. Pharm. Bull.* **1987**, 35, 849.

[8] Shibutani, S. et al.:*Chem. Pharm. Bull.* **1981**, 29, 874; Nishizawa, M. et al.:*ibid.* **1983**, 31, 2593.

[T. Kimura]

44.　　　*Paeonia suffruticosa* **Andrews** (= *Paeonia moutan* Sims)　(Paeoniaceae)

Mu-dan (C), Mou-dan (H), Botan (J), Mo-Ran (K)

Root bark　(CP, JP, KP)

Local Drug Name: Mu-dan-pi (C), Mou-dan-pai (H), Bo-tan-pi (J), Mok-Dan-Pi (K).

Processing: Take off the central cylindar and dry under the sun (J).

Method of Administration: Oral (decoction or powder: C, H, J, K).

Folk Medicinal Uses:

　　　　　　　1) Women's diseases (C, J, K).

　　　　　　　2) Blood circulation disorder (C, J, K).

　　　　　　　3) Bleeding (C, J, K).

　　　　　　　4) Fever (C, J, K).

　　　　　　　5) Appendicitis (J).

　　　　　　　6) Amenorrhea (H).

　　　　　　　7) Convulsion (H).

　　　　　　　8) Hematemesis, epistaxis (H).

　　　　　　　9) Lumbago (H).

　　　　　　　10) Eruption in epidemic diseases (C).

　　　　　　　11) Carbuncles and sores (C).

　　　　　　　12) Traumatic injuries (C).

Scientific Researches:

Chemistry

　1) Phenolic compounds: paeonol, paeonolide, paeonoside [1, 2, 3].

　2) Monoterpene glycosides: paeoniflorin [4] and oxypaeoniflorin derivatives [5, 6].

3) Tannins [7].

Pharmacology

  1) Antibacterial (paeonol) [8].

  2) Sedative (paeonol) [9].

  3) Central antipyretic analgesic (paeonol) [9].

  4) Central antispasmodic (paeonol) [9]. Muscle antispasmodic [10].

  5) Antiinflammatory (paeonol) [10].

  6) Antiulcer (paeonol) [10].

  7) Blood coaguration depressing (paeonol) [11, 12].

  8) Diuretic (paeonol) [13].

  9) Antiviral (tannins) [14].

Literatures:

1) Kariyone T. et al.:*Yakugaku Zasshi* **1956**, 76, 917, 927.

2) Nagai N.: *Yakugaku Zasshi* **1887**, 8, 288, 495.

3) Yu, Jin, et al.:*Yaoxue Xuebao* **1987**, 21, 191.

4) Shibata, S., Nakahara, M., Aimi, N.:*Chem. Pharm. Bull.* **1963**, 11, 379.

5) Kaneda, M., et al.: *Tetrahedron* **1972**, 28, 4309.

6) Kitagawa I. et al.:*Shoyakugaku Zasshi* **1979**, 33, 171.

7) Nonaka, G. et al.:*99th Ann. Meeting Jap. Soc. Pharmacy, Abstr.* **1979**, p153.

8) Ohta, T. et al.:*Shoyakugaku Zasshi* **1960**, 14, 100.

9) Harada, M. et al.:*Yakugaku Zasshi* **1969**, 89, 1205; Suzuki, Y. et al.:*Nippon Yakurigaku Zasshi,* **1981**, 78, 48.

10) Harada, M. et al.: *Yakugaku Zasshi* **1972**, 92, 750.

11) Ishida, H., et al.:*Chem. Pharm. Bull.* **1987**, 35, 846.

12) Kubo, M. et al.:*Shoyakugaku Zasshi* **1982**, 36, 70.

13) Kawashima, K. et al.:*Planta Med.* **1985**, 51, 187.

14) Takechi, M. et al.:*Planta Med.* **1982**, 45, 252.

[T. Kimura]

45.   *Corydalis turtschaninovii* Besser forma *yanhusuo* Y. H. Chou et C. C.Hsu
(Papaveraceae)

Yan-hu (C), Yin-woo-sok (H)

Related plants: *Corydalis ternata* Nakai (= *C. nakai* Ishidoya): Korai-engosaku (J), Deul-Hyun-Ho-Saek (K)

Rhizome (CP, JP, KP)

  Local Drug Name: Yan-hu-suo (C), Yin-woo-sok (H), En-go-saku (J), Hyun-Ho-Saek (K).

  Processing: 1) Dry under the sun (J, K). 2) Soak in vinegar and stir-fry until slightly dry, then dry under the sun (C).

  Method of Administration: 1) Oral (decoction or powder: C, H, J, K). 2) External (C).

  Folk Medicinal Uses:

      1) Pain, abdominal pain, headache, menorralgia (C, H, J, K).

      2) Convulsive diseases (J).

      3) Anorexia, dyspepsia (J).

      4) Traumatic injury (C, H).

      5) Menstrual disorder (H).

      6) Lochia (H).

      7) Rheumatalgia (H).

Scientific Researches:
Chemistry
  1) Alkaloids: *l*–corydaline, protopine, bulbocapnine, *d*–tetrahydropalmatine, *l*–canadine, coptisine,
                dehydrocorydaline, *l*–tetrahydrocolumbamine, α–allocryptopine, *l*–tetrahydrocoptisine [1].
Pharmacology
  1) Antispasmodic (alkaloids) [2].
  2) Anti–ulcer (dehydrocorydaline) [3, 4].
  3) Blood coaguration depressing (protopine, *d*–corydaline, *l*–tetrahydro-
    columbamine, glaucine) [5, 6, 7].
  4) Central analgesic and sedative (tetrahydropalmatine) [8].

Literatures:

[1] Imazeki I. et al.: *Yakugaku Zasshi* **1962**, 82, 1214; Takemoto T. et al.:*ibid.* **1964**, 84, 721; Iwasa, J.
    et al.: *ibid.* **1966**, 86, 396, 437; **1967**, 87, 1382; Kiryakov, H. G. et al.:*Planta Med.* **1984**, 50, 136.
[2] Kitabatake Y. et al.:*Yakugaku Zasshi* **1964**, 84, 73.
[3] Shoji, Y. et al.:*Nippon Yakurigaku Zasshi* **1969**, 65, 196.
[4] Shoji, Y. et al.:*Nippon Yakurigaku Zasshi* **1974**, 70, 425; Watanabe, K. et al.:*Oyo Yakuri* **1974**, 8,
    1105.
[5] Kosuge T. et al.:*Yakugaku Zasshi* **1984**, 104, 1050.
[6] Matsuda, H. et al.:*Planta Med.* **1988**, 54, 27, 498.
[7] Shiomoto, H. et al.:*Chem. Pharm. Bull.* **1990**, 38, 2320.
[8] Hsu, B. et al.:*Arch. Int. Pharmacodyn.* **1962**, 139, 318.

[T. Kimura]

46.   *Capsella bursa–pastoris* **(L.) Medic.** (Cruciferae)

Ji–cai (C), Chai–choi (H), Nazuna (J), Naeng–i (K)

Whole plant
Local Drug Name: Ji–cai (C), Chai–choi (H), Sei–sai (J), Je–chae (K).
Processing: Dry under the sun or use fresh.
Method of Administration: Oral (decoction: C, H, J, K).
Folk Medicinal Uses:
           1) Hematuria in renal tuberculosis (H).
           2) Hemoptysis from pulmonary tuberculosis (H, K).
           3) Nephritis edema (C, H, K).
           4) Urolithiasis (H).
           5) Chyluria (C, H).
           6) Uterine bleeding (C, H, K).
           7) Menorrhagia, metrorrhagia (C, H, J).
           8) Common cold and fever (H, K).
           9) Hypertension (H).
           10) Sore eyes (C, H, J).
           11) Dysentery (C, K).
           12) Diarrhea (J).
           13) Stomachache (J).
Seed
Local Drug Name: Ji–cai–zi (C), Je–chae–ja (K).
Method of Administration: Oral (decoction: C).
Folk Medicinal Uses:
           1) Anthelmintic (C).

Flower
 Local Drug Name: Ji–cai–hua (C), Je–chae–hwa (K).
 Method of Administration: Oral (decoction: C).
 Folk Medicinal Uses:
>   1) Dysentery (C).
>   2) Uterine hemorrhage (C).

Scientific Researches:
 Chemistry
   1) Alkaloid: brucine.
   2) Flavonoids: rutin, hesperidin, luteolin–7–rutinoside, dihydrofisetin, diosmin, robinetin,
        quercetin–3–methylether, sinigrin.
 Pharmacology
   1) Hemostatic effects.
   2) Hypotensive effects.
   3) Sedative effects.
   4) Antiinflammatory effects.
   5) Antipyretic effects.
   6) Antimicrobial effects [1].
   7) Antineoplastic effects [2].
   8) Antitoxic effects [2].
   9) Uterotonic effects [3].

Literatures:
[1] El–Abyad, M.S. et al.:*Microbios* **1990**, 62(250), 47.
[2] Kuroda, K. et al.:*Gann* **1981**, 72, 777.
[3] Shipochliev, T.:*Vet. Med. Nauki.* **1981**, 18, 94.

[P.P.H. But]

47.   *Rorippa indica* (L.) **Hieron**   (Cruciferae)

Jiang–jian–dao–cao (C), Tong–got–choi (H), Inugarashi (J), Gae–gat–naeng–i (K)

Related Plant: *Rorippa montana* (Wall.) Small: Han–cai (C).

Herb
 Local Drug Name: Han–cai (C), Tong–got–choi (H), Kan–sai (J), Han–chae(K).
 Processing: Dry under the sun (C).
 Methed of Administration: Oral (decoction: C, H). Topical (paste of fresh herb: C, H).
 Folk Medicinal Uses:
>   1) Chronic tracheitis (C).
>   2) Emaciation due to blood disorders, abdominal distention (C).
>   3) Toothache due to pathogenic wind–cold, sore throat (C, H).
>   4) Carbuncles and boils, scald burn (C).
>   5) Acute bronchitis (H).
>   6) Sore throat (H).
>   7) Cough (H).
>   8) Rheumatic arthritis (H).
>   9) Hepatitis (H).
>   10) Oliguria (H).
 Contraindications: Not to use with leaf of *Vitex negundo*.

Scientific Resarches:
  Chemistry
    1) Cyanogenic compounds: rorifone [1].
    2) Organic acids [1].
  Pharmacology
    1) Expectorant effect (rorifone) [2].
    2) Bacteriostatic effect (rorifone) [2].

Literatures:

[1] Shanghai Institute of Materia Medica:*Zhongcaoyao Tongxun* **1972**, (4), 27.
[2] Nanjing College of Pharmacy: *"Zhongcaoyao Xue"* Vol. 2, **1976**, 372.

[J.X. Guo]

48   *Agrimonia pilosa* Ledeb. var. *japonica* (Miq.) Nakai (Rosaceae)

Long–yia–cao(C), Sin–hock–cho(H), Kinmizuhiki(J), Jip–sin–na–mul(K)

Related plant: *Agrimonia pilosa* Ledeb.: Shu–mao–long–yia–cao (C; CP).

Herb (CP)
  Local Drug Name: Xian–he–cao (C), Sin–hock–cho (H), Sen–kaku–so, Ryu–ga–so (J), Yong–a–cho (K).
  Processing: Cut into sections and dry under the sun (C, H, J, K).
  Method of Administration: Oral (decoction: C, H, J, K); Gargle (decoction: J); Topical (decoction or
            electuary: C).
  Folk Medicinal Uses:
            1) Hematuria (C, H).
            2) Hematemesis (C, H).
            3) Leukorrhea (C, H).
            4) Taenia (C, K).
            5) Boil (C, K).
            6) Traumatic injury (C).
            7) Diarrhea (J).
            8) Stomatitis (J).
            9) Tonsillitis (J).
            10) Eczema (K).
            11) Hemoptysis (C).
            12) Hematochezia (C).
            13) Gastroenteritis (C).
            14) Enteric trichomoniasis (C).
            15) Vaginal trichomoniasis (C).

Rhizome with adventitious bud
  Local Drug Name: Xian–he–cao–gan–ya (C).
  Processing: Dry under the sun (C).
  Method of Administration: Oral (decoction: C).
  Folk Medicinal Uses:
            1) Taenia (C).

Scientific Researches:
  Chemistry
    1) Phenols: agrimol A, B [1, 2, 5], C[13], D, E [1, 2, 5], F, G [13], ellagic acid, gallic acid [4],

49

agrimophol [7, 8, 14], (R)–(–)–agrimol B [14], pseudoaspidin [14].

2) Tannins: agrimoniin [3, 9, 10, 11], potentillin [3], pedunculagin [3].

3) Isocoumarins: agrimonolide [6], agrimonolide 6-O-β-D-glucopyranoside [14].

4) Phenylpropanoids: caffeic acid [4], $trans$–p–Hydroxycinnamic esters of n–C_{22}, n–C_{24-32}, n–C_{34} alcohols [14].

5) Flavonoids: luteolin–7–glucoside, apigenin–7–glucoside, quercetin [4], (2S,3S)–(–)–taxifolin–3-O-β-D-glucopyranoside [15].

6) Triterpenoids: 2,19–dihydroxyursolic acid–(28–1)-β-D-glucopyranoside, 1,2,3,19–tetrahydroxy–urs–12–en–28–oic acid, 1,2,3,19–tetrahydroxy–urs–12–en–28–oic acid [12].

7) Hydrocarbons: n–nonacosane [14].

8) Sterols: β–sitosterol [14].

Pharmacology

1) Antitumor activity (agrimoniin) [9, 10].

2) Dysentery (flavonoid mixture) [4].

3) Bacteristatic action (luteolin–7–glucoside, apigenin–7–glucoside, ellagic acid, gallic acid) [4].

4) Immune stimulating action (agrimoniin) [11].

Literatures:

[1] Cheng, C. L. et al.: *Huaxue Xuebao* **1978,** 36, 35.

[2] Shian Ho Tasao Working group: *Kexue Tongbao*, **1974,** 19, 479.

[3] Okuda, T. et al.: *J. Chem. Soc., Chem. Commun.* **1982,** 163.

[4] Su, G. et al.: *Senyang Yaoxueyuan Xuebao* **1984,** 1(1), 44.

[5] Li, L. C. et al.: *Hua Hsueh Hsueh Pao* **1978,** 36(1), 43.

[6] Yamato, M. et al.: *Chem. Pharm. Bull.* **1976,** 24(2), 200.

[7] Shenyang College of Pharmacy: *Hua Hsueh Hsueh Pao* **1977,** 35(1–2), 87.

[8] Sha, Shi–Yan: *Yao Hsueh Tung Pao* **1980,** 15(7), 6.

[9] Miyamoto, K. et al.: *Chem. Pharm. Bull.* **1985,** 33, 3977.

[10] Miyamoto, K. et al.: *Jpn. J. Pharmacol.* **1987,** 43(2), 187.

[11] Miyamoto, K. et al.: *Cancer Immunol. Immunother.* **1988,** 27(1), 59.

[12] Kouno, I. et al.: *Phytochemistry* **1988,** 27(1), 29.

[13] Yamaki, M. et al.: *Planta Med.* **1989,** 55(2), 169.

[14] Pei, Y. H. et al.: *Yaoxue Xuebao* **1989,** 24(11), 837.

[15] Pei, Y. H. et al.: *Yaoxue Xuebao* **1990,** 25(4), 267.

[C.K. Sung]

49. *Chaenomeles sinensis* **(Thouin) Koehne** (Rosaceae)
(= *Pseudocydonia sinensis* (Thouin) Schneid.)

Mu–gua (C), Muk–gwa (H), Karin (J), Mo–gwa–na–mu (K)

Fruit

Local Drug Name: Mu–gua (C), Muk–gwa (H), Mei–sa, Wa–mok–ka (J), Mo–gwa (K).

Processing: Treat with boiling water for five to ten minutes, cut in half with copper knife, dry under the sun (C, J).

Method of Administration: Oral (decoction or spirit: C, H, J, K).

Folk Medicinal Uses:

1) Pain due to pathogenic wind–dampness (C, H).

2) Systremma due to vomiting and diarrhea (C, K).

3) Edema and weakness of the legs (C, H, K).

4) Rheumatalgia (H).

5) Cough (J, K).
6) Low back pain (J).
7) Common cold (K).
8) Harsh throat (K).

Scientific Researches:
Chemistry
1) Organic acids: malic acid, tartaric acid, citric acid, ascorbic acid [1].
Pharmacology
1) Anthydropic effect [2].

Literatures:
[1] Yu, D. W.: *Zhongyao Tiyao* **1954**, 24, 172.
[2] Nanjiing College of Pharmacy:*Yaoxue Xuebao*, **1966**, 13, 94.

[J.X. Guo]

50.   *Chaenomeles speciosa*(Sweet) **Nakai**   (Rosaceae)

Tie–geng–hai–tang (C), Boke (J), Myeong–ja–ggot (K)

Fruit (CP)
Local Drug Name: Mu–gua (C), Muk–gwa (H), Mok–ka (J), Mo–gwa (K).
Processing: Wash clean, soften or steam thoroughly, cut into thin slices and dry under the sun (C, J).
Method of Administration: Oral (decoction: C, H, J); (liquor: J).
Folk Medicinal Uses:
1) Arthritis with ankylosis, aching and heaviness sensation of the loins and knees
   (C, H, J).
2) Systremma due to vomiting and diarrhea (C).
3) Edema and weakness of the legs (C, H, J).
4) Rheumatalgia (H).
5) Insomnia (J).
6) Hypotonia (J).
7) Feeling of cold (J).

Scientific Researches:
Chemistry
1) Organic acids: malic acid, tartaric acid, citric acid, vitamin C [1].
2) Triterpenes: oleanolic acid [2].
3) Others: saponins, flavonoids, tannins [1].
Pharmacology
1) Anthydropic effect [3].
2) Antitumer effect [4].

Literatures:
[1] *"Zhongcaoyao Youxiaochengfen Yanjiu"* **1972**, Vol.1, 435.
[2] Luo, J. F.: *Zhongcaoyao* **1983**, 14, 48.
[3] Nanjing College of Pharmacy:*Yaoxue Xuebao* **1966**, 13, 94.
[4] Jin, Z. R.:*Zhongcaoyao Tongxun***1975**, 6, 18.

[J.X. Guo]

51.   *Eriobotrya japonica* **Lindl.**   (Rosaceae)

Pi–pa (C), Pay–par (H), Biwa (J)

Fruit
Local Drug Name: Pi–pa (C), Pay–par–gwo (H), Bi–wa (J).
Method of Administration: Oral (fresh).
Folk Medicinal Uses:
        1) Hematemesis (C).
        2) Hemorrhinia (C).
        3) Hiccup (C).
        4) Coughing and sputum (C, H).
Contraindications: Spleen deficiency.

Leaf (CP)
Local Drug Name: Pi–pa–ye (C), Pay–par–yip (H), Bi–wa–yo (J).
Processing: 1) Eliminate hairs, moisten with water, cut into slivers and dry (C).
               2) Stir–fry slivers with honey until not sticky to fingers (C).
Method of Administration: Oral or topical wash (decoction: C, H, J).
Folk Medicinal Uses:
        1) Bronchitis, cough (C, H, J).
        2) Gastritis (C, H, J).
        3) Antiemetic (H, J).
        4) Coughing and sputum (C, H).
        5) Summer heat diseases (J).
        6) Eczema (J).
        7) Prickly heat (J).
Contraindications: Vomitting in cold stomach disease.

Flower
Local Drug Name: Pi–pa–hua (C), Bi–pa–hwa (K), Bi–wa–ka (J).
Method of Administration: Oral (decoction: C).
Folk Medicinal Uses:
        1) Common cold (C).
        2) Sore throat (C).
        3) Coughing (C).

Seed
Local Drug Name: Pi–pa–he (C), Pay–par–wat (H), Bi–wa–kaku (J), Bi–pa–haek (K).
Method of Administration: Oral (Water extract, C, H).
Folk Medicinal Uses:
        1) Coughing and sputum (C, H).
        2) Hernia (C, H).
        3) Edema (C).
        4) Scrofula (C).
        5) Lymphoid tuberculosis (H).

Root
Local Drug Name: Pi–pa–gen (C), Pay–par–gun (H), Bi–wa–kon (J), Bi–pa–geun (K).
Method of Administration: Oral (decoction: C, H).
Folk Medicinal Uses:
        1) Consumptive coughing (C, H).
        2) Rheumatalgia (C, H).
        3) Hepatitis (C, H).

Scientific Researches:

Chemistry

1) Leaf contains nerolidol, farnesol, amygdalin, ursolic acid, oleanolic acid [1]α-, β-pinene, camphene, β-myrcene, *p*-cymene, *cis*-β,γ-hexenol, *trans*-linaloöloxide, *cis*-linaloöloxide, linaloöl, camphor, α-ylangene, β-farnesene, α-farnesene, nerol, geraniol,*cis*-nerolidol,*trans*-nerolidol, elemol, α-cadinene, *trans,cis*-farnesol,*trans,trans*-farnesol [2].

2) Seed contains amygdalin, ceryl alcohol [1], 4–methyleneproline [3].

Literatures:

[1] Arthur, H.R. et al.:*J. Chem. Soc.* **1954**, 2782.

[2] Suemitsu, R. et al.:*Shoyakugaku Zasshi* **1973**, 27, 7.

[3] Gray, D.O. et al.:*Nature* **1962**, 163, 1285.

[P.P.H. But]

---

52.   *Prunus armeniaca* **Linn.**   (Rosaceae)

Xing (C), Heng–sue (H), Hon anzu (J)

Related plant: *Prunus armeniaca* L. *var. ansu* Maxim.: Shan–xing (C), Anzu (J), Sal–gu (K);

                   P. sibirica L.: Xi–bo–li–ya–xing (C), Mouko anzu (J);

                   P. mandshurica Koene: Dong–bei–xing, Liao–xing (C), Manshu anzu (J)

Seed   (CP, JP, KP)

Local Drug Name: Ku–xing–ren (C), Heng–yan (H), Kyo–nin (J), Haeng–in (K).

Processing: 1) Dry under the sun (J, K). 2) Rinsed in boiling matter (C). 3) Stir–fry (C).

Method of Administration: 1) Oral (decoction or powder: H, J, K). 2) Oral (Apricot kernel water: J).

                         3) To be added when the decoction is nearly done (C).

Folk Medicinal Uses:

             1) Common cold (H, J, K).

             2) Cough (C, H, J, K).

             3) Phlegm (C, H, J, K).

             4) Constipation due to deficiency of blood and fluid (C).

Side Effects: Toxic on overdose.

Scientific Researches:

Chemistry

      1) Cyanhydrin glycoside: amygdalin [1].

      2) Enzyme: emulsinase [2].

Pharmacology

      1) Antitussive (amygdalin) [3, 4].

      2) Antipyretic (decoction) [3].

      3) Toxicity (amygdalin) [5].

Literatures:

[1] Nagoshi, Y. et al.:*Shoyakugaku Zasshi* **1976**, 30, 42.

[2] Nagamoto N. et al.:*Shoyakugaku Zasshi* **1988**, 42, 81.

[3] Goto K. et al.:*Wakan Iyaku Gakkaishi* **1984**, 1, 126.

[4] Miyagoshi, M. et al.:*Planta Med.* **1986**, 52, 275.

[5] Reitnauer, P. G.:*Arzneim. Forsch.* **1972**, 22, 1347.

[T. Kimura]

53.   *Prunus persica* Batsch   (Rosaceae)

Tao (C), Toe–sue (H), Momo (J), Bok–sung–a–na–mu (K)

Related plant: *Prunus davidiana* Franch. (= *P. persica* Batsch var. *davidiana* Max.):
Shan–tao (C), Nomomo (J), San–bok–sung–a–na–mu (K).

Seed   (CP, JP, KP)
Local Drug Name: Tao–ren (C), Toe–yan (H), To–nin (J), Do–in (K).
Processing: 1) Dry under the sun (J). 2) Rinsed in boiling water and dry (C). 3)Stir–fry (C).
Method of Administration: Oral (decoction or powder: C, H, J, K).
Folk Medicinal Uses:

> 1) Women's disease (C, J, K).
> 2) Dysmenorrhea, amenorrhea (H).
> 3) Blood circulation disorder (C, J).
> 4) Mass formation in the abdomen (C).
> 5) Constipation (C, H, J, K).
> 6) Traumatic injury (C).
> 7) Hematoma (H).
> 8) Contusion (H).

Side Effects: Toxic on overdose (J).

Leaf
Local Drug Name: Tao–ye (C), Toe–yip (H), To–yo (J).
Processing: Dry under the sun or fresh (J).
Method of Administration: Oral (decoction: H, J).
Folk Medicinal Uses:

> 1) Malaria (H).
> 2) Furunculosis (H).
> 3) Hemorrhoid (H).
> 4) Eczema (H).
> 5) Vaginal trichomoniasis (H).
> 6) Dermatitis with lacquer (J).

Flower
Local Drug Name: Tao–hua (C), Toe–fa (H), Haku–to–ka (J).
Processing: Collect the flower buds, and dry under the sun (J).
Method of Administration: Oral (decoction: H, J).
Folk Medicinal Uses:

> 1) Edema (H, J).
> 2) Ascites (H).
> 3) Constipation (H, J).

Scientific Researches:
Chemistry
1) Cyanhydrin glycoside: amygdalin [1].
2) Enzyme: emulsinase [1].
3) Steroids [2].
4) Proteine [3].
Pharmacology
1) Antiinflammatory (proteine) [3].
2) Platelet coaguration depressing [4].
3) Vasodilator activity [5].
4) Toxicity (amygdalin) [6].

Literatures:

[1] Nagoshi, T. et al.:*Shoyakugaku Zasshi* **1946**, 30, 42; Nagamoto, N. et al.:*ibid.* **1988**, 42, 81.

[2] Mori H. et al.: *Shoyakugaku Zasshi* **1983**, 37, 46.

[3] Arichi S. et al.:*Shoyakugaku Zasshi* **1986**, 40, 129.

[4] Kosuge, T. et al.:*Chem. Pharm. Bull.* **1985**, 33, 1496; Yun–Choi, H. S., et al.:*J. Nat. Prod.* **1985**, 48, 363.

[5] Watanabe K. et al.:*Wakan Iyaku Gakkaishi***1987**, 4, 274.

[6] Reitnauer, P. G.:*Arzneim. Forsch.* **1972**, 22, 1347.

[T. Kimura]

54.   *Rosa cymosa* Tratt.   (Rosaceae)

Xiao–guo–qiang–wei (C)

Root, Leaf

Local Drug Name: Xiao–guo–qiang–wei (C), Sho–kin–ou (J).

Processing: Wash clean, dry under the sun (C).

Method of Administration: Oral (decoction: C); Topical (appropriate quantity of the fresh leaves to be pounded into paste: C).

Folk Medicinal Uses:

1) Rheumatic arthritis, traumatic injury (C).

2) Abnomal uterine bleeding, boils and sores (C).

3) Traumatic bleeding (C).

Scientific Researches

Chemistry

1) Tannins: ellagic acid [1].

2) Others: organic acids, saponins, resins, carbohydrates, proteins, inorganic salts, etc.[2].

Pharmacology

1) Styptic effect [1].

2) Bacteriostatic effect [1].

Literatures:

[1] Nanijing College of Pharmacy: *"Zhongcaoyao Xue"*, Vol. 2, **1976**, 421.

[2] *"Quanguo Zhongcaoyao Huibian"* **1975**, Vol. 1, 93.

[J.X. Guo]

55.   *Rosa multiflora* Thunb. (= *R. polyantha* Sieb. et Zucc.) (Rosaceae)

Shan–ci–mei (C), Noibara (J), Jjil–re–na–mu (K)

Fruit   (JP)

Local Drug Name: Ci–mei, Ying–shi (C), Ei–jitsu (J), Yeong–sil (K).

Processing: 1) Dry under the sun (C, J, K). 2) Dry in the shade or use in fresh (C).

Method of Administration: Oral (decoction: C, J, K); Powder: J, K).

Folk Medicinal Uses:

1) Constipation (J, K).

2) Articular pain (J, K).

3) Myalgia (J).
4) Dyspepsia (C).
5) Irregular menstruation (C).
Side Effects: Nausea, stomach ache (J).

Scientific Research:
Chemistry
1) Flavonoid glycoside: multiflorin A, B, multinoside A, B, quercetin glucorhamnoside, kaempferol–glucorhamnoside, quercitrin, afzelin [1].
2) Phenolic compounds: methyl gallate [1].
3) Carotenoids: lycopin.
Pharmacology
1) Purgative: multiflorin A [1, 2].

Literatures:
[1] Takagi S. et al.: *Yakugaku Zasshi* **1976**, 96, 284, 1217; **1980**, 100, 466.
[2] Ando S.: *Kyoto Igakkashi* **1912**, 9, 91.

[T. Kimura]

56   *Sanguisorba officinalis* **L.**   (Rosaceae)

Di–yu (C), Day–yue (H)

Related Plant: *Sanguisorba officinalis* L. var. *carnea* Regel: Waremoko (J), O–i–pul (K).

Root and rhizome
Local Drug Name: Di–yu (H), Ji–yu (J), Ji–yu (K).
Processing: Dry under the sun (J, K).
Method of Administration: Oral (decoction: C, H, J, K); Topical (J).
Folk Medicinal Uses:
1) Boils (H, K).
2) Abscess (H, K).
3) Hemostyptic (J, K).
4) Hematemesis (J, K).
5) Arthritis (K).
6) Neuralgia (K).
7) Leukorrhea (K).
8) Indigestion due to hot weather (K).
9) Frost–bite (K).
10) Syphilis (K).
11) Pus (K).
12) Snake bite (K).
13) Tympanitis (K).
14) Burns (H).
15) Antiphlogistic (K).
16) Menostasis (K).
17) Dysentery (H, K).
18) Gonorrhea (K).
19) Endometritis (K).
20) Blood leukorrhea (K).
21) Hemoptysis (J).

22) Melena (J).
23) Menorrhagia (J).
24) Burn, eczema, boil, dermatitis (topical:J).
25) Epistaxis (H).
26) Hemorrhoid (H).
27) Eczema (H).
28) Knife wound (H).

Scientific Researches:
Chemistry
1) Tannins: sanguiin H$_4$, methyl 6– O–galloyl β –D–glucoside, 3–O–galloylprocyanidin [1], ellagitannins [2], 2',5–di–O–galloylhamamelose (hamamelitannin), 2',3,5–tri–O–galloyl–,1,2'–di–O–galloyl–, 5–O–galloyl–, 1,2',5–tri–O–galloyl–1,2',3,5–tetra–O–galloyl–D–hamamelofuranose [3], 3,3',4–tri–O–methylellagic acid [4], gambiriin A–1, B–3 [7], sanguiin H–1, H–2, H–3, H–6, H–11 [14–16].
2) Catechols: (+)–catechol, (+)–gallocatechol [5].

Pharmacology
1) Anti–periodontal disease [6].
2) Increasing action of the endurance of the animals subjected to stress [5].
3) Anticoagulant activity (polysaccharide) [8].
4) Skin–lightening effect [9].
5) Antihemorrhagic action (3,3',4–tri-O–methylellagic acid) [4, 10, 11].
6) Promotion of healing and anti–inflammatory [12].
7) Anti–inflammatory action [13].
8) Protease inhibitory effect (tannin) [17].

Literatures:
[1] Nippon Shinyaku Co.:*Jpn. Kokai Tokkyo Koho* JP58,154,571, 14 Sep. **1983**.
[2] Sunstar, Inc:*Jpn. Kokai Tokkyo Koho* JP58,38,208, 05 Mar. **1983**.
[3] Nonaka, G. et al.:*Chem. Pharm. Bull.* **1984,** 32(2), 483.
[4] Hokuriku Pharmaceutical Co., Ltd.:*Jpn. Kokai Tokkyo Koho* JP57,145,879, 09, Sep. **1982**.
[5] Azovtsev, G. R. et al.:*Izv. Sib. Otd. Akad. Nauk SSSR Ser. Biol. Nauk,***1985,** 41.
[6] Sunstar, Inc.:*Jpn. Kokai Tokkyo Koho* 80,120,509, 17 Sep. **1980**.
[7] Tanaka, T. et al.:*Phytochem.* **1983,** 22(11), 2575.
[8] Han, Y. N. et al.:*Yakhak Hoechi* **1984,** 28(2), 69.
[9] Mori, K. et al.:*Jpn. Kokai Tokkyo Koho* JP63,303,910, 12 Dec. **1988**.
[10] Ishida, H. et al.:*Yakugaku Zasshi* **1989,** 109(3), 179.
[11] Kosuge, T. et al.:*Chem. Pharm. Bull.* **1984,** 32(11), 4478.
[12] Lou, B. et al.:*Faming Zhuanli Shenqing Gongkai Shuomingshu CN*1,032,294, 12 Apr. **1989**.
[13] Sunstar, Inc.:*Jpn. Kokai Tokkyo Koho* JP58,38,209, 05 Mar. **1983**.
[14] Nonaka, G. et al.:*J. Chem. Soc., Perkin Trans.* I, **1982**(4), 1067.
[15] Nonaka, G. et al.:*Chem. Pharm. Bull.***1982,** 30(6), 2255.
[16] Tanaka, T. et al.:*J. Chem. Res., Synop.*, **1985**(6), 176.
[17] Okuda, T. et al.:*Wakanyaku Shinpojumu, [Kiroku]***1982,** 15, 111.

[C.K. Sung]

57. *Albizia julibrissin* **Durazz.** (Leguminosae)

He–huan (C), Hup–foon (H), Nemunoki (J), Ja–gwi–na–mu (K).

Bark (CP)

Local Drug Name: He–huan–pi (C), Hup–foon–pay (H), Go–kan–pi (J), Hap–hwan–pi (K).
Processing: Eliminate foreign matter, wash clean, soften thoroughly, cut into slices or pieces, and dry.
Method of Administration: Oral (decoction: C, H, J, K); Topical (decoction: J).
Folk Medicinal Uses:

> 1) Insomnia (C, H, K).
> 2) Pruritus (C).
> 3) Scrofula (C).
> 4) Traumatic injury (C).
> 5) Anthelmintic (C).
> 6) Coughing and sputum (C, K).
> 7) Sprain (J).
> 8) Articular pain (J).
> 9) Low back pain (J).

Flower (CP)

Local Drug Name: He–huan–hua (C), Hup–foon–fa (H), Go–kan–ka (J), Hap–hwan–hwa (K).
Method of Administration: Oral (decoction: C, H).
Folk Medicinal Uses:

> 1) Insomnia (C, H).
> 2) Chest distention (C).
> 3) Conjunctivitis (C).
> 4) Sore throat (C).
> 5) Traumatic injury (C).

Scientific Researches:

Chemistry

1) Glycosides: albizzin, albiside [3], (−)–syringaresinol–4–*O*–β–D–glucopyranoside, 4,4'–bis–*O*–β–D–glucopyranoside, (−)–syringaresinol–4–*O*–β–D–apiofuranosy–l(1→2)–β–D–gluco–pyranoside, (−)–syringaresinol–4–*O*–β–D–apiofuranosyl–(1→2)–β–D–glucopyranosyl–4'–*O*–β–D–glucopyranoside, (−)–syringaresinol–4,4'–bis–*O*–β–D–apiofuranosyl–(1→2)–β–D–gluco–pyranoside [4], syringic acid methyl ester 4–*O*–β–D–apiofuranosyl–(1→2)–β–D–gluco–pyranoside, glaberide I 4–*O*–β–D–glucopyranoside, glaberide I 4–*O*–β–D–apiofuranosyl–(1→2)–β–D–glucopyranoside, (+)–5,5'–dimethoxylaricresinol–4–*O*–β–D–apiofuranosy–(1→2)–β–D–glucopyranoside, 5,5'–dimethoxy–7–oxolariciresinol 4'– *O*–β–D–apiofuranosyl–(1→2)–β–D–glucopyranoside [5], icariside E$_5$, 3,4,5–trimethoxyphenol 1–*O*–β–D–apiofuranosy–(1→2)–β–D–glucopyranoside, vomifoiol 3'–*O*–β–D–apiofuranosyl–(1→6)–β–D–glucopyranoside, (+)–lyoni–resinol 9'–*O*–β–D–glucopyranosyl–(1→4)–β–D–glucopyranoside, (+)–lyoniresinol 4,9'–di–*O*–β–D–glucopyranoside [6], julibrines I–II [7], 3–hydroxy–5–hydroxymethyl–methoxymethyl–2–methylpyridine 3–*O*–β–D–glucopyranoside [7], and julibrosides A$_1$–A$_4$, B$_1$, and C$_1$ [8].

2) Serotonin, norepinephrine [1]
3) 4,6–dimethoxyphthalide, (+)–pinitol, α–spinasterol, α–spinasterone [2].
4) Sapogenols: julibrogenins B, C [8].
5) Lactone: julibrotriterpenoidal lactone A [9].
6) Willardiine, isowillardiine [10].

Pharmacology

1) Oxytocic effects
2) Sedative effects
3) Arrhythmic effects (julibrine II) [7]

Literatures:

[1] Applewhite, P.B.:*Phytochem.* **1973**, 12, 191.

[2] Nakano, Y. et al.:*Mokuzai Gakkaishi* **1975**, 21, 577.

[3] Sergienko, T.V. et al.:*Khim. Prir. Soedin.* **1977**, 13, 708.

[4] Kinjo, J. et al.: *Chem. Pharm. Bull.* **1991**, 39, 1623.

[5] Kinjo, J. et al.: *Chem. Pharm. Bull.* **1991**, 39, 2952.

[6] Higuchi, H. et al.:*Chem. Pharm. Bull.* **1992**, 40, 534.

[7] Higuchi, H. et al.:*Chem. Pharm. Bull.* **1992**, 40, 829.

[8] Kinjo, J. et al.: *Chem. Pharm. Bull.* **1992**, 40, 3269.

[9] Kang, S.W. et al.:*Zhongguo Zhongyao Zazhi* **1992**, 17, 357.

[10] Murakoshi, I. et al.:*Phytochem.* **1978**, 17, 1571.

[11] Kaneta, M. et al.:*Agric. Biol. Chem.* **1980**, 44, 1407.

[P.P.H. But]

58.   *Astragalus membranaceus* **Bunge** (Leguminosae)

Mo–jia–huang–qi (C), Wong–kay (H), Kibana–ogi (J), Hwang–gi (K)

Related plant: *Astragalus mongholicus* Bunge: Meng–gu–huang–qi (C), Naimo–ogi (J);

Root (CP, JP, KP)

Local Drug Name: Huang–qi (C), Wonng–kay (H), O–gi (J), Hwang–gi (K).

Processing: 1) Dry under the sun (J). 2) Eliminate foreign matter, wash clean, soften thoroughly, cut into thick slices, and dry (C). 3) Stir–fry with honey (C, H).

Method of Administration: Oral (decoction or powder: C, H, J, K).

Folk Medicinal Uses:

1) Gastrointestinal disorder (C, J, K).

2) Weakness (C, J, K). Debility (stir fryed/honey; H).

3) Hypertension (J).

4) Edema (H). Edema with articular pain (C, J).

5) Night sweat (H). Spontaneous sweating due to weakened superficial resistance (C).

6) Abscess difficult to burst or to heal (C). Carbuncle (H).

7) Anemia (C).

8) Diabetes caused by internal Heat (C).

9) Albuminuria in chronic nephritis (C).

10) Diabetes mellitus (C).

11) Arthralgia due to blood–deficiency (H).

12) Diarrhea (stir fryed/honey; H).

13) Prolapse of rectum (stir fryed/honey; H).

14) Leucorrhea (stir fryed).

Scientific Researches:

Chemistry

1) Isoflavonoids: 2',4'–dihydroxy–5,6–dimethoxyisoflavone [1], astraisoflavan, astraisoflavan–7–O–β–D–glucoside, astrapterocarpan [2].

2) Saponins: astragaloside I ~ IV [3].

3) Amino acids: γ –amino butyric acid [4].

4) Phenolic glycosides[5].

Pharmacology

1) Antihypertensive (γ –amino butyric acid [4, 6, 7, 8], saponins[9]).

2) Diuretic (decoction) [10].

3) Antiinflammatory (saponins) [9].
4) Serum cyclic AMP increasing [9].
5) Macropharge stimulation [11, 12].

Literatures:

[1] Kuarabayashi, M. et al.:*Ann. Meeting Jap. Soc. Pharmacy* **1969**.
[2] Yu, J. et al.:*Zhongyao Tongbao* **1986**, 11, 550.
[3] Kitagawa, I. et al.: *Chem. Pharm. Bull.* **1983**, 31, 689, 698, 709, 716.
[4] Hikino, H. et al.:*Planta Med.* **1976**, 30, 297; Cao, Z. et al.:*Huaxue Xuebao* **1985**, 43, 581.
[5] Takai, M. et al.:*100th Ann. Meeting, Jap. Soc. Pharm., Abstr.* **1980**, p.214.
[6] Terada, B. et al.:*Nippon Yakubutsugaku Zasshi* **1934**, 18, 40; **1938**, 25, 27.
[7] Fujita, M.:*Shikoku Igaku Zasshi* **1959**, 14, 513.
[8] Takahashi, T. et al.:*Nippon Yakurigaku Zasshi* **1959**, 55, 51.
[9] Zhang, Y. D. et al.:*Yaoxue Xuebao* **1984**, 19, 333, 619.
[10] Huang, H. K. et al.:*Yaoxue Xuebao* **1965**, 12, 319.
[11] Lau, B. H. S. et al.:*Phytother. Res.* **1989**, 3, 148.
[12] Wang, J. et al.:*Japan. J. Pharmacol.* **1989**, 51, 432.

[T. Kimura]

59   *Caragana sinica* (Buehoz) Rehd.(= *C. chamlagu* Lam.)   (Leguminosae)

Jin–ji–er, Jin–que–hua (C), Muresuzume (J), Gol–dam–cho (K)

Root
  Local Drug Name: Jin–ji–er (C), Geum–jak–geun (K).
  Processing: Dry under the sun (C, K).
  Method of Administration: Oral (Decoction or tablet, C, K. Sweet drink made from rice, sprouted barley
                 and this drug, K)
  Folk Medicinal Uses:
           1) Edema, hypogalactia (C).
           2) Traumatic injury (C).
           3) Arthralgia due to pathogenic wind–dampness (C).
           4) Hypertension (C).
           5) Irregular menstruation (C).
           6) Arthritis (K).
           7) Neuralgia (K).
           8) Bone–weakness (K).
           9) Diarrhea (K).
  Side Effects: Diarrhea (K).

Scientific Researches:
  Chemistry
    1) Saponins: caraganoside A, kalopanax–saponin F, hemsloside Ma3, uraloside A [1].
  Pharmacology
    1) Bacteriostatic effect [2].
    2) Antihypertensive effect [2].

Literatures:

[1] Lee, Y.B. et al.:*Arch. Pharmacal. Res.* **1992**, 15, 62.
[2] Nanjing College of Pharmacy:*"Zhongcaoyao Xue"*, **1976**, Vol.2, 459.

[J.X. Guo]

60.   Cassia tora L.   (Leguminosae)

Xiao–jue–ming (C), Kuet–ming (H), Hosomi–ebisugusa (J), Gyul–myung–cha (K)

Related plant: *Cassia obtusifolia* L.: Jue–ming (C), Kuet–ming (H), Ebisugusa (J).
                     C. torosa Cavanilles: Habuso (J), Seok–Gyul–Myung (K).

Seed   (CP, JP, KP)
  Local Drug Name: Jue–ming–zi (C), Kuet–ming–gee (H), Ketsu–mei–shi (J), Gyul–myung–ja (K).
  Processing: 1) Dry under the sun (C, J). 2) Stir–fry (C, J).
  Method of Administration: Oral (decoction: C, J, K); Herb tea or powder (J, K).
  Folk Medicinal Uses:
                  1) Gastrointestinal disorder (J, K).
                  2) Constipation (C, H, J, K).
                  3) Glaucoma, nyctalopia (C, H, J, K).
                  4) Edema (J, K).
                  5) Headache, dizziness (C).
                  6) Conjunctivitis (H).
                  7) Hepatitis (H).
                  8) Hypertension (H).
                  9) Ascites (H).
                  10) Inflammation of the eye with pain (C).
                  11) Photophobia and lacrimination (C).

Scientific Researches:
  Chemistry
    1) Anthraquinones: Chrysophanol, emodin, obtusifolin, obtusin, chryso–obtusin,
                aurantio–obtusin [1].
    2) Naphthopyrones: rubrofusarin, nor–rubrofusarin [2].
  Pharmacology
    1) Gastric secretion increasing [3].
    2) Antibacterial (emodin, isotoralactone, toralactone) [4].
    3) Cyclic AMP phospho–diesterase inhibition (emodin, obtusin) [5].
    4) Platelet coaguration depressing (glucosides of obtusifolin, chryso–obtusifolin and
                aurantio–obtusifolin) [6].
    5) Hepatotonic (cassiaside, rubrofusarin–6–β–gentiobiose) [7].

Literatures:
[1] Takido M.: *Chem. Pharm. Bull.* **1958**, 6, 398, **1960**, 8, 246; Kitanaka, S. et al.:*Chem. Pharm. Bull.* **1984**, 32, 860; **1985**, 33, 1274; Wong, S. M. et al.:*Phytochem.* **1988**, 28, 211.
[2] Kimura Y. et al.:*Yakugaku Zasshi* **1966**, 86,   1087; Shibata S. et al.:*Chem. Pharm. Bull.* **1969**, 17, 454, 458; Kitanaka, S., et al.:*Chem. Pharm. Bull.* **1988**, 36, 3980.
[3] Sato I.: *Kyoto Furitsu Ikadaigaku Zasshi***1936**, 16, 443.
[4] Kitanaka S., Takido M.:*Yakugaku Zasshi* **1986**, 106, 302.
[5] Nikaido, T. et al.:*Chem. Pharm. Bull.* **1984**, 32, 3075.
[6] Yun–Choi, H. S., et al.:*J. Nat. Prod.* **1990**, 53, 630.
[7] Wong, S.–M., et al. :*Planta Med.* **1989**, 55, 276.

                                                                   [T. Kimura]

61. *Desmodium pulchellum* (L.) Benth.   (Leguminosae)

Pai–qian–cao (C), Pie–chin–cho (H)

Root and Leaf
Local Drug Name: Pai–qian–cao (C), Pie–chin–cho (H), Hai–sen–so (J).
Processing: Dry under the sun (C).
Method of Administration: Oral (decoction: C, H).
Folk Medicinal Uses:
  1) Influenza with fever (C, H).
  2) Malaria, hepatosplenomegaly (C, H).
  3) Pain due to pathogenic wind–dampness, traumatic injury (C, H).
  4) Endometrorrhagia (C).
Contraindications: Pregnancy (H).

Scientific Researches:
Chemistry
  1) Alkaloids: bufotenine–*O*–methyl ether, 5–methoxy–*N,N*–dimethyl–tryptamine–oxide, bufotenine, nigerin, *N,N*–dimethyltryptamine oxide, 5–methoxyl–*N*–methyltryptamine, gramine [1].
Pharmacology
  1) Alternating blood pressure (gramine) [2].
  2) Excitatory effect on CNS (gramine) [2].
  3) Excitatory effect on extracorporeal womb (gramine) [2].

Literatures:
[1] Ghosal, S. et al.: Chem. & Ind.**1964**, 1800; **1965**, 793.
[2] Henry, T.A.: "The Plant Alkaloids",**1949**, 485.

[J.X. Guo]

62. *Desmodium triquetrum* (L.) DC.   (Leguminosae)

Hu–lu–cha (C), Woo–lo–cha (H)

Herb
Local Drug Name: Hu–lu–cha (C), Woo–lo–cha (H).
Processing: Dry under the sun or use in fresh (C).
Method of Administration: Oral (decoction: C, H).
Folk Medicinal Uses:
  1) Pulmonary abscess (C, H).
  2) Hepatitis, nephritic edema, inflammatory diarrhea (C, H).
  3) Malnutrition of children due to impairment of the spleen and stomach caused by improper feeding, manifested by sallowness, emaciation and insomnia (C, H).
  4) Non–healing of boils (C).
  5) Vomiting during pregnancy (C).
  6) Tonsillitis (H).
  7) Pyorrhea (H).
  8) Parotitis (H).
  9) Hookworms (H).
  10) Tuberculosis of bone (H).
  11) Lymphadenitis (H).
  12) Trichomonal vaginitis (H).

62

13) Scleroderma (H).

Scientific Researches:
Chemistry
  1) Triterpenoids: friedelin, epi–friedelin [1].
  2) Steroids: stigmasterol [1].
  3) Others: coumarins, phenols, organic acids, tannins [2].
Pharmacology
  1) Bacteriostatic effect [2].

Literatures:
[1] Yang, Q.W. et al.:*Zhiwu Xuebao* **1978**, 31(2), 128.
[2] Nanjing College of Pharmacy: "*Zhongcaoyao Xue*", Vol. 2, **1976**, 467.

[J.X. Guo]

63.   *Glycine max* (L.) **Merr.**   (Leguminosae)

Da–dou (C), Die–dou (H), Dai–zu (J)

Seed (CP)
Local Drug Name: Da–dou, Hei–da–dou (C), Die Dou (H), Daizu, Kuro–mame (J).
Processing: (1) Dry under the sun. (2) Ferment in various combinations with other herbs.
Method of Administration: Oral (decoction: C, H, J, K).
Folk Medicinal Uses:
         1) Edema (C, H, J).
         2) Beriberi (C, H).
         3) Jaundice (C).
         4) Rheumatalgia (C).
         5) Pruitus (C, K).
         6) Poisoning (C, J, K).
         7) Chills, fever, headache in colds and influenza (C, H).
         8) Vexation, oppressed feelings in the chest (C).
         9) Insomnia (C).
         10) Cough (J).
         11) Frost–bite (K).
Contraindications: Not for patients taking seed of *Ricinus communis* or bark of *Magnolia officinalis.*

Leaf
Local Drug Name: Hei–da–dou–ye (C), Heuk–dae–du–yeop (K).
Method of Administration: Oral (juice or decoction: C).
Folk Medicinal Uses:
         1) Snake bite (C).

Seed coat
Local Drug Name: Hei–da–dou–pi (C), Heuk–dae–du–pi (K).
Method of Administration: Oral (decoction: C).
Folk Medicinal Uses:
         1) Headache (C).

Scientific Researches:
Chemistry

1) Flavonoids: daidzin, genistin, afrormosin, glycitein 7–O–β–D–(6"–O–acetyl)–glucopyranoside [1].
2) Saponins: soyasaponin I–IV, A_3, soyasapogenol A, B, E, acetylsoyasaponins A_{1-6} [2].
3) Others: glycinoprenol–10 [3], soya–cerebroside I, II [4].
Pharmacology
1) Estrogenic effect.

Literatures:

[1] Carballero, P. et al.:*J. Nat. Prod.***1986**, 49, 1126; Kudou, S. et al.:*Agric. Biol. Chem.* **1991**, 55, 859.
[2] Burrows, J. C. et al.:*Phytochem.* **1987**, 26, 1214; Curl, C. L. et al.:*J. Nat. Prod.* **1988,** 51, 122;
   Massiot, G. et al.:*J. Nat. Prod.* **1992**, 55, 1339–42; Kitagawa, I. et al.:*Chem. Pharm. Bull.* **1988**, 36, 153;
   2819, 2829; Shiraiwa, M. et al.:*Agric. Biol. Chem.***1991**, 55, 315, 323, 911.
[3] Suga, T. et al.:*J. Org. Chem.* **1989**, 54, 3390.
[4] Shibuya, H. et al.:*Chem. Pharm. Bull.* **1990**, 38, 2933.

[P.P.H. But]

64.   *Glycyrrhiza uralensis* Fisher (Leguminosae)

Gan–cao (C), Gum–cho (H), Urarukanzo (J), Gam–cho (K)

Related plant: *Glycyrrhiza glabra* L.: Guang–guo–gan–cao (C), Supeinkanzo (J), Mi–gam–cho (K);
                  G. inflata Batal.: Zhang–guo–gan–cao (C).

Root and stolon (CP, JP, KP)
 Local Drug Name: Gancao (C), Gum–cho (H), Kan–zo (J), Gam–cho (K).
 Processing: 1) Dry under the sun (J). Cut into thick pieces and dry (C).
                   2) Stir–fry with honey (C, H, J, K).
 Method of Administration: Oral (decoction or powder: C, H, J, K).
 Folk Medicinal Uses:
  [Rough dried] 1) Sore throat (C, H).
                 2) Digestive ulcer (C, H, J, K).
                 3) Carbuncle (C, H).
                 4) Poisoning (C, H, J, K).
  [Stir–fried]   1) Pain, abdominal pain (C, H, J, K).
                 2) Convulsive diseases (C, J).
                 3) Ulcer (J, K).
                 4) Hepatitis (J).
                 5) Phlegm (C, H, J, K).
                 6) Common cold (C, J, K).
                 7) Gastrointestinal disorder (J, K).
                 8) Palpitation and breath disorder (C, H).
                 9) Arrhythmia (C).
                 10) Epilepsy (H).
                 11) Reduce the toxic or drastic actions of other drug (C, H, J, K).
 Contraindications: Incompatible with Radix Euphorbiae Pekinensis, Flos Genkwa and Radix Kansui (C).
 Side Effects: Edema, hypertension, hypokalemia on overdose.

Scientific Researches
 Chemistry
  1) Triterpenoids: glycyrrhizin (= glycyrrhizic acid) [1], glabric acid [2].
  2) Flavonoids: liquiritin, liquiritigenin [3], isoliquiritin, isoliquiritigenin [4], licoricidin [5], formononetin,
       licoricone [6].

3) Polysaccharides: glycyrrhizan UA, UB, UC [7].

Pharmacology

1) Anti–ulcer [8, 9, 10].
2) Antispasmodic [9].
3) Corticoid activity (glycyrrhizin) [11, 12].
4) Anti–inflammatic (glycyrrhizin) [13].
5) Antitussive (glycyrrhizin) [14].
6) Antiallergic (glycyrrhizin) [15].
7) Antidote (glycyrrhizin) [16].

Literatures:

[1] Beaton, M. et al.:*J. Chem. Soc.* **1956**, 2417.
[2] Shibata, S. et al.: *Taisha* **1973**, 10, supplment, 157; Zhang, R. et al.:*Yaoxue Xuebao* **1986**, 21, 510; Shu, Y. et al.:*ibid.* **1987**, 22, 512.
[3] Shinoda, J. et al.:*Yakugaku Zasshi* **1934**, 54, 707; Nakanishi, T. et al.:*Phytochem.* **1985,** 24, 339.
[4] Puri, R. et al.:*J. Sci. Ind. Res.* **1954**, 13, 475; Miething, H. et al.:*Arch. Pharm.* **1989**, 322, 141 (1989).
[5] Shibata, S. et al.: *Chem. Pharm. Bull.* **1968**, 16, 1932 (1968).
[6] Kaneda, M. et al.: *Chem. Pharm. Bull.* **1973**, 21, 1338.
[7] Tomoda M. et al.:*Chem. Pharm. Bull.* **1990**, 38, 1667, 3069.
[8] Revers, F. E.:*Ned. Tijdschr. Geneesk* **1946**, 90, 135 , **1948**, 92, 2963; Schulze, E. et al.:*Dtsch. Med. Wschr.* **1951**, 76, 988.
[9] Desmarez, J. J.:*C. R. Soc. Biol.* **1956**, 150, 1022; Nomura, H.:*Fukuoka Igaku Zasshi* **1959**, 50, 354; Takagi, K. et al.:*Arzneim.–Forsch.* **1967**, 17, 1544.
[10] Schulze E. et al.:*Dtsch. Med. Wschr.* **1954**, 79, 716; Nishiyama T.:*Igaku Kenkyu* **1955**, 25, 366; Doll R. et al.:*Lancet* **1962**, 793; Tewari, S. N. et al.:*Gut,* **1968**, 9, 48; Takagi K. et al.:*Japan. J. Pharmacol.* **1969**, 19, 418; Aarsen P. N.:*Arzneim.–Forsch.* **1973**, 23, 1346; Okabe S. et al.:*Oyo Yakuri* **1979**, 469.
[11] Louis L. H. et al.:*J. Lab. Clin. Med.* **1956**, 47, 20; Kraus S. D.:*J. Exptl. Med.* **1957**, 106, 415; Atherden, L. M.:*Biochem. J.* **1958**, 69, 75: Ulmann A. et al.:*Endocrinoloogy* **1975**, 97, 46; Armanini D. et al.:*Clin. Endocrinol.* **1983**, 19, 609; Mackenzie, M. A. et al.:*J. Clin. Endocrinol. Metab.* **1990**, 70, 1637.
[12] Kumagai A. et al.:*Endocrinol. Japon* **1957**, 4, 17; Yano S.:*Nihon Naibunpi Gakkai Zasshi***1958**, 34, 745.
[13] Finney, R. S. H. et al.:*J. Pharm. Pharmacol.* **1958**, 10, 613; Tangri, K. K. et al.:*Biochem. Pharmacol.* **1965**, 14, 1277; Colin–Jones, E.:*Br. Med. J.* **1956**, 1305, **1957**, 161.
[14] Anderson, D. M. et al.:*J. Pharm. Pharmacol.* **1961**, 13, 396.
[15] Miyake Y.:*Allergy* **1961**, 10, 131; Banyanagi, T. et al:*ibid.* **1966**, 15, 67.
[16] Miyoshi H.: *Nisshin Igaku* **39**, 358; Shindo C. et al.:*Allergy* **1954**, 2, 332.

[T. Kimura]

65.   *Pueraria lobata* **Ohwi**   (Leguminosae)
              (= *P. hirsuta Matsum., P. thunbergiana*Benth.)

Ye–ge (C), Got–gun (H), Kuzu (J), Chik (K)

Root   (CP, JP, KP)
Local Drug Name: Ge–gen (C), Got–gun (H), Kak–kon (J), Gal–geun (K).
Processing: Cut into thick pieces and dry under the sun (J).
Method of Administration: Oral (decoction: C, H, J, K).
Folk Medicinal Uses:

1) Fever (C, H, J, K).
2) Pain (C, J, K).
3) Myalgia (C, J, K).
4) Common cold (J, K).
5) Headache and stiffness of the nape in exogenous affection (C, J).
6) Thirst caused by diabetes (C).
7) Early measles (H). Measles with inadequate eruption (C).
8) Angina pectoris (H).
9) Enteritis (H). Acute dysentery or diarrhea (C, H).
10) Acute gastritis (K).
11) Hypertension (C, H).
12) Alcoholism (K).

Flower
Local Drug Name: Got–fa (H), Kak–ka (J), Gal–hwa (K).
Processing: Dry under the sun.
Method of Administration: Oral (decoction: H, K).
Folk medicinal Uses:
       1) Drunkeness (H, K).
       2) Hemorrhoid (H).

Scientific Researches:
Chemistry
  1) Flavonoids: daizin, daizein, puerarin, puerarin xyloside [1].
  2) Saponin [2].
Pharmacology
  1) Antipyretic [3].
  2) Antispasmodic (daizein) [4].
  3) Antihypertensive [5].
  4) β–Blocking activity [6].

Literatures:
[1] Shibata, S. et al.: *Yakugaku Zasshi* **1959**, 79, 757; Murakami, T. et al.: *Bull. Chem. Soc. Japan* **1960**, 8, 688; Ohshima, Y., et al.: *Planta Medica* **1988**, 54, 250.
[2] Kinjo, J., et al. : *Chem. Pharm. Bull.* **1985**, 33, 1293.
[3] Tanno, Y.: *Nippon Yakubutsugaku Zasshi* **1941**, 33, 263; Noguchi, M.: *Shoyakugaku Zasshi* **1967**, 21, 17.
[4] Shibata, S. et al.: *Yakugaku Zasshi* **1959**, 79, 863.
[5] Zeng, G.-Y. et al.: *Zhonghua Yixue Zazhi* **1974**, 54, 265.
[6] Lu, X.-R. et al.: *Yaoxue Xuebao* **1980**, 15, 218.

[T. Kimura]

66.   *Sophora flavescens* **Aiton**   (Leguminosae)
                      (= *S. flavescens* Ait. var. *angustifolia* Kitagawa)

Ku–shen (C), Fu–sum (H), Kurara (J), Go–sam (K)

Root (CP, JP, KP)
Local Drug Name: Ku–shen (C), Fu–sum (H), Ku–jin (J), Go–sam (K).
Processing: Dry under the sun (C, J, K).
Method of Administration: Oral or Topical (decoction or powder: C, H, J, K).
Folk Medicinal Uses:

1) Diarrhea (H, J, K).
2) Gastrointestinal disorder (J, K).
3) Fever (J).
4) Pain (J, K).
5) Skin parasite, crab louse (C, J).
6) Dermatomycosis (C, J).
7) Acute dysentery with bloody stools (C).
8) Jaundice with oliguria (C, H).
9) Bloody and purulent leukorrhea (C, H).
10) Pudendal swelling and itching (C).
11) Tonsilitis (H).
12) Prolapse of rectum (H).
13) Tinea, boils, furunculosis (H).
14) Burns (H).

Side Effects: Toxic (J).

Scientific Researches:

Chemistry

1) Alkaloids: matrine, oxymatrine, sophoranol, anagyrine, isomatrine [1]
2) Flavonoids: kurarinol, kurarinone [2].
3) Saponins [2].

Pharmacology

1) Inhibition of stress ulcer outbreak (50% methanol extract, water extract, matrine, oxymatrine) [3]. Antiulcer (vexibinol) [4].
2) Cholagogue effect (methanol extract) [5].
3) Antipyretic (matrine) [6].
4) Stomach movement decreasing [7].
5) Central nervous system depressing [8].
6) Decreasing of ventricular fibrillation and arythmia [9].
7) Antibacterial (kurarinone and other flavonoids) [10].
8) Antidermatophytes (l-maackiain) [11].
9) Antifungal (kurarinone) [12].
10) Inhibition of cyclic AMP phospho-diesterase activity (kurarinone, kushenol A, kuraridin) [13].
11) Others [14].

Literatures:

[1] Ueno, A. et al.:*Chem. Pharm. Bull.* **1975**, 23, 2560.
[2] Komatsu, M. et al.:*Yakugaku Zasshi* **1970**, 90, 463; *Chem. Pharm. Bull.* **1971**, 19, 2126; **1973**, 21, 2733; Wu, L. J. et al.:*Chem. Pharm. Bull.* **1985**, 33, 3231; Yoshikawa, M. et al.:*Chem. Pharm. Bull.* **1985**, 33, 4267; Wu, L.-J. al.:*Yakugaku Zasshi* **1985**, 105, 736, 1034; **1986**, 106, 22.
[3] Yamahara, J. et al.:*Shoyakugaku Zasshi* **1974**, 28, 33; Yamazaki, M. et al.:*ibid.* **1981**, 35, 96.
[4] Yamahara, J. et al.:*Chem. Pharm. Bull.* **1990**, 38, 1039.
[5] Miura, M. et al.:*Yakugaku Zasshi* **1987**, 107, 992.
[6] Cho, C. H. et al.:*Planta Med.* **1986**, 52, 343.
[7] Yamazaki, M. et al.:*J. Pharmacobio-Dyn.* **1985**, 8, 513.
[8] Yamazaki, M. et al.:*Yakugaku Zasshi* **1984**, 104, 293.
[9] Zhang, P. et al.:*Yaoxue Xuebao* **1979**, 14, 449.
[10] Yamaki, M. et al.:*Phytother. Res.* **1990**, 4, 235.
[11] Honda, G. et al.:*Planta Med.* **1982**, 46, 122.
[12] Yagi, A. et al.:*Shoyakugaku Zasshi* **1989**, 43, 343.
[13] Ohmoto, T., et al. :*Chem. Pharm. Bull.* **1986**, 34, 2094.
[14] Ishida, M. et al.:*Brit. J. Pharmacol.* **1984**, 82, 523; Kimura, M., et al.: Phytother. Res.**1989**, 3, 101.

[T. Kimura]

67.   *Sophora japonica* **L.**   (Leguminosae)

Huai (C), Why–sue (H), Enju (J), Hoe–hwa–na–mu (K).

Flower and flower bud(CP)
Local Drug Name: Huai–hua (C), Why–fa (H), Kai–ka (J), Goe–hwa (K).
Processing: 1) Eliminate foreign matter and dry. 2) Stir–fry until dark yellow or charred brown.
Method of Administration: Oral (decoction: C, H, J).
Folk Medicinal Uses:

1) Hematuria (C, H, J).
2) Hemorrhinia (C, H).
3) Conjunctivitis (C, H).
4) Hemorrhoid (C, H, J).
5) Leukorrhea (C).
6) Uterine or intestinal hemorrhage (C, J).
7) Pyodermas (C).
8) Metrorrhagia (J).
9) Arteriosclerosis (J).
10) Hypertension (J).

Contraindications: Spleen and stomach deficiency.
Side Effects: Anaphylactic response causing rashes.

Fruit (CP)
Local Drug Name: Huai–jiao (C), Why–gok (H), Kai–jitsu (J), Goe–gak (K).
Processing: Stir–fry with honey until lustrous and unsticky.
Method of Administration: Oral (decoction: C, H,).
Folk Medicinal Uses:

1) Hemorrhoid (C, H).
2) Dysentery (C, H).
3) Hematochezia (C).
4) Headache, dizziness and congestion of the eyes due to heat in the liver (C).

Contraindications: pregnancy, spleen and stomach cold–deficiency.

Root
Local Drug Name: Huai–gen (C), Goe–geun (K).
Method of Administration: Oral (decoction: C).
Folk Medicinal Uses:

1) Pruitus (C).
2) Hemorrhoid (C).
3) Ascaridiasis (C).

Contraindications: Cold disease.

Resin
Local Drug Name: Huai–jiao (C), Goe–gyo (K).
Method of Administration: Oral (powder: C).
Folk Medicinal Uses:

1) Rheumatism (C).

Contraindications: Blood deficiency, Qi–stagnant.

Twig
Local Drug Name: Huai–zhi (C), Goe–ji (K).
Method of Administration: Oral (decoction: C).
Folk Medicinal Uses:

1) Pyodermas (C).

2) Hemorrhoid (C).

3) Conjunctivitis (C).

Scientific Researches:

Chemistry

1) Sophorabioside, kaempferol glucoside, sophoraflavonoloside, *dl*–maackiain, *d*–maackiain–mono–
β–D–glucoside, genistein, kaempferol, rutin, sophoricoside, betulin, sophoradiol, glucuronic acid, isorhamnetin [12, 13, 23, 24].

2) Lectin [5–6,18–20].

3) Anhydropisatin (=flemichapparin B), irisolidone, biochannin A, 5,7–dihydroxy–3'4'–methylenedioxy–
isoflavone [4].

4) Rutoside [10].

5) Kaikasaponins I–III [15].

6) Sophoraside A, puerol A, puerol B [17].

7) Cytisine,*N*–methylcytisine, sophocarpine, matrine [22].

Pharmacology

1) Antiinflammatory effects.

2) Antihemorrhagic effects (isorhamnetin, quercetin) [1, 12–14, 21].

3) Anti–arteriosclerosis and antithrombosis [2].

4) Antifertility effect (fruit): genistein and kaempferol exhibited anti–implantation activity in mice, and genistein and sophoricoside interrupted early pregnancy in mice [3].

5) Protective effects against lipid peroxidation [9].

6) Skin–care uses [11].

7) Antioxidant effects [16].

8) Inhibitory effects on ^{3}H–ethylketocycloazocine receptors (puerol A) [17].

9) Hemagglutinating effects [20].

Literatures:

[1] Wang, A.F.: *Zhongyi Zazhi* **1982**, 23, 81.

[2] Zhou, W.Q.: *Shanghai J. Trad. Chin. Med.* **1983**, 12, 25.

[3] Kong, Y.C. et al.: *J. Ethnopharm.* **1986**, 15, 1.

[4] Komatsu, M. et al.: *Yakugaku Zasshi* **1976**, 96, 254.

[5] Baba, K.: *Wood Res.* **1991**, 78, 74.

[6] Ueno, M. et al.: *J. Chromatogr.* **1992**, 597, 197.

[7] Sabirov, K.A. et al.: *Uzb. Biol. Zh.* **1991**, (4), 60.

[8] Ji, D.Z.: *Sichuan Daxue Xuebao*, Ziran Kexueban **1991**, 28, 265.

[9] Sokol'chik, I.G. et al.: *Zdravookhr. Beloruss.* **1991**, (10), 31.

[10] Djordjevic, S. et al.: *Herba Hung.* **1991**, 30(1–2), 11.

[11] Tsukumo, K.: *Jpn. Kokai Tokkyo Koho* JP 03, 255,015 [91, 255,015] **1991**.

[12] Ishida, H. et al.: *Chem. Pharm. Bull.* **1989**, 37, 1616.

[13] Ishida, H. et al.: *Yakugaku Zasshi* **1989**, 109, 179.

[14] Ishida, H. et al.: *Jpn. Kokai Tokkyo Koho* JP 02, 72,116 [92, 72,116] **1990**.

[15] Kitagawa, I. et al.: *Yakugaku Zasshi* **1988**, 108, 538.

[16] Ohta, S.: *Fragrance J.* **1988**, 16, 57.

[17] Shirataki, Y.: *Chem. Pharm. Bull.* **1987**, 35, 1637.

[18] Fournet, B. et al.: *Eur. J. Biochem.* **1987**, 166, 321.

[19] McPherson, A. et al.: *J. Biol. Chem.* **1987**, 262, 1791.

[20] Ito, Y.: *Plant Sci. (Limerick, Irel.)* **1986**, 47, 77.

[21] Ishida, H. et al.: *Chem. Pharm. Bull.* **1987**, 35, 857.

[22] Abdusalamov, B.A. et al.: *Khim. Prir. Soedin.* **1972**, 8, 658.

[23] Farkas, L. et al.: *Tetrahedron Lett.* **1964**, 3919.

[24] Balbaa, S.I. et al.: *Planta Med.* **1974**, 25, 325.

[P.P.H. But]

Wisteria floribunda DC. (Leguminosae)

Fuji (J), Deung (K)

Stem
Method of Administration: Oral (decoction: K).
Folk Medicinal Uses:
1) Pain of the stapes (K).
2) Apoplexy (K).
3) Weakness (K).
4) Gonorrhoea (K).

Stem knot
Local drug Name: Fuji–kobu, To–ryu (J).
Processing: Dry under the sun (J).
Method of Administration: Oral (decoction: J).
Folk Medicinal Uses:
1) Diarrhea (J).
2) Stomatitis, gingivitis (J).
3) Tonsillitis (J).
4) Gastric cancer (J).

Scientific Researches:
Chemistry
1) Flavonoids: luteol–7–glucorhamnoside, luteolol–7–rhamnoglucoside (loniceroside), apigenol–
7–rhamnoglucoside [1].
2) Triterpenes: α–amyrin, betulin, betulinic acid, afromosin, ursolic acid [8].
3) Lecitins [2, 3].
4) Polysaccharides [4].
5) Trypsin and chymotrypsin inhibiting protein: WTI–I [5].
6) Cysteine proeinase inhibitor: WTI–A, –B, –C [6], cystatin [7].
7) Sterols: β–sitosterol 3–O–β–D–glucoside [8].
Pharmacology
1) Antitumor activity (polyscaccharide) [4].
2) Hemagglutinating activity (lectin) [3].
3) Mitogenic activity [9].
4) Activation of adenylate cyclase [10].

Literatures:
[1] Torck, M. et al.:*Bull. Soc. Pharm. Lille* **1970**(3–4), 179.
[2] Kurokawa, T. et al.:*J. Biol. Chem.* **1976**, 251(18), 5686.
[3] Cheung, G. et al.:*Biochemistry* **1979**, 18(9), 1646.
[4] Kosuge, T. et al.:*Jpn. Kokai Tokkyo Koho* JP 60 84,301, 13 May **1985**.
[5] Norimura, H. et al.:*Agric. Biol. Chem.* **1990**, 54(11), 3029.
[6] Hirayama, K. et al.:*Mem. Fac. Sci., Kyushu Univ., Ser. C,* **1989**, 17(1), 878.
[7] Hirashiki, I. et al.:*J. Biochem.(Tokyo)* **1990**, 108(4), 604.
[8] Tanaka, I. et al.:*Yakugaku Zasshi* **1975**, 95(11), 1388.
[9] Kaladas, P. M. et al.:*Biochemistry* **1979**, 18(22), 4806.
[10] Van Heyningen, S.:*FEBS Lett.* **1983**, 164(1), 132.

[C.K. Sung]

69. *Geranium thunbergii* Sieb. et Zucc. (Geraniaceae)

Gennoshoko (J), I–jil–pul (K)

Herb (JP, KP)
Local Drug Name: Lao–guan–cao (C), Gennoshoko (J), Hyun–cho (K).
Processing: Dry under the sun (J, K).
Method of Administration: Oral or topical (decoction or herb tea: J, K).
Folk Medicinal Uses:

        1) Diarrhea, dysentery (J, K).
        2) Acute and chronic catarrh (J, K).
        3) Chronic constipation (J).
        4) Gastric ulcer (J, K).
        5) Swelling, frostbite (J).

Scientific Researches
Chemistry
  1) Tannins: geraniin [1].
  2) Flavonoids: quercetin, kaempferitrin [2].
Pharmacology
  1) Antidiarreic [3].
  2) Bowel movement stimuration [4].

Literatures:
[1] Okuda, T. et al.:*Yakugaku Zasshi* **1976**, 96, 1143; *Phytochemistry* **1978**, 14, 1877; *Yakugaku Zasshi* **1975**, 95, 1462; *Tetrahedron Letters* **1976**, 3721; *Chem. Pharm. Bull.* **1977**, 25, 1862; *Tetrahedron Letters* **1977**, 4421; *J. Chromatography* **1977**, 171, 313; *Phytochem.* **1982**, 21, 2871; *Yakugaku Zasshi* **1977**, 97, 1267, 1273; *ibid.* **1979**, 99, 505; *Chem. Pharm. Bull.* **1982**, 30, 1113; *ibid.* **1986**, 34, 4076; Nonaka, G. et al.: *ibid.* **1986**, 34, 941; Mizobuchi, K.:*Yakugaku Zasshi* **1954**, 74, 1224.
[2] Nishimoto, Y. et al.:*Shoyakugaku Zasshi* **1980**, 34, 122, 127, 131.
[3] Sone, Y. : *Tohoku J. Exptl. Med.* **1936**, 29, 218.
[4] Murao, S.: *Osaka Igakkai Zasshi* **1943**, 42, 1176, 1385.

[T. Kimura]

70. *Euphorbia pekinensis* Rupr. (Euphorbiaceae)

Da–ji (C), Takatodai (J), Dae–geuk (K)

Root (CP)
Local Drug Name: Jing–da–ji (C), Dai–geki (J), Dae–geuk (K).
Processing: 1) Wash, soften thoroughly, cut into thick slices and dry (C).
             2) Process with vineger(C).
Method of Administration: Oral (decoction: C, J).
Folk Medicinal Uses:

        1) Anasarca (C, J).
        2) Hydrothorax and ascites with dyspnea (C, J).
        3) Constipation and oliguria (C, J).
Contraindications:

        1) Pregnancy (C).
        2) Incompatible with Radix Glycyrrhizae (C).

Scientific Researches:
 Chemistry
  1) Triterpenes: euphornin [1].
  2) Pigments: euphorbia A, B, C [2].
  3) Alkaloids [2].
 Pharmacology
  1) Lapactic effect [3].
  2) Expassing peripheral blood vessels [3].
  3) Exciting extracorporeal womb [3].
  4) Counteracting to hypertension due to adrenalin [3].

Literatures:
[1] Junzo, A. et al.:*J. Chem. Soc.* **1928**, 49, 252.
[2] *"Quanguo Zhongcaoyao Huibian"* Vol. 1, **1975**, 470.
[3] *Igaku Chuo Zasshi* **1966**, 218, 567.

[J.X. Guo]

71. *Mallotus apelta* (**Lour.**) **Muell.–Arg.** (Euphorbiaceae)

Bai–bei–ye (C), Bak–bui–yip (H)

Root and Leaf
 Local Drug Name: Bai–bei–ye (C), Bak–bui–yip (H), Haku–hai–yo (J).
 Processing: 1) Root: Cut into slices, and dry under the sun (C).
         2) Leaf: Mostly used in fresh, or dry under the sun (C).
 Method of Administration: Oral (decoction or powder: C, H).
 Folk Medicinal Uses:
         1) Chronic hepatitis (C, H).
         2) Inflammatory diarrhea (C, H).
         3) Pyogenic tympanitis (C, H).
         4) Prostatitis (C).
         5) Cervicitis (C).
         6) Hepatosplenomegaly (H).
         7) Prolapse of uterus and rectum (H).
         8) Leukorrhea (H).
         9) Edema in pregnancy (H).
         10) Furuncles (H).
         11) Traumatic injury (H).

Scientific Researches:
 Chemistry
  1) Triterpenes: erythordiol–3–acetate, 3β–29–dihydroxy–lupane, ursolic acid acetate [1].
  2) Steroides: β–sitosterol [1].
 Pharmacology
  1) Antibacterial effect (EtOH extract and the above compounds.) [1].

Literature:
[1] Shan, X. Q. et al.:*Zhiwu Xuebao*, **1985**, 27(2), 192.

[J.X. Guo]

72. *Sapium sebiferum* (L.) Roxb. (Euphorbiaceae)

Wu–jiu (C), Woo–kou (H), Nankinhaze (J), Jo–gu–na–mu (H)

Root bark and leaf
Local Drug Name: Wu–jiu (C), Woo–kou (H), U–kyu–boku–kon–pi (J), Jo–gu–mok–geun–pi (K).
Processing: Dry under the sun (C).
Method of Administration: Oral (decoction: C, H); Topical (fresh leaf: C, H).
Folk Medicinal Uses:
        1) Schistosomiasis (C, H).
        2) Sore, mastitis, snake bites and insect stings (C, H).
        3) Scabies, eczema, dermatitis (C).
        4) Edema, oligusia (H).
        5) Constipation (H).
        6) Ascites, cirrhosis (H).
        7) Infectious hepatitis (H).
        8) Arsenic poisoning (H).
Side Effects: Severe vomiting, weakness.

Scientific Researches:
Chemistry
  1) Aromatic compounds: xanthoxylin (from root bark) [1].
  2) Triterpenes: moretenone (from root bark) [2].
  3) Phenolic compounds: corilagin, gallic acid, ellagic acid, shikimic acid (from fresh leaf) [3].
  4) Flavonoids: isoquercetin (from fresh leaf) [3].
Pharmacology
  1) Purgative effect (decoction) [4].
  2) Vermicidal effect (xanthoxylin) [4].
  3) Antibacterial effect (50% decoction of leaf) [5].
  4) Leptospinostatic effect [5].
  5) Carcinogenic effect [6].

Literatures:
[1] Zhu, Y.L.: *Yaoxue Xuebao* **1985**, 6, 51.
[2] Wu, Z.X. et al.: *Zhongcaoyao* **1992**, 23(1), 34.
[3] Arthur, H.R.: *Symposium on Phytochemisty* **1964**, 164.
[4] Liu, Z.J.: *Huaxue Xuebao* **1957**, 23, 259.
[5] Nanjing College of Pharmacy: *'Zhongcaoyao Xue''*, Vol. 2, **1976**, 597.
[6] Ji, Z. W. et al.: *Cancer (China)* **1989**, 8(5), 350; Wang, Z. J. et al.: *Tumor (China)* **1989**, 9(5), 214.

[J.X. Guo]

73. *Citrus aurantium* L. (Rutaceae)

Suan–cheng (C), Jik–sut (H), Gwang–gyul–na–mu (K)

Related plant: *Poncirus trifoliata* Raf.: Gou–ju (C), Karatachi (J),
                  Citrus aurantium L. var. *daidai* Makino: Daidai (J),
                  C. natsudaidai Hayata: Natsumikan (J), *C. wilsonii* Tanaka; Xiang–yuang (C)

Pericarp (JP, KP)
Local Drug Name: To–hi (J), Deung–pi (K).

Processing: Dry the pericarps of ripe fruits, under the sun (J, K).
Method of Administration: Oral (decoction or powder: J, K).
Folk Medicinal Uses:
        1) Dyspepsia, gastrointestinal disorder (J, K).
        2) Common cold (K).

Young fruit (CP, JP, KP)

Local Drug Name: Zhi–shi (C), Jik–sut (H), Ki–jitsu (J).
Processing: Cut the very young fruits picked in May to June, into 2–3 pieces, and dry under the sun.
Method of Administration: Oral (decoction: C, H, J, K).
Folk Medicinal Uses:
        1) Dyspepsia (C, H, J, K).
        2) Edema (H).
        3) Stagnation of qi (air) marked by feeling of stuffiness and distending pain, tenesmus in dysentery or constipation (C), Constipation (H, J).
        4) Gastroptosis, prolapse of stomach, rectum and uterus (C, H).
        5) Tenderness and feeling of fullness in the costal, epigastrium or lower abdomen regions, accompanied by constipation (C, J).
        6) Pectoral pain and stuffiness sensation due to stagnation of phlegm and qi (C, J). Chest distention (H).
        7) Phlegm (H).
Contraindications: Weak constitution and woman in pregnancy.

Immature fruit (CP)

Local Drug Name: Zhi–qiao (C), Ki–koku (J).
Processing: Slice the unripe and middle size fruit, take seeds away and dry.
Method of Administration: Oral (decoction: C, H, J, K).
Folk Medicinal Uses: Same as the immature fruit, but the activity is moderate in compare with it.

Scientific Researches:

Chemistry
    1) Essential Oil: *d*–limonene.
    2) Flavonoids: hesperidin, naringin, neohesperidin, rhoifolin [1–4].
    3) Triterpenoids: limonin.
Pharmacology
    1) Choleretic (ethanol extract [5], limonene [6]).
    2) Sedative (limonene) [7].
    3) Angiotonic (limonene) [6].

Literatures:

[1] Kolle, F. et al.: *Pharm. Zentralhall.* **1936**, 77, 421.
[2] Hattori, S., et al. : *J. Am. Chem. Soc.* **1952**, 74, 3614.
[3] Nakabayashi, T.: *Nogei Kagaku Zasshi* **1961**, 35, 945.
[4] Nishiura, M., et al. : *Agr. Biol. Chem.* **1969**, 33, 1109.
[5] Miura, M. et al.: *Yakugaku Zasshi* **1987**, 107, 992.
[6] Tsuji, M.: *Oyo Yakuri* **1974**, 8, 1439; **1975**, 10, 187; Ariyoshi, T. et al.: *Xenobiotica* **1975**, 5, 33; Kodama, R. et al.: *Life Sci.* **1976**, 19, 1559.
[7] Wagner, H. et al.: *Deut. Apoth. –Ztg.* **1973**, 113, 1159.

                                        [T. Kimura]

74.   *Citrus unshiu* Markovich   (Rutaceae)

Chan–pay (H), Mikan, Unshu–mikan (J), Gyul (K)

Related plant: *Citrus reticulata* Blanco (= *C. nobilis* Lour.); *C. tangerina* Hort.

Pericarp (JP, KP)
  Local Drug Name: Chen pi, Qing–pi (C), Chan–pay (H), Chin–pi (J), Jin–pi (K).
  Processing: Dry under the sun.
  Method of Administration: Oral. (decoction or powder: H, J, K).
  Folk Medicinal Uses:
                1) Dyspepsia (H, J, K).
                2) Cough (H, J, K).
                3) Phlegm (H, J, K).
                4) Common cold (K).
                5) Annorexia (H).
                6) Vomiting (H).

Scientific Researches:
  Chemistry
    1) Essential oil: *d*–limonene.
    2) Flavonoids: hesperidin.
    3) Phenolic amines: synephrine [1].
  Pharmacology
    1) Gastric secretion increasing [2].
    2) Gastric movement stimuration [3].
    3) Anaphylaxis depression [4].
    4) Serotonin antagonism [1].

Literatures:
  [1] Kinoshita, T. et al:*Shoyakugaku Zasshi* **1979**, 33, 146.
  [2] Ikuta, M.: *Osaka Igakkai Zasshi* **1940**, 39, 2072; **1941**, 40, 711, 727.
  [3] Suga, S.: *Osaka Igakkai Zasshi* **1942**, 41, 649.
  [4] Goda, S.: *Nippon Yakurigaku Zasshi* **1973**, 69, 88.

                                                                    [T. Kimura]

75.   *Tetradium ruticarpum* (Benth.) **Hartley**   (Rutaceae)
                   (= *Euodia (Evodia) rutaecarpa* Benth.)

Wu–zhu–yu (C), Ng–tsue–yue (H), Goshuyu, Nise goshuyu (J)

Related plant: *E. officinalis* Dode (= *E. rutaecarpa* Benth. var. *officinalis* Huang): Shi–hu (C),
                   Hon goshuyu (J), O–su–yu (K); *E. danielli* Hemsl.; Chosen goshuyu (J), Swi–na–mu (K).

Fruit (CP, JP, KP)
  Local Drug Name: Wu–zhu–yu (C), Ng–tsue–yue (H), Go–shu–yu (J), O–su–yu (K).
  Processing: 1) Dry under the sun. 2) Soak in a decoction of Glycyrrhizae Radix entirely, and dry under
                the sun (C).
  Method of Administration: Oral or topical (decoction: C, H, J, K).
   Folk Medicinal Uses:
                1) Gastrointestinal disorder (C, H, J, K).

2) Feeling of chill (C, H, J, K).

3) Pain (C, J, K). Abdominal pain (H).

4) Toothache (H).

5) Vertigo (C, J).

6) Weakness and edema of legs (C).

7) Hypertension (C).

8) Stomachitis (external, C).

9) Hernia (H).

10) Beriberi (H).

11) Eczema (H).

Scientific Researches:

Chemistry

1) Alkaloids: evodiamine, rutaecarpine, higenamine, dehydroevodiamine [1], evocarpine [2].

2) Aromatic amines:*N,N*–dimethyl–5–methoxytryptamine, *N*–methylanthranylamide, synephrine [3].

3) Triterpenoids: limonin.

4) Essential oil.

Pharmacology

1) Analgesic [4].

2) Serotonin antagonism [5].

3) Brain dopamine receptor inhibition [6].

4) Cardiotonic (evodiamine, hygenamine) [7].

5) Antihypertensive (dehydroevodiamine) [8].

Literatures:

[1] King, C. L., et al.:*J. Nat. Prod.* **1980**, 43, 577.

[2] Tscheshe, R. et al.: *Tetrahedron* **1967**, 23, 1873.

[3] Takagi, S.: *Shoyakugaku Zasshi* **1979**, 33, 30, 35.

[4] Yamada, Y.: *Gifu Ikadagaku Kiyo* **1957**, 5, 269, 278, **1958**, 6, 360.

[5] Kinoshita, T. et al.: *Shoyakugaku Zasshi* **1979**, 33, 146.

[6] Sumida, T.: *Yakugaku Zasshi* **1988**, 108, 450.

[7] Shoji, N., et al.:*J. Pharm. Sci.* **1986**, 75, 612.

[8] Yang, M. C. M., et al.:*Eur. J. Pharmacol* **1990**, 182, 537.

[T. Kimura]

76.   *Murraya paniculata*(L.) Jack (=*M. exotica* L.)   (Rutaceae)

Jiu–li–xiang (C); Gou–lee–heung (H); Gekkitsu (J)

Leaf

Local Drug Name: Jiu–li–xiang (C), Gou–lee–heung (H).

Processing: Fresh or dry in shade.

Method of Administration: Oral or topical (decoction: C, H).

Folk Medicinal Uses:

1) Traumatic injury (C, H).

2) Rheumatalgia (C, H).

3) Ulcer pain, toothache (C, H).

4) Stomach ache (C).

5) Epidemic encepahlitis B (C, H).

6) Absecess (C).

7) Pruritus (C).

8) Eczema (C)

Root
Local Drug Name: Jiu–li–xiang–gen (C); Gou–lee–heung–gun (H).
Processing: Dry under the sun.
Method of Administration: Oral or topical (decoction: C, H).
Folk Medicinal Uses:
                1) Rheumatalgia (C, H).
                2) Lumbago (C)
                3) Traumatic injury (C)
                4) Tinea (C).
                5) Eczema (C).
                6) Bronchitis (C).

Scientific Researches:
Chemistry
1) Leaf contains volatile oil composed predominantly of sesquiterpenoids [1].
2) Alkaloids: Noracronycine, de–*N*,*N*–methylnoracronycine, de–*N*–methylacronycine, skimmianine,
        mahanimbine, murrayazoline, yuehchukene (root), paniculol (leaf) [13–16, 35].
3) Aurantiamide acetate (stem bark) [12].
4) Coumarins: Phebalosin, paniculatin, murrayone, aurapten, murralongin, murrangatin, meragin hydrate,
        imperatorin, murralonginol isovalerate, isomurralonginol isovalerate, murrangatin isovalerate,
        minumicrolin isovalerate, chloculol, paniculonol isovalerate, isomurralonginol nicotinate,
        panial, *cis*–osthenon, paniculin, murpaniculol, paniculal, coumurrin (leaf of *M. paniculata*)
        [4, 6, 9, 14, 20, 22, 35]; murrayanone, murraculatin (leaf of *M. paniculata* var. *omphalo–*
        carpa) [7]; peroxyauraptenol, cis–dehydroosthol, murraol, murranganon, isomurranganon
        senecioate, murrangatin acetate, isomurralonginol acetate, chlotical, peroxymurraol,
        murraxocin, aurapten, osthol, (+)–erythromurangatin, (–)–minumicrolin, murralongin (leaf of
        M. exotica) [6, 8, 23, 25, 32, 33]; paniculidines A, B and C, murralongin, osthol, 3–(1,1–
        dimethylallyl)xanthyletin (root bark) [10, 27].
5) Murrayacarine, 3–formylindole, imphalocarpin, 5,7–dimethoxy–8–(3'–methyl–2'–oxobutyl) coumarin,
        coumurrayin, murragleinin, omphamurin, murraol, murracarpin, mupanidin, mexoticin,
        murrangatin, ferulyl esters (root bark of *M. paniculata* var. *omphalocarpa*) [5].
6) From flower of *M. paniculata* var. *omphalocarpa*: omphalocarpin, (–)–murracarpin, murrayacarpin–A
        and –B, scopolin, scopoletin, 5,7–dimethoxy–8–(3'–methyl–2'–oxobutyl)coumarin,
        (±)–murracarpin, mupanidin [11].
7) Sitosterol–β–D–galactoside [24]; colensenone, colensanone [26].
8) Glycoprotein, polysaccharide [28, 34].
9) Flavonoids: 3,5,6,7,8,3',4',5'–octamethoxyflavone, 3,5,6,7,3',4',5'–heptamethoxyflavone, 5,6,7,3',4',5'–
        hexamethoxyflavone, 5,6,7,3',4'–pentamethoxyflavone, 3,5,7,3',4',5'–hexamethoxyflavone,
        3,5,7,8,3',4',5'–heptamethoxyflavone [29].
10) Protein polysaccharide [31].
11) Cycloartenols: lupeol, 3–epi–cycloaudenol [33].
Pharmacology
1) Anti–implantation effects [2,13–14].
2) Antithyroid effects [3].
3) LD50 of methanol–water extract of bark and leaf are both >1 g/kg i.p. in mice [17].
4) Abortifacient effects [18–19, 34].
5) Antiinflammatory effects [31].
6) Anticoagulant effects [31].
7) Antifertility effects [31].
8) LD50 of protein polysaccharide = 462 mg/kg i.p. in mice [31].
9) Antimicrobial effects [32].

Literatures:

[1] Li, Q. et al.:*Biochem. Syst. Ecol.* **1988**, 16, 491.

[2] Kong, Y.C. et al.:*Planta Med.* **1985**, 304.

[3] Upadhyay, S.C.:*Proc. 42th Indian Pharm. Cong.***1990**, E06:39.

[4] Imai, F. et al.: *Chem. Pharm. Bull.* **1989**, 37, 358.

[5] Wu, T.S. et al.:*Phytochem.* **1989**, 28, 2873.

[6] Ito, C. et al.: *Chem. Pharm. Bull.* **1989**, 37, 819.

[7] Wu, T.S.: *Phytochem.* **1988**, 27, 2357.

[8] Ito, C. et al.: *Chem. Pharm. Bull.* **1987**, 35, 4277.

[9] Imai, F. et al.: *Shoyakugaku Zasshi* **1987**, 41, 157.

[10] Kinoshita, T. et al.:*Phytochem.* **1989**, 28, 147.

[11] Wu, T.S. et al.:*Phytochem.* **1989**, 28, 293.

[12] Kong, Y.C. et al.:*Planta Med.* **1987**, 53, 393.

[13] Kong, Y.C. et al.:*J. Chem. Soc., Chem. Comm.***1985**, 47.

[14] Kong, Y.C. et al.:*J. Ethnopharm.* **1986**, 15, 195.

[15] But, P.P.H. et al.:*Acta Phytotaxon. Sin.* **1986**, 24, 186.

[16] Kong, Y.C. et al.:*Biochem. System. Ecol.* **1986**, 14, 491.

[17] Nakanishi, K. et al.:*Chem. Pharm. Bull.* **1965**, 13, 882.

[18] Chen, Q.H. et al.:*Zhongguo Yaoke Daxue Xuebao***1987**, 18, 213.

[19] Wang, S.R. et al.:*Zhongguo Yaoke Daxue Xuebao***1987**, 18, 183.

[20] Cuca Suarez, L.E. et al.:*Rev. Latinoam. Quim.* **1991**, 22, 38.

[21] Waterman, P.G.:*Fitoterapia* **1987**, 58, 333.

[22] Ito, C. et al.:*Heterocycles* **1987**, 26, 2959.

[23] Barik, B.R. et al.:*Phytochem.* **1987**, 26, 3319.

[24] Ahmad, Z.A. et al.:*Planta Med.* **1987**, 53, 579.

[25] Ito, C. et al.:*Heterocycles* **1987**, 26, 1731.

[26] Ahmad, Z.A. et al.:*Indian Drugs* **1987**, 24, 322.

[27] Ahmad, Z.A. et al.:*Indian Drugs* **1986**, 24, 64.

[28] Liu, J.L. et al.: *Shengwu Huaxue Zazhi* **1989**, 5, 33.

[29] Bishay, DW. et al.:*Bull. Pharm. Sci., Aasiut Univ.***1987**, 10, 55.

[30] Imai, F. et al.:*Chem. Pharm. Bull.* **1989**, 37, 119.

[31] Liu, J.L. et al.: *Shengwu Huaxue Zazhi* **1989**, 5, 119.

[32] Bishay, D.W. et al.:*Bull. Pharm. Sci., Aasuit Univ.***1988**, 11, 88.

[33] Bishay, D.W. et al.:*Bull. Pharm. Sci., Aasuit Univ.***1988**, 11, 105.

[34] Zhang, Z.Y. et al.:*Zhongguo Yaoke Daxue Xuebao***1989**, 20, 283.

[35] Ito, C. et al.:*J. Chem. Soc., Perkin Trans. 1,* **1990**, 2047.

[P.P.H. But]

77.   *Phellodendron amurense***Ruprecht** (Rutaceae)

Huang–bi (C), Wong–pak (H), Kihada (J), Hwang–byuk–na–mu (K)

Related plant: *Phellodendron amurense* Ruprecht var. *sachalinense* Fr. Schmidt; Hirohano kihada (J),
P. amurense Ruprecht var. *japonicum* Ohwi; Obanokihada (J),
P. amurense Ruprecht var. *lavallei* Sprague; Miyamakihada (J),
P. chinense Schneider: Huang–pi–shu (C).

Bark (CP, JP, KP)
Local Drug Name: Huang–bai (C), Wong–pak (H), O–baku (J), Hwang–baek (K).
Processing: 1) Dry under the sun. 2) Stir–fry with salt water (C). 3) Stir–fry until carbonized (C).
Method of Administration: Oral or external. Decoction or powder (C, H, J, K).

Folk Medicinal Uses:
>1) Gastrointestinal disorder (C, J, K).
>2) Diarrhea (C, H, J, K).
>3) Food intoxication (J, K).
>4) Swelling (C, J, K).
>5) Urinary infection (C).
>6) Consumptive fever and night sweating (C).
>7) Eczema with itching (C).
>8) Jaundice (H).
>9) Spermatorrhea (H).
>10) Dysuria (H).
>11) Leukorrhea (H).
>12) Ulcer (K).
>13) Sore throat (H).
>12) Conjunctivitis (H).
>13) Bruise (external, J).

Scientific Researches:

Chemistry
1) Alkaloids: berberine, palmatine [1], magnoflorine, phellodendrine, jateorrhizine [2].
2) Triterpenoids: obakunone [3], limonin (obakulactone) [4].
3) Butenolide [5].

Pharmacology
1) Antiinflammatory (berberine) [6, 7, 8, 9].
2) Antiulcer [10].
3) Antibacterial (berberine) [11].
4) Antihypertensive (berberine) [12].
5) Central nervous system depressing (berberine) [13].
6) Antipyretic (berberine) [14].
7) Choleretic (berberine) [15].
8) Serum cholesterol [16] and blood sugar [17] lowering (berberine).
9) Acetylcholine stimulation (berberine) [18].
10) Others [19].

Literatures:

[1] Murayama, Y. et al.:*Yakugaku Zasshi* **1926**, 46, 299.
[2] Tomita, M. et al.:*Chem. Pharm. Bull.* **1957**, 5, 10; Idem.: *Yakugaku Zasshi* **1960**, 80, 880, 885, 1238, 1300.
[3] Murayama, Y. et al.:*Yakugaku Zasshi* **1927**, 47, 1035; Kubota, T., et al.:*Tetrahedron Letters* **1961**, 325.
[4] Fujita, A. et al.:*Yakugaku Zasshi* **1931**, 51, 506; **1935**, 55, 291; Barton, D. H. R. et al.:*J. Chem. Soc.* **1961**, 255.
[5] Kondo, Y. et al.: *Yakugaku Zasshi* **1985**, 105, 742.
[6] Mase, A. et al.: *Wakan Iyaku Gakkaishi* **1985**, 2, 634.
[7] Fujimura, H. et al.:*Yakugaku Zasshi* **1970**, 90, 782.
[8] Uchiyama, T. et al.:*Wakan Iyaku Gakkaishi* **1989**, 6, 158.
[9] Takase, H., et al.:*Japan. J. Pharmacol.* **1989**, 49, 301.
[10] Uchiyama, T. et al.:*Yakugaku Zasshi* **1989**, 109, 672.
[11] Ukita, T. et al.: *Penishirin* **1949**, 2, 534; Amin, A. H. et al.:*Can. J. Microbiol.* **1969**, 15, 1067; Sun, D. C. et al.:*Antimicrob. Agents Chemother.* **1988**, 32, 1370; Higaki, S. et al.:*Wakan Iyaku Gakkaishi* **1987**, 4, 458; Lahiri, S. C. et al.:*J. Indian Med. Assoc.* **1967**, 48, 1; Dutta, N. K.et al.:*Br. J. Pharmacol.* **1972**, 44, 153; Sabir, M. et al.:*Indian J. Med. Res.* **1977**, 65, 305; Sun, D., Abraham, S. N. et al.:*Antimicrob. Agents Chemother.* **1988**, 32, 1274; Kuwano, S. et al.:*Chem. Pharm. Bull.*

1960, 8, 491, 497; Idem.:*ibid.* **1961**, 9, 651.

[12] Arakawa, K. et al.:*Shoyakugaku Zasshi* **1985**, 39, 162; Suzuki, S.:*Tohoku J. Exptl. Med.* **1939**, 36, 134.

[13] Shanbhag, S. M. et al.:*Japan. J. Pharmacol.* **1970**, 20, 482.

[14] Sabir, M. et al.:*Indian J. Physiol. Pharmacol.***1978**, 22, 9.

[15] Oshiba, S. et al.:*Nihon Univ. J. Med.* **1974**, 16, 69; Chan, M. Y.:*Comp. Med. East West***1977**, 5, 161.

[16] Vad, B. G. et al.:*Indian J. Pharm.* **1971**, 33, 23.

[17] Chen, Q. M. et al.: *Yaoxue Xuebao* **1986**, 21, 401; **1987**, 22, 161.

[18] Uchizumi, S.:*Nippon Yakurigaku Zasshi***1957**, 53, 63; Shimamoto, T. et al.:*ibid.* **1957**, 53, 75.

[19] Nishino, H. et al.:*Oncology* **43**, 131 (1986); Anan, S.:*Nagasaki Igakkai Zasshi***1927**, 5, 243, 363.; Hano, K. et al.: *Yakugaku Kenkyu* **1960**, 32, 836; Chopra, L. R. N. et al.:*Indian J. Med. Res.* **1932**, 19, 1193; Kulkarni, S. K. et al.:*Japan. J. Pharmacol.***1972**, 22, 11; Eaker, E. Y. et al.:*Gastroentero-logy* **1989**, 96, 1506; Swabb, E. A. et al.:*Am. J. Physiol.* **1981**, 241, G248; Zhu, B. et al.:*Am. J. Vet. Res.* **1982**, 43, 1594; Wada, K. et al.:*Chem. Pharm. Bull.* **1990**, 38, 2332.

[T. Kimura]

78   *Poncirus trifoliata* **DC.**   (Rutaceae)

Gou–ju (C), Gou–gwut (H), Karatachi (J), Taeng–ja–na–mu (K)

Fruit

Local Drug Name: Zhi–ke, Zhi–shi (C), Gou–gwut (H), Ki–koku, Ki–jitsu (J), Ji–gak (K).

Processing: Cut immature fruits and dry under the sun (J, K).

Method of Administration: Oral (decoction: extract) (H, J, K), Bathing (J).

Folk Medicinal Uses:

       1) Gastritis (K).

       2) Perspiration (J, K).

       3) Apepsia (J, K).

       4) Hernia (C, H).

       5) Traumatic injury (C, H).

       6) Abdominal pain (K).

       7) Sputum remedy (K).

       8) Common cold (K).

       9) Diarrhea (K).

       10) Itching (K).

       11) Infant beri–beri (K).

       12) Neuralgia (K).

       13) Contusion (K).

       14) Urticaria (K).

       15) Sinusitis (K).

       16) Rhagadia (J).

       17) Thirst (J).

       18) Uterine prolaopse (C).

Contraindications: In pregnancy. "Spleen" and "stomach" indeficiency.

Scientific Researches:

Chemistry

   1) Flavonoids: hesperidin [1].

   2) Coumarins: 7–geranyloxycoumarin, bergapten, poncimarin I, isoponcimarin [2, 15], khelmarin A [13], aurapten [3], poncitrin [4, 8], isopimpinellin, prangenin [6], heraclenin, impertonin [9],

ponfolin [14].

3) Amino acids: proline, alanine,γ –aminobutyric acid, asparagine, etc.[5].

4) Fatty acids: palmitic, stearic, oleic, linoleic, linolenic acids [7].

5) Essential oils: β –myrcene, β –phellandrene, caryophyllene [10], limonin, marmesin [11], limonol,
    deoxylimonol, 7α –obacunol [12].

6) Alkaloids: acridone [16].

Literatures:

[1] Kanao, M. et al.: *Yakugaku Zasshi* **1978,** 98(2), 245.

[2] Guiotto, A. et al.: *Phytochem.* **1977,** 16(8), 1257.

[3] Guiotto, A. et al.: *Z. Naturforsch., Teil C.* **1974,** 29(5–6), 201.

[4] Tomimatsu, T. et al.: *Tetrahedron* **1974,** 30(8), 939.

[5] Nobile, L. et al.: *Cl. Sci. Fis., Rend* **1970–1971,** 8(1), 121.

[6] Guiotto, A. et al.: *Z. Naturforsch., Teil C* **1973,** 28(5–6), 260.

[7] Aburano, S. et al.: *Yakugaku Zasshi* **1972,** 92(10), 1298.

[8] Tomimatsu, T. et al.: *Tetrahedron* **1972,** 28(7), 2003.

[9] Weinstein, B. et al.: *Phytochem.* **1972,** 11(4), 1530.

[10] Kamiyama, S.: *Bull. Brew. Sci.* **1970,** 16, 1.

[11] Tomimatsu, T. et al.: *Shoyakugaku Zasshi* **1970,** 24(2), 122.

[12] Benett, R. D. et al.: *Phytochem.* **1982,** 21(9), 2349.

[13] Ito, C. et al.: *Chem. Pharm. Bull.* **1990,** 38(5), 1230.

[14] Furukawa, H. et al.: *Chem. Pharm. Bull.* **1986,** 34(9), 3922.

[15] Guiotto, A. et al.: *Phytochem.* **1976,** 15(2), 348.

[16] Wu, T. et al.: *J. Nat. Prod.* **1986,** 49(6), 1154.

[C.K. Sung]

79.   *Zanthoxylum nitidum* (Roxb.)DC.   (Rutaceae)

Guang–ye–hua–jiao (C), Leung–min–jum (H).

Root

Local Drug Name: Ru–di–jin–niu (C), Leung–min–jum (H), Ryo–men–shin (J).

Method of Administration: Oral or topical (decoction: C, H).

Folk Medicinal Uses:

1) Rheumatalgia (C, H).

2) Traumatic injury (C, H).

3) Epigastric pain (C, H).

4) Toothache (C, H).

5) Sorethroat (C, H).

6) Snake bite (C, H).

7) Pyodermas, dermatitis (H).

8) Burns (C).

9) Mumps (C).

Contraindications: Sour foods, pregnancy.

Side Effects: Dizziness, vomiting, abdominal pain. Injections of extracts caused anaphyletic response in one
    case.

Scientific Researches:

Chemistry

1) Nitidine, oxynitidine, diosmin.

2) 7–Demethyl–6–methoxy–5,6–dihydrochelerythrine, 6–methoxy–5,6–dihydrochele⁻

81

thrine, 6–ethoxy–5,6–dihydrochelerythrine [4].

Pharmacology
1) Analgesic effects [1–2].
2) Antispasmodic effects [2].
3) Antineoplastic effect by nititine.
4) Crystal–8 caused catalepsy in rats and mice [3].

Literatures:

[1] Hong, G.X. et al.:*Yao Hsueh Hsueh Pao* **1983**, 18, 227.
[2] Zeng, X.Y. et al.:*Yao Hsueh Hsueh Pao* **1982**, 17, 253.
[3] Zeng, X.Y.: *Zhongcaoyao* **1988**, 19, 266.
[4] Chen, Y.Z. et al.:*Huaxue Xuebao* **1989**, 47, 1048.

[P.P.H. But]

80.   *Zanthoxylum piperitum* DC.   (Rutaceae)

Sansho (J), Cho–pi–na–mu (K)

Related plant: *Zanthoxylum bungeanum* Maxim.: Hua–jiao (C);*Z. schnifolium*
Z. piperitum DC. var. *inerme* Makino: Asakura–zansho (J)

Pericarp   (JP, KP)
Local Drug Name: San–sho (J), San–cho (K).
Processing: Dry under the sun. Eliminate seeds as much as possible (J, K).
Method of Administration: Oral (decoction or powder: J, K).
Folk Medicinal Uses:
1) Stomachic, dyspepsia (J, K).
2) Anthelmintic (J, K).

Scientific Researches:
Chemistry
1) Essential oil: dipentene, citronellal, β–phellandrene, geraniol, citronellol, citral [1].
2) Acid amides: α–sanshool, γ–sanshool, hydroxy α–sanshool, hydroxy γ–sanshool, sanshoamide [2].
3) Flavonoids: quercitrin, afzelin, hesperidin.
Pharmacology
1) Anthelmintic [3].
2) Local hypesthesia (amides) [4].
3) Antifungal (methanol extract) [5].
4) Others [6].

Literatures:

[1] Sakai, T. et al.:*Bull. Chem. Soc.* **1968**, 41, 1945; Yasuda, I. et al.:*Shoyakugaku Zasshi* **1982**, 36, 301.
[2] Aihara, D.:*Yakugaku Zasshi* **1950**, 70, 405, 409; **1951**, 71, 1112, 1323; Crombie, L. et al.:*J. Chem. Soc.* **1957**, 2760; Yasuda, I. et al.:*Chem. Pharm. Bull.* **1981**, 29, 1791;*Phytochem.* **1982**, 21, 1295.
[3] Kiuchi, F. et al.:*Shoyakugaku Zasshi* **1989**, 43, 279; Kubota, H. et al.:*Nippon Yakubutsugaku Zasshi* **1935**, 20, 29; Bando, T. et al.:*Nippon Yakurigaku Zasshi* **1956**, 52, 76.
[4] Izeki, M. et al.:*Nippon Yakurigaku Zasshi* **1949**, 44, 9.
[5] Jain, S. R. et al.:*Planta Med.* **1972**, 22, 136.
[6] Ohmoto, T. et al.:*Shoyakugaku Zasshi* **1985**, 39, 28; Kinoshita, T. et al.:*ibid.* **1979**, 33, 146; Aihara, D. et al.:*Yakugaku Zasshi* **1951**, 71, 1323.
[T. Kimura]

81.   *Ailanthus altissima* (Mill.) Swingle   (Simaroubaceae)

Chou–chun (C), Tzou–chun (H), Niwaurushi, Sinju (J), Ga–juk–na–mu (K)

Root Bark and Stem Bark   (CP)
Local Drug Name: Chun–pi, Chu–bai–pi (C), Tzou–chun–pay (H), Jeo–geun–baek–pi (K).
Processing: 1) Cut into slivers or sections, and dry (C, K).
                 2) Stir–fry the slivers with bran until turning slightly yellow (C).
Method of Administration: Oral (decoction: C, H, K).
Folk Medicinal Uses:
                 1) Morbid leukorrhea (C, H).
                 2) Diarrhea caused by damp–heat (C).
                 3) Chronic diarrhea, chronic dysentery (C, H, K).
                 4) Hematochezia, abnormal uterine bleeding (C).
                 5) Ascariasis (H).

Scientific Researches:
Chemistry
   1) Lactones: amarolide, amarolide–11–acetate[1–3], shinudilactone [3].
   2) Organic acids: syringic acid, vanillic acid, azelaic acid [3].
   3) Steroids: β–sitosterol [3].
Pharmacology
                 1) Anticancer effect (shinudilactone) [3].

Literatures:
[1] Gasinovi, C.G. et al.:*Tetrahedron Letters* **1964**, 3991; **1965**, 2273.
[2] Stocklin, W. et al.:*ibid.* **1970**, 2399
[3] Guo, Y. Z. et al.:*Zhongcaoyao* **1985**, 11(7), 46.

[J.X. Guo]

82.   *Picrasma quassioides* (D. Don) Bennet   (Simarubaceae)

Kumu (C), Fu–muk (H), Nigaki (J), So–tae–na–mu (K)

Stem and Leaf (CP), **Wood** (JP, KP)
Local Drug Name: Ku–mu (C), Fu–muk (H), Niga–ki (J), Go–mok (K).
Processing: Slice and dry under the sun.
Method of Administration: Oral or topical (decoction or powder: C, H, J, K).
Folk Medicinal Uses:
                 1) Bitter stomachic (C, H, J, K).
                 2) Chronic dyspepsia (C, J, K).
                 3) Enteritis (H).
                 4) Colds (C).
                 5) Acute tonsillitis (C).
                 6) Pharyngitis (C).
                 7) Eczema (C, H).
                 8) Bacillary dysentery (C, H).
                 9) Tinea (H).
                 10) Burns (H).
                 11) Boils (C).
                 12) Ascariasis (H).

13) Venomous snake bite (C).

14) Insecticide (J).

Contraindications: Woman in pregnancy.

Scientific Researches:

Chemistry

1) Diterpenoids: quassin (= nigakilactone D), nigakilactone A–C [1], E–N, picrasin B–G [2].

2) Alkaloids: nigakinone, methylnigakinone [3].

3) Others: nigakihemiacetal, 2,6–dimethoxy–p–benzoquinone [4, 5].

Pharmacology

1) Gastric secretion [6, 7].

2) Insecticide (quassin) [8].

3) Antihypertensive (alkaloids) [9].

4) Inhibition of cyclic AMP phospho diesterase activity (alkaloids) [10].

5) Gastric and intestinal blood flow increasing (alkaloids) [11].

6) Antiviral for herpes (alkaloids) [11].

Literatures:

[1] Takahashi, T. et al.:*Tetrahedron Letters* **1969**, 3013; *Chem. Pharm. Bull.* **1979**, 18, 2590; Hikino, H. et al.: *Chem. Pharm. Bull.* **1971**, 19, 213; Murae, T. et al.:*Chem. Pharm. Bull.* **1971**, 19, 2426; *Tetrahedron* **1971**, 27, 5147; **1973**, 29, 1515.

[2] Hikino, H. et al.:*Phytochem.* **1975**, 14, 2473.

[3] Kimura, Y. et al.:*Yakugaku Zasshi* **1967**, 87, 1371; Kondo, Y. et al.:*Chem. Pharm. Bull.* **1973**, 21, 837; Ohmoto, T. et al.:*Chem. Pharm. Bull.* **1982**, 30, 1204; **1983**, 31, 3198; **1984**, 32, 3579, **1985**, 33, 4901; Luo, W. et al.:*Yaowu Fenxi Zazhi* **1985**, 5, 11; Yang, J. S. et al.:*Yaoxue Xuebao* **1988**, 23, 267; Koike, K. et al.:*Phytochem.* **1988**, 27, 3029; Luo, S. R. et al.:*Yaoxue Xuebao* **1988**, 23, 906.

[4] Murae, T. et al.:*Chem. Pharm. Bull.* **1975**, 23, 2188.

[5] Niimi, Y. et al.:*Chem. Pharm. Bull.* **1989**, 37, 57 (1989).

[6] Sone, Y.: *Tohoku J. Exptl. Med.* **1936**, 29, 321.

[7] Esaki, T.:*Nippon Yakurigaku Zasshi* **1954**, 50, 103; **1955**, 51, 62.

[8] Park, M. H., et al.:*Chem. Pharm. Bull.* **1987**, 35, 3082.

[9] Ma, S. D. et al.:*Yaoxue Xuebao* **1982**, 17, 327.

[10] Sung, Y.–I. et al.:*Chem. Pharm. Bull.* **1984**, 32, 1872; Ohmoto, T., et al.:*Chem. Pharm. Bull.* **1988**, 36, 4588.

[11] Ohmoto, T., et al.:*Shoyakugaku Zasshi* **1985**, 39, 28; **1988**, 42, 160.

[T. Kimura]

83.   *Melia toosendan* **Sieb. et Zucc.**   (Meliaceae)

Chuan–lian (C), Chuan–lin (H), Tosendan (J), Dang–meol–gu–seul–na–mu (K)

Related Plant: *Melia azedarach L.*: Lian (C).

Bark (CP)

Local Drug Name: Ku–lian–pi (C), Fu–lin–pay (H), Ku–ren–pi (J), Go–ryun–pi (K).

Processing: Eliminate foreign matter, wash clean, cut into slices and dry.

Method of Administration: Oral (decoction: C, H, J, K).

Folk Medicinal Uses:

        1) Ascariasis, hookworm infestation, oxyuriasis (C, H, J, K).

        2) Tinea capitis, scabies, eczema, urticaria (C, H).

        3) Trichomonal vaginitis (C, H).

4) Impetigo, ringworm infestation, boils, dermatitis (C, H, J).

Contraindications: Debility, spleen and stomach cold–deficiency, hepatitis, nephritis.
Side Effects: Dizziness, vomiting, abdominal pain, malaise, numbness of extremities.

Fruit (CP)
Local Drug Name: Chuan–lian–zi (C), Chuan–lin–gee (H), Sen–ren–shi (J), Cheon–ryun–ja (K).
Processing: Clean and dry; or cut into slices or pulverize into powder, stir–fry until the outer surface turns brown.
Method of Administration: Oral (decoction: C, H, J, K).
Folk Medicinal Uses:
1) Ascariasis, hookworm infestation, oxyuriasis (C, H, J, K).
2) Hernia (C, H).
3) Diuretic (C, H).
4) Distending pain in the chest, hypochondrium and epigastrium (C).
Contraindications: Spleen and stomach cold–deficiency.
Side Effects: Dizziness, vomiting, abdominal pain, malaise, numbness of extremities.

Leaf
Local Drug Name: Lian–ye (C), Yeon–yeop (K).
Method of Administration: Oral (decoction: C).
Folk Medicinal Uses:
1) Ascariasis (C).
2) Traumatic injury (C).
3) Boils, eczema (C).
Side Effects: Dizziness, vomiting, abdominal pain, malaise, numbness of extremities.

Flower
Local Drug Name: Lian–hua (C).
Method of Administration: Topical (powder: C).
Folk Medicinal Uses: 1) Pruritus (C).

Scientific Researches:
Chemistry
1) Glucosides: toosendanoside [2], melia–ionosides A and B (leaf) [3, 10].
2) Steroids: toosendansterols A and B (leaf) [4].
3) Terpenoid: loliolide (leaf) [4].
4) Triterpenoid: lipomelianol, melianone, 21–O–methyltoosendapentol (fruit) [5–6, 11].
5) Limonoid: toosenadanin (bark) [7–8], isotoosendanin [9].
Pharmacology
1) Anthelmintic effect.

Literatures:
[1] Zang, Q.Z. In: Chang HM, But PPH (Eds): "*Pharmacology and Applications of Chinese Materia Medica*" World Scientific, Singapore,**1987**, 2, 778–80.
[2] Nakanishi, T. et al.:*Chem. Pharm. Bull.* **1988**, 36, 4148.
[3] Nakanishi, T. et al.:*Chem. Pharm. Bull.* **1991**, 39, 2529.
[4] Inada, A. et al.:*Chem. Pharm. Bull.* **1988**, 36, 609.
[5] Nakanishi, T. et al.:*Chem. Pharm. Bull.* **1986**, 34, 100.
[6] Nakanishi, T. et al.:*Chem. Lett.* **1986**, 69.
[7] Chung C.C., et al.:*Hua Hsueh Hsueh Pao* **1975**, 33, 35.
[8] Shu G.X. et al.:*Hua Hsueh Hsueh Pao* **1980**, 38, 196.
[9] Xie J.X. et al.: *Yueh Hsueh Tung Pao* **1984**, 19, 369.
[10] Nakanishi, T. et al.:*Chem. Pharm. Bull.* **1990**, 38, 830.

[11] Inada, A. et al.:*Heterocycles* **1989**, 28, 383.

[P.P.H. But]

84.   *Polygala tenuifolia* **Willdenow** (Polygalaceae)

Yuan–zhi (C), Yuan–gee (H), Itohimehagi (J), Weon–ji

Root (CP, JP, KP)

Local Drug Name: Yuan–zhi (C), Yuan–gee (H), On–ji (J), Weon–ji (K).

Processing: 1) Dry under the sun. 2) Boil down gently with a decoction of Glycyrrhiae Radix until exhausted, and dry (C).

Method of Administration: Oral (decoction: C, H, J, K; or powder: J, K).

Folk Medicinal Uses:

        1) Palpitation (C, H, J).
        2) Anxiety, insomnia (C, H, J).
        3) Phlegm (C, H, J, K).
        4) Cough (C, H, J).
        5) Amnesia (K).
        6) Swelling and pain in the breast (C).
        7) Boils and sores (C).
        8) Carbuncle (H).

Scientific Researches:

Chemistry

  1) Saponins: senegin III, IV, onjisaponin C, D, E, F, G [1].

Pharmacology

  1) Expectorant (water extract) [2].
  2) Congestion edema lowering (water extract) [3].
  3) Diuretic (water extract) [3].
  4) Anti–stress ulcer (water extract) [4].
  5) Cyclic AMP inhibition (saponins) [5].

Literatures:

[1] Sakuma, S. et al.:*Chem. Pharm. Bull.* **1981**, 29, 2431; **1982**, 30, 810.
[2] Igarashi, K.: *Sogo Igaku* **1951**, 8, 526.
[3] Yamahara, J. et al.: *Chem. Pharm. Bull.* **1979**, 27, 1464.
[4] Yamazaki, M. et al.:*Shoyakygaku Zasshi* **1981**, 35, 96.
[5] Nikaido, T. et al.:*Chem. Pharm. Bull.* **1982**, 30, 2020.

[T. Kimura]

85.   *Impatiens balsamina* **L.** (Balsaminaceae)

Feng–xian–hua (C), Fung–sin–fa (H), Hosenka (J), Bong–seon–hwa (K)

Seed

Local Drug Name: Ji–xing–zi (C), Gup–sing–gee (H), Kyu–sei–shi (J), Bong–seon–ja (K).

Processing: Dry under the sun (C).

Method of Administration: Oral (decoction: C).

Folk Medicinal Uses:
        1) Masses (C).
        2) Amenorrhea (C, H, J).
        3) Dysphagia (C, J).
        4) Neoplasm (H).
        5) Constipation (J).
        6) Gastroatony (J).
        7) Acute gastritis (K).
Contraindications: Use with caution in pregnancy (C, H).

Flower
Local Drug Name: Fung–sin–fa (H).
Method of Administration: Oral (decoction: H).
Folk Medicinal Uses:
        1) Amenorrhea (H).
        2) Traumatic injury (H).
        3) Hematoma (H).
        4) Rheumatalgia (H).
        5) Furunculosis (H).
        6) Snake bites (H).
        7) Ringworm (H).

Herb
Local Drug Name: Ho–sen–ka (J), Bong–seon (K).
Processing: Dry under the sun (J, K).
Method of Administration: Oral (decoction: J, K); Topical (decoction, J).
Folk Medicinal Uses:
        1) Articular rheumatism (J).
        2) Bruise (J).
        3) Menstrual disorder (J).
        4) Scrofula (J).
        5) Carbuncle (J).
        6) Leukorrhea (K).
        7) Apepsia (K).
        8) Menoxenia (K).

Scientific Researches:
Chemistry
  1) Fatty oil: parinaric acid, balsaminasterol, spinasterol, β–sitosterol [1], (–)–(R,Z)–glycerol 1–9–
        octadecenoate [2].
  2) Flavonoids: apigenin–4'-O–β–D–glucopyranoside [3].
Pharmacology
  1) Excitatory effect on ulterus [4].
  2) Antifertility effect (Antinidatory effect) [4].

Literatures:
[1] Nanjing College of Pharmacy: "*Zhongcaoyao Xue*", Vol. 2, **1976**, 634.
[2] Patra, A. et al.:*J. Indian Chem. Soc.* **1988**, 65(5), 367.
[3] Yadlava, R.N. et al.:*Fitoterapia* **1992**, 63(2), 188.
[4] Wang, Y.S. et al.: "*Zhongyao Yaoli Yu Yingyong*", **1983**, 799.

                                          [J.X. Guo]

86.   *Ilex pubescens* Hook. et Arn.   (Aquifoliaceae)

Mao–dong–qing (C), Mo–dung–ching (H), Mo–dong–cheong (K)

Root and Leaf
Local Drug Name: Mao–pi–shu (C), Mo–dung–ching (H), Mo–to–sei (J), Mo–dong–cheong (K).
Processing: Root: cut into slices and dry under the sun (C). Leaf: use in fresh (C).
Method of Administration: Oral (decoction: C, H, J); Topical (decoction: C, H).
Folk Medicinal Uses:
      1) Coronary arteriosclerotic cardiopathy (C, H, K).
      2) Acute myocardial infarction (C, H).
      3) Thrombotic angiitis (C, H, K).
      4) Infantile pneumonia (C, H).
      5) Central retinopathy (C, H).
      6) Burn (C, H).
      7) Cold, cough, tonsillar (C).
      8) Tonsillitis, pharyngitis (H).
      9) Cerebral thrombosis (H).

Scientific Researches:
Chemistry
  1) Tritepenes: ilexgenin A [1], ilexonin [2], ursolic acid, oleanolic acid [3].
  2) Saponins: ilexsaponin A1 [1], ilexsaponin B1, B2, B3 [4]. Peduculoside, ilexsaponin B [5],
     ilexolide A [6].
  3) Flavonoids [7].
Pharmacology
  1) Expectorant effect [8].
  2) Effect on cardiovasculor system (flavonoids) [9].
    a. Expanding coronary artery.
    b. Decreasing oxygen consumption of myocardium.
    c. Acting on the smooth muscle of pheripheral blood vasculars directly, making the blood vasculars
      expand.
  3) Bacteriostasis effect (flavonoids) [7, 8].
  4) Antithrombotic activity (ilexonin A [10], ilexoside A, D [11]).

Literatures:
[1] Hidaka, K. et al.,*Phytochem.*,**1987**, 26(7), 2023.
[2] Sha, J. Z. et al., *Yaoxue Tongbao* **1984,** 19(2), 23.
[3] Arthur, H.R. et al.: *J. Chem. Soc.,* **1965,** 1461.
[4] Hidaka, K. et al.,*Chem. Phrm. Bull.* **1987,** 35(2), 524.
[5] Jiang, Z.F.,*Zhongcaoyao* **1991,** 22(7), 291.
[6] Zeng, L.M. et al., *Chem. Nat. Prod. Prec Sino–Am Symp,* **1980** (pub, 1982), p.280.
[7] The Third Pharmaceutical Factory, *Zhongcaoyao Tongxun* **1971**(2), 48; **1974**,(4), 35.
[8] Nanjing College of Pharmacy: "*Zhongcaoyao Xue*", Vol. 2, **1976**, 615.
[9] The Second Teaching Hospital of Zhongshan Medicial College:*Zhonghua Yixue Zazhi,* **1973**(1), 64.
[10] Liu, G.D. et al.:*Zhongguo Yaoli Xuebao* **1984,** 5(3), 185.
[11] Han, Y.N. et al.:*U.S.* us 4987125 (cl.514–33; A 61k 31170), 22 Jan. 1991, Appl, 213, 232, 29 Jun
   1988.

[J.X. Guo]

87. *Euonymus alatus* **Sieb.**   (Celastraceae)

Wei–mao (C), Gwai–jin–yu (H), Nishikigi (J), Hwa–sal–na–mu (K)

Bark
Local Drug Name: Gui–jian–yu (C), Ki–sen–u (J), Gywi–myun–u (K)
Processing: Dry under the sun (J).
Method of Administration: Oral (decoction: J).
Folk Medicinal Uses:
  1) Taenia (H, K).
  2) Amenorrhea (C, H).
  3) Cancer (K).
  4) Menstrual disorder (J).
  5) Thorn sticking (J).
  6) Anemia (C).
  7) Abdominal pain due to verminosis (C).
  8) Leukorrhagia (C).
  9) Allergic dermatitis (C).
  10) Sty (K).
Contraindications: In pregnancy (C).

Scientific Researches:
Chemistry
  1) Flavonoids: kaempferol, quercetin [1], kaempferol 3–rhamnosylxyloside (deuonymin) [5, 6].
  2) Alkaloids: evonine, euonymine, wilfordine, alatamine [2], neoevonine [7].
  3) Sesquiterpenes: euolalin [3], alatol, alatolin [4, 8].
  4) Steroids: stigmast–4–en–3–one, stigmast–4–ene–3,6–dione, β–sitosterol, 6–hydroxystigmast–
          4–ene–3–one [9].
  5) Catechins: Dehydrodicatechin A, aromadendrin,D–catechin [10].

Literatures:
1) Olechnowicz–Stepien, W.:*Diss. Pharm. Pharmacol.* **1971,** 23(3), 231.
2) Shizuri, Y. et al.: *Tetrahedron Lett.,* **1973**(10), 741.
3) Sugiura, K. et al.: *Chem. Lett.,* **1975**(5), 471.
4) Sugiura, K. et al.: *Tetrahedron Lett.,* **1975**(27), 2307.
5) Ishikura, N. et al.: *Phytochemistry* **1976,** 15(7), 1183.
6) Ishikura, N. et al.: *Bot. Mag.* **1977,** 90(1018), 83.
7) Yamada, K. et al.: *Tetrahedron* **1978,** 34(12), 1915.
8) Sugiura, K. et al.: *Tetrahedron* **1982,** 38(23), 3465.
9) Chen, K. et al.: *Zhongcaoyao* **1983,** 14(9), 385.
10) Chen, K. et al.: *Zhongcaoyao* **1986,** 17(3), 97.

[C.K. Sung]

88. *Berchemia racemosa* **Sieb. et Zucc.**   (Rhamnaceae)

Gou–er–cha (C), Kumayanagi (J), Cheong–sa–cho (K)

Stem and leaf
Local Drug Name: Gou–er–cha (C), Kuma–yanagi (J).
Processing: Dry under the sun (J).
Method of Administration: Oral (decoction: J).

Folk Medicinal Uses:
> 1) Gastrointestinal disorder (J).
> 2) Gallstone (J).
> 3) Stomatitis (J).

Scientific Researches:
Chemistry
1) Quinones: 2,6–dimethoxy–*p*–benzoquinone [1].
2) Aromatic glycosides: nudiposide, isotachioside, β–D–glucopyranosyl syringate, methoxyhydroquinone–
>> 4–*O*–β–D–glucopyranoside [2].
3) Monoterpene glycosides: (+)–angelicoidenol–2–*O*–β–D–glucopyranoside, (–)–angelicoidenol–2–*O*–
>> β–D–glucopyranoside, isoarborinol [3].
4) Lignans: (–)–berchemol [4, 5], secoisolariciresinol, (–)–secoisolariciresinol–*O*– β–D–glucopyranoside
>> [2].

Pharmacology
1) Inhibition of mast cell histamine release (2,6–dimethoxy–*p*–benzoquinone) [1].

Literatures:
[1] Inoshiri, S. et al.:*Chem. Pharm. Bull.* **1986,** 34(3), 1333.
[2] Inoshiri, S. et al.:*Phytochemistry* **1987,** 26(10), 2811.
[3] Inoshiri, S. et al.:*Phytochemistry* **1988,** 27(9), 2869.
[4] Sakurai, N. et al.:*Chem. Pharm. Bull.* **1989,** 37(12), 3311.
[5] *Idem: ibid* **1990,** 38(6), 1801.

[C.K. Sung]

89.   *Hovenia dulcis* **Thunb.**   (Rhamnaceae)

Zhi–ju (C), Gee–qui (H), Kenponashi (J), Hut–gae–na–mu (K)

Fruit
Local Drug Name: Zhi–ju–zi (C), Gee–qui–gee (H), Ki–gu–shi (J), Ji–gu–ja (K).
Processing: Dry under the sun (J, K).
Method of Administration: Oral (decoction: C, J, K).
Folk Medicinal Uses:
> 1) Vomiting (C, H, J).
> 2) Rheumatism (H, C).
> 3) Hiccup (C, H).
> 4) Unconsciousness caused by alcohol intoxication (C).
> 5) Drunkenness (H). Hang over (J, K).
> 6) Thirst caused by heat (C).
> 7) Oliguria (C).
> 8) Infantile epilepsy (C).

Contraindications: "Spleen" and "stomach" cold and insufficiency.

Scientific Researches:
Chemistry
1) Peptide alkaloids: frangulanine, hovenine A, B [1].
2) Saponins: hovenoside G [2–6], hodulcin [7].
3) Alkaloids(seed): perlolyrine [8].

Pharmacology
1) Sweetness–reducing activity (hodulcin) [7].

Literatures:

[1] Takai, M. et al.:*Phytochemistry* **1973,** 12(12), 2985.

[2] Kawai, K. et al.:*Phytochemistry* **1974,** 13(12), 2829.

[3] Inoue, O. et al.:*J. Chem. Soc., Perkin Trans.* **1978,** 1(11), 1289.

[4] Kimura, Y. et al.:*J. Chem. Soc., Perkin Trans.* I, **1981**(7), 1923.

[5] Kobayashi, Y. et al.:*J. Chem. Soc., Perkin Trans.* I. **1982**(12), 2795.

[6] Ogihara, Y. et al.:*Chem. Pharm. Bull.* **1987,** 35(6), 2574.

[7] Kennedy, L. M. et al.:*Chem. Senses* **1988,** 13(4), 529.

[C.K. Sung]

90.   *Ziziphus jujuba* **Mill. var.** *spinosa* **(Bunge) Hu ex H.F. Chou**   (Rhamnaceae)
(= *Z. vulagris* Lamark var. *spinosa* Bunge, *Z. spinosa* Hu)

Suan–zao (C), Suan–jo (H), Sanebuto–natsume (J), Moet–dae–chu–na–mu (K)

Seed (CP)

Local Drug Name: Suan–zao–ren (C), Suan–jo–yan (H), San–so–nin (J). San–jo–in (K).

Processing: 1) Pounding to pieces before use (C, K). 2) Stir–fry the clean seed to slilghtly inflated and the colour slightly darken. Pound to pieces before use (C, K).

Method of Administration: Oral (decoction: C. K).

Folk Medicinal Uses:

         1) Insomnia (C, H, J, K).

         2) Irritability (C, H, J, K).

Contraindications: 1) Severe diarrhea (C). 2) Excess heat (C).

Side Effects: Fever and joint pain (one case reported in 1989, C).

Scinentific Researches:

Chemistry

   1) Saponins: jujuboside A, B, B1, XI [1].

   2) Triterpenes: betulin [2], betulinic acid [3], jujubogenin.

   3) Peptide alkaoids: sanjuinine a–j [4].

   4) Flavonoids: zivulgarin, swertisin and its derivatives.

   5) Organic acids: ferulic acid, ceanoshic acid, alphitolic acid.

Pharmacology

   1) Sedative effect (sanjoinine a–j).

   2) Hypnotic effect (sanjoinine a–j).

   3) Antiarrhythmic effect (Water extract) [5].

   4) Myocardium protective effect (total saponins) [6].

   5) Immuno–enhancement [7].

Literatures:

[1] Kawai, K. et al.:*Phytochem.,* **1974,** 13, 2829: Shibata, S. et al.:*ibid,* **1970,** 9, 677.

[2] Kawaguchi, R., et al.:*Yakugaku Zasshi,* **1940,** 60(6), 343.

[3] Kawaguchi, R., et al.:*ibid,* **1940,** 60(11), 595.

[4] Han, B.H. et al.:*Kor. Pharm. J.,* **1985,** 39(3), 36.

[5] Xu, S.R. et al.:*Zhongcaoyao* **1987,** 18(12), 18.

[6] Chen, X.J. et al.:*Zhongguo Yaoli Xuebao***1990,** 11(2), 153.

[7] Lang, X.C.:*Zhongyao Tongbao* **1988,**13(11).

[J.X. Guo]

91.   *Zizyphus jujuba* Miller var. *inermis* Rehder (= *Z. jujuba* Mill.) (Rhamnaceae)

Zao (C), Die–jo (H), Natsume (J), Dae–chu–na–mu (K)

Fruit (CP, JP, KP)
Local Drug Name: Da–zao (C), Die–jo (H), Tai–so (J), Dae–chu (K).
Processing: Dry under the sun. Cut or remove the kernel before use (C). Boil for a short time then dry
under the sun (J, K).
Method of Administration: Oral. (decoction: C, H, J, K).
Folk Medicinal Uses:
1) Pain (J, K).
2) Myargia (J).
3) Cough, pharyngitis, bronchitis (H, J).
4) Bronchial asthma (J).
5) Anorexia (C, H, K).
6) Lassitude and loose stools in deficiency syndromes of spleen (C, H).
7) Hysteria (C).
8) Palpitation (H).
9) Dysosmia (K).
10) Cholelithiasis (K).
11) Corn of foot (K).
Side Effects: Allergic reaction, rashes (H).

Scientific Researches:
Chemistry
1) Saponins: zizyphussaponin I , II , III , jujuboside B [1].
2) Triterpenoids: oleanolic acid, betulinic acid, ursolic acid, maslinic acid, maslinic acid–3-O–*trans*–p–
coumaroylate, maslinic acid–3–O–*cis*–p–coumaroylate, alphitolic acid p–coumaroulate [1].
3) Aromatic compounds: zizybeoside I , II , vomifoliol and its glycoside [1].
4) Flavonoids: rutin [2]. Swertisin [12], spinosin [13].
5) Alkaloids: Stepharine, N–nornuciforine, asimilobine [11].
5) Others: Zizyphus–arabinan, cyclic AMP [3,4].
Pharmacology
1) Antiallergic (water extract, ethyl α–D–fructofuranoside) [5,6].
2) Complement activity inhibition (zizyphus–arabinan) [6].
3) Anti–stress ulcer (50% methanol extract) [7].
4) Serum urea nitrogen inhibition (water extract) [8].
5) Cyclic AMP effect [10, 14].
6) Central inhibition [10].
7) Liver–protective effect [10].
8) Others [9].

Literatures:
[1] Yagi, A. et al.:*Chem. Pharm. Bull.* **1978**, 26, 1798, 3075; Okamura, et al.:*Chem. Pharm. Bull.* **1981**,
29, 676, 3507.
[2] Tomoda, S.: *Gendai Toyo Igaku* **1984**, 5, 47.
[3] Tomoda, S. et al.:*Shoyakugaku Zasshi* **1969**, 23, 45; **1981**, 35, 194; *Chem. Pharm. Bull.* **1983**, 31, 499;
1985, 33, 4017.
[4] Cyong, J.–C. et al.:*Phytochem.* **1980**,19, 2747; **1982**, 21, 1871.
[5] Koda, A. et al.:*Nippon Yakurigaku Zasshi* **1973**, 69, 88; **1982**, 80, 31; Yagi, A. et al.:*Yakugaku
Zasshi* **1981**, 101, 700.
[6] Yamada, H. et al.:*Carbohydr. Res.* **1985**, 144, 101.
[7] Yamahara, J. et al.:*Shoyakugaku Zasshi* **1974**, 28, 33.

[8] Hattori, T. et al.:*Japan. J. Pharmacol.* **1989**, 50, 477.
[9] Kohda, H. et al.:*Planta Med.* **1986**, 52, 119.
[10] Li, S. Z. et al.: *Zhongcaoyao* **1983**, 14(10), 39.
[11] Khokhai, I. et al.:*Pak. J. Sci. Res.* **1978**, 30, 81.
[12] Inoue, O. et al:*Nagoya Shiritsu Daigaku Yakugakubu Kenkyu Nenpo***1974**, 22, 36.
[13] Woo, W. S. et al.:*Phytochem.* **1979**, 18(2), 353.
[14] Hanabusa, K. et al.:*Planta Med.* **1981**, 42, 380.

[T. Kimura, J.X. Guo]

92. *Althaea officinalis* L.   (Malvaceae)

Yao–shu–kui (C), Usubenitachiaoi (J), Seo–yang–chok–gyu–hwa (K)

Related plant:*Althaea rosea* (L.) Cav.: Shu–kui (C), Tachiaoi (J).

Root
Local Drug Name: Arutea–kon (J).
Processing: Dry under the sun (J).
Method of Administration: Gargle (decoction: J).
Folk Medicinal Uses:
      1) Pharyngitis (J).
      2) Gastritis (J).

Scientific Researches:
Chemistry
  1) Polysaccharide: althaea–mucilage OL [1, 7], L–arabinofuranan [3], glucan [5, 8], L–arbinan [6],
          mucopolysaccharide [9].
  2) Glycopeptides: PS1, PS2 [12].
  3) Phenylpropanoids:*p*–coumaric acid, caffeic acid, ferulic acid [2].
  4) Aromatic acids: salicylic acid,*p*–hydroxybenzoic acid, vanillic acid, syringic acid, p–hydroxy–
          phenylacetic acid [2].
  5) Flavonoids: kaempferol 3–glucoside, kaempferol 3-β–D–(6"–*O*–*p*–hydroxycinnamoyl)–glucoside,
          quercetin–3–glucoside, 8–hydroxydiosmetin–8–glucoside, K salt of 3'–sulfo–8–hydroxy–
          diosmetin–8–glucoside [2, 10]. Hypoletin–8–glucoside, hypoletin–8– β–gentiobioside [14].
  6) Steroids: β–sitosterol, stigmasterol [4].
  7) Fatty acids: palmitic acid, myristic acid, stearic acid, oleic acid, linoleic acid [4].
  8) Coumarins: scopolin [11].
Pharmacology
  1) Immunostimulating action (glucomacropeptide) [12, 13].

Literatures:
[1] Tomoda, M. et al.:*Chem. Pharm. Bull.* **1981,** 29(8), 2277.
[2] Gudej, J.:*Acta Pol. Pharm.* **1981,** 38(3), 385.
[3] Locis, P. et al.:*Bioorg. Khim.* **1983,** 9(2), 240.
[4] Karawya, M. S. et al.:*Egypt. J. Pharm. Sci.* **1979,** 20(1–4), 291.
[5] Kardosova, A. et al.:*Collect. Czech. Chem. Commun.* **1983,** 48(7), 2082.
[6] Capek, P. et al.:*Carbohydr. Res.* **1983,** 117, 133.
[7] Rosik, J. et al.:*Cesk. Farm.* **1984,** 33(2), 689.
[8] Capek, P. et al.:*Collect. Czech. Chem. Commun.* **1984,** 49(11), 2674.
[9] Capek, P. et al.:*Czech. OS* 227,759, 01 Nov. **1985**.
[10] Gudej, J.:*Acta Pol. Pharm.* **1985,** 42(2), 192.

93

[11] Koleva, M. et al.:*Farmatsiya(Sofia)* **1986,** 36(3), 15.
[12] Marinova, S. et al.:*Ann. Immunol. Hung.* **1986,** 26(2), 859.
[13] Marinova, S. et al.:*Probl. Farmakol. Farm.* **1987,** 1, 101.
[14] Gudej, J.:*Acta Pol. Pharm.* **1987,** 44(3–4), 369.
[15] Gudej, J.:*Planta Med.* **1991,** 57(3), 284.

[C.K. Sung]

93.   *Hibiscus syriacus* L.   (Malvaceae)

Mu–jin (C), Muk–gun (H), Mukuge (J), Mu–gung–hwa (K)

Flower
Local Drug Name: Mu–jin–hua (C), Muk–gun–fa (H), Moku–kin–ka (J), Mu–gung–hwa (K)
Processing: Dry under the sun.
Method of Administration: Oral (decoction: C, H, J, K); Topical (H).
Folk Medicinal Uses:
        1) Dysentery (H, J, K).
        2) Leukorrhea (H).
        3) Hemorrhoid (H).
        4) Boils, pyodermas (topical) (H).
        5) Scalds (topical) (H).

Root bark
Local Drug Name: Chuan–jin–pi (C), Muk–gun–pay (H), Mok–geun–pi (K).
Processing: Dry under the sun.
Method of Administration: Oral (decoction: C, H, J, K); topical (decoction or powder: C; tincture: C, H).
Folk Medicinal Uses:
        1) Dysentery (H, J, K).
        2) Ringworm (C, K).
        3) Abdominal pain (J, K).
        4) Leukorrhea(H, K).
        5) Neuralgia (K).
        6) Sputum (K).
        7) Omalgia (K).
        8) Headache (J).
        9) Intestinal hemorrhege (J).
        10) Gastroenteritis (J).
        11) Vomiting (J).
        12) Water eczema (topical)(J).
        13) Eczema with itching (C).
        14) Traumatic bleeding (C).
        15) Pruritus (H).
        16) Oliguria (H).
        17) Scrotal eczema (H).
        18) Tinea flava, Tinea pedis (tincture or vinegar extract) (H).

Fruit
Local drug Name: Mu–jin–zi (C), Chiu–tin–gee (H).
Processing: Dry under the sun.
Method of Administration: Oral (decoction: H).
Folk Medicinal Uses:

1) Cough or wheezing (H).
2) Neuritic headache (H).

Scientific Researches:
Chemistry
  1) Mucilages: hibiscus–mucilage SL [6, 7].
  2) Carotenoids: β–carotene, lutein, lutein 5,6–epoxide, cryptoxanthin, chrysanthemaxanthin, anthera–
      xanthin [1], 3,4–dihydroxy–β–carotene [4].
  3) Essential oils [2].
  4) Fatty acid (seeds): malvic acid, sterculinic acid [3].
  5) Sterols: β–sitosterol, campesterol.
  6) Vitamin E: α–, β–, γ–tocopherol [4].
  7) Alkaloids: canthin–6–one [5].
  8) Anthocyanidins: anthocyanidin–3–glucoside, 3–*O*–malonylglucoside of delphinidin, cyanidin, petunidin,
      pelargonidin, peonidin, malvidin [8, 9].
Pharmacology
  1) Antifungal activity (canthin–6–one) [5].
  2) Anticomplementary activity [10].
  3) Hypoglycemic activity [10].

Literatures:
[1] Hanny, B. et al.:*J. Agr. Food Chem.* **1972,** 20(4), 914.
[2] Hanny, B. et al.:*J. Agr. Food Chem.* **1973,** 21(6), AY.
[3] Chernenko, T. V. et al.:*Khim. Prir. Soedin.* **1973**(6), 719.
[4] Chernenko, T. V. et al.:*Khim. Prir. Soedin.* **1974**(5), 652.
[5] Yokota M. et al.:*Yakugaku Zasshi* **1978,** 98(11), 508.
[6] Shimizu, N. et al.:*Chem. Pharm. Bull.* **1986,** 34(10), 4133.
[7] Tomoda, M. et al.:*Chem. Pharm. Bull.* **1987,** 35(6), 2360.
[8] Kim, J. H. et al.:*J. Fac. Agric., Kyushu Univ.* **1989,** 33(3–4), 243.
[9] Kim, J. H. et al.:*Phytochem.* **1989,** 28(5), 1503.
[10] Tomoda, M. et al.:*Carbohydr. Res.* **1989,** 190(2), 323.

[C.K. Sung]

94.   *Malva verticillata* L.   (Malvaceae)

Dong–kui (C), Dung–kwai (H), Fuyuaoi (J), A–uk (K)

Fruit (CP) or Seed
Local Drug Name: Dong–kui–zi (C), Dung–kwai–gee (H), To–ki–shi (J), Dong–gyu–ja (K)
Processing: Dry in the shade (C, K).
Method of Administration: Oral (decoction: C, H, J, K).
Folk Medicinal Uses:
              1) Postpartum fever(K).
              2) Poisoned dermatitis with lacquer (K).
              3) Constipation (J).
              4) Lactation deficiency (J).
              5) Urinary infection with oliguria (C).
              6) Thirst (C).
              7) Oliguria (C).
              8) Edema (C).
              9) Galactosemia (C).

Contraindications: In "spleen" deficiency, caution in pregnancy.

Scientific Researches:
Chemistry
  1) Mucilage [1].
  2) Polysaccharides: MVS–1 (seed) [2], MVS–IIA, MVS–IIG [3], MVS–V [4], IVA [5].
Pharmacology
  1) Reticuloendothelial system potentiating activity (MVS–IVA) [5, 6, 8].
  2) Anti–complementary activity (MVS) [7].
  3) Hypoglycemic activity (MVS) [7].

Literatures:
[1] Racz, G. and Mathe, I.:*Farmacia (Bucharest)* **1981,** 29(3), 153.
[2] Shimizu, N. et al.:*Chem. Pharm. Bull.* **1987,** 35(12), 4981.
[3] Shimizu, N. et al.:*Chem. Pharm. Bull.* **1988,** 36(8), 2778.
[4] Gonda, R. et al.:*Chem. Pharm. Bull.* **1988,** 36(8), 2790.
[5] Gonda, R. et al.:*Planta Med.* **1990,** 56(1), 73.
[6] Tomoda, M. et al.:*Phytochem.* **1989,** 28(10), 2609.
[7] Tomoda, H. et al.:*Planta Med.* **1990,** 56(2), 168.
[8] Gonda, R. et al.:*Chem. Pharm. Bull.* **1990,** 38(10), 2771.

[C.K. Sung]

95.   *Viola mandshurica* **W. Beck.**   (Violaceae)

Sumire (J), Je–bi–ggot (K)

Related plant: *Viola yedoensis* Makino: Di–ding (C), Nojisumire (J).

Herb
Local Drug Name: Di–ding (C), Shi–ka–ji–cho (J), Ji–jeong (K).
Processing: Dry under the sun (K).
Method of Administration: Oral (decoction: J, K); topical (fresh juice: J).
Folk Medicinal Uses:
         1) Hemorrhoid (J, K).
         2) Swelling (J, K).
         3) Boil (J, K).
         4) Abscess (K).
         5) Neuralgia(K).
         6) Arthritis (K).
         7) Insonia (K).
         8) Distorsion (K).
         9) Antitussive (K).
        10) Limbs pain (K).
Contraindications: In cold and deficiency symptom.

Scientific Researches:
Chemistry
  1) Essential oils (*Viola* spp.): ionones, acetylenic acid esters, 2,6–nonadienal, 2,6–nonadienol [1].

Literature:
[1] Bedoukian, P. Z.:*Fragrance Chem.: Sci. Sense Smell,* **1982,** 285.
                                            [C.K. Sung]

Carica papaya L. (Caricaceae)

Fan–mu–gua (C), Muk–gwa (H), Papaia (J), Pa–pa–i–a (K)

Fruit
Local Drug Name: Fan–mu–gua (C), Muk–gwa (H).
Method of Administration: Oral (Fresh or decoction: C, H).
Folk Medicinal Uses:
1) Gastralgia (C).
2) Dysentery (C).
3) Rheumatalgia (C).
4) Constipation (C).
5) Hypogalactia in parturients (C, H).

Leaf
Local Drug Name: Fan–mu–gua–ye (C).
Method of Administration: Topical (juice: C).
Folk Medicinal Uses:
1) Ulcer (C).

Scientific Researches:
Chemistry
1) Fruit contains carpaine, papain, rennin.
2) Seed contains carposide.
3) Leaf contains carpaine, pseudocarpaine.
4) Chymopapain, a polypeptide of 218 amino acid residues and structurally similar with papain and papaya proteinase omega, including conservation of the catalytic site and of the disulphide bonding [1].
5) Volatile acids and terpenes [16, 17].
Pharmacology
1) Antineoplastic effects.
2) Antimicrobial effects [2, 10, 19].
3) Fertility–reducing effects in male albino rats [3, 14].
4) Use for traumatic injury or surgery [4–6, 8].
5) Anthelmintic effects [7, 9].
6) Abortifacient effects [12].
7) Androgenic effect on vas deferens of rats [13].
8) Beneficial effects in treating vertebral disc hernias by chemonucleolysis because of the enzymatic properties of chymopapain [15].
9) Antisickling effects [18].
10) Inhibitory effects on central nervous system (carpaine) [15].

Literatures:
[1] Watson, D.C. et al.:*Biochem. J.* **1990**, 266, 75.
[2] Giordani, R. et al.:*Mycoses* **1991**, 34, 469.
[3] Lohiya, N.K. et al.:*Indian J. Exp. Biol.* **1992**, 30, 1051.
[4] Holt, H.T.: *Curr. Ther. Res. Clin. Exp.* **1969**, 11, 621.
[5] Vallis, C.P.: *Curr. Ther. Res. Clin. Exp.* **1969**, 11, 356.
[6] Lund, M.H. et al.:*Arch. Surg.* **1969**, 98, 180.
[7] Mehta, R.K. et al.:*Indian Vet. J.* **1966**, 43, 744.
[8] Kapur, B.M. et al.:*Arch. Surg.* **1972**, 105, 761.
[9] Lal, J. et al.:*Indian J. Physiol. Pharmacol.* **1976**, 20, 64.
[10] Jimenez Misas, C.A. et al.:*Rev. Cubana Med. Trop.* **1979**, 31, 21.

[11] Boum, B. et al.:*Toxicol. Appl. Pharmacol.* **1978**, 46, 353.
[12] Gopalakrishnan, M. et al.:*Indian J. Physiol. Pharmacol.***1978**, 22, 66.
[13] Chinoy, N.J. et al.:*Acta Eur. Fertil.* **1984**, 15, 59.
[14] Chinoy, N.J. et al.:*Acta Eur. Fertil.* **1983**, 14, 425.
[15] Moneret–Vautrin, D.A. et al.:*Ann. Fr. Anesth. Reanim.* **1985**, 4, 313.
[16] Idstein, H. et al.:*Z. Lebensm. Unters. Forsch.* **1985**, 180, 394.
[17] Schreier, P. et al.:*Z. Lebensm. Unters. Forsch.* **1985**, 180, 297.
[18] Thomas, K.D. et al.:*Trans. R. Soc. Trop. Med. Hyg.* **1987**, 81, 510.
[19] Le Grand, A.:*J. Ethnopharmacol.* **1989**, 25, 315.

[P.P.H. But]

97. *Benincasa hispida* (Thunb.) Cogn. (= *B. cerifera* Savi) (Cucurbitaceae)

Dong–gua (C), Dung–gwa (H), Toga (J), Dong–gwa (K)

Exocarp (CP)
Local Drug Name: Dong–gua–pi (C), Dung–gwa–pay (H).
Processing: Dry under the sun.
Method of Administration: Oral (decoction: H).
Folk Medicinal Uses:
  1) Edema (H). Edema with oliguria (C).
  2) Diarrhea (H).
  3) Boils (H).
  4) Thirst and oliguria due to summer–heat (C).

Fruit
Local Drug Name: Dung–gwa (H), Dung–gwa (K).
Processing: Dry under the sun (K).
Method of Administration: Oral (decoction: H, K).
Folk Medicinal Uses:
  1) Nephritis (K).
  2) Freckle (K).
  3) Edema (H).
  4) Beriberi (H).
  5) Sputum (H).
  6) Thirst (H).
  7) Diarrhea (H).
  8) Boils (H).
  9) Hemorrhoid (H).
Contraindications: In cold symptom.

Seed
Local Drug Name: Dong–gua–zi (C), To–ga–shi (J), Dong–gwa–ja (K).
Processing: Dry under the sun (J, K).
Method of Administration: Oral (decoction: J, K).
Folk Medicinal Uses:
  1) Stomachache (J, K).
  2) Nephritis (J, K).
  3) Hepatopathy (K).
  4) Anasarca (J).

Scientific Researches:

Chemistry

1) Triterpenes: cucurbitacin B [1], cucurbita–5,24–dienol [3], isomultiflorenol acetate [5].
2) Sterols: β–sitosterol, campesterol, stigmasterol [2].
3) Lipids [2].
4) Volatile compds.: E–2–hexenal, n–hexanal, n–hexyl formate, 2,5–dimethyl–pyrazine, 2,6–dimethyl–pyrazine, 2,3,5–trimethylpyrazine, 2–methylpyrazine [4].

Literatures:

[1] Silapa–Archa, W. et al.:*Varasarn Paesachasarthara* **1981,** 8(1), 5.
[2] Tsuyuki, H. et al.:*Nihon Daigaku No–Juigakubu Gakujutsu Kenkyu Hokoku* **1982**(39), 75.
[3] Akihisa, T. et al.: *Yukagaku* **1986,** 35(12), 1036.
[4] Wu, C. M. et al.:*J. Food Sci.* **1987,** 52(1), 132.
[5] Wolleweber, E. et al.:*Indian Drugs* **1991,** 28(10), 458.

[C.K. Sung]

98.   *Cucurbita moschata* **Duch.**
C. moschata **Duch. var.** *toonas* **Makino**   (Cucurbitaceae)

Nan–gua (C), Nam–gwa (H), Kabocha (J), Ho–bak (K)

Fruit

Local Drug Name: Nan–gua (C), Nam–gwa (H), Nan–ga (J), Nam–gwa (K).
Method of Administration: Oral (fresh or decoction: C, H, J, K).
Folk Medicinal Uses:

1) Inflammation (C).
2) Pain (C).
3) Morphine poisoning (C).
4) Ascariasis (C).
5) Intercostal neuralgia (J).
6) Pleurisy (J).
7) Postpartum edema (K).
8) Debility after sickness or child–birth (K).

Contraindications: Qi–stagnant, wetness–blocked.

Seed

Local Drug Name: Nan–gua–zi (C), Nam–gua–gee (H), Nan–ga–nin, Nan–ga–shi (J), Nam–gwa–ja (K).
Processing: Dry under the sun.
Method of Administration: Oral (decoction: C, H, J, K).
Folk Medicinal Uses:

1) Taeniasis (C, H, J).
2) Schistosomiasis (C).
3) Whooping cough (C, J, K).
4) Postpartum edema (C, J, K).
5) Hemorrhoid (C, J).

Side Effects: Dizziness, nausea, vomiting, gastric distention, anorexia, diarrhea and borborygmus.

Root

Local Drug Name: Nan–gua–gen (C), Nam–gwa–geun (K).
Method of Administration: Oral (decoction: C).
Folk Medicinal Uses:

1) Jaundice (C).
2) Dysentery (C).

Tendril
Local Drug Name: Nan–gua–xu (C); Nam–gwa–su (K).
Method of Administration: Oral (decoction: C).
Folk Medicinal Uses:
1) Withdrawn nipple (C).

Flower
Local Drug Name: Nan–gua–hua (C), Nam–gwa–hwa (K).
Method of Administration: Oral (decoction: C, K).
Folk Medicinal Uses:
1) Jaundice (C).
2) Dysentery (C).
3) Coughing (C).
4) Pyodermas (C).
5) Bee–bite (K).

Pedicel
Local Drug Name: Nan–gua–di (C), Nan–ga–tei (J).
Processing: Collect when green, dry under the sun.
Method of Administration: Oral (decoction: C, J).
Folk Medicinal Uses:
1) Boils (C, J).
2) Burns (C).
3) Sputum (C).
4) Eczema (J).
5) Abdominal distention due to retention of food (C).
6) Icterohepatitis, chronic hepatitis, cirrhosis (C).

Vine
Local Drug Name: Nan–gua–teng (C), Nam–gwa–deung (K).
Method of Administration: Oral (decoction: C, K).
Folk Medicinal Uses:
1) Tuberculosis (C).
2) Gastralgia (C).
3) Irregular menses (C, K).

Scientific Researches:
Chemistry
1) Cucurbitine, cucurbitacine, avenasterol.
Pharmacology
1) Anthelmintic effects (seed, cucurbitine) [1].
2) Antischistosomal effects (seed).

Literature:
[1] Zheng, Z.Y. In: Chang H.M., But, P.P.H. (Eds): *"Pharmacology and Applications of Chinese Materia Medica"* World Scientific, Singapore, **1987**, 2, 857.

[P.P.H. But]

99. *Luffa cylindrica* **(L.) Roem.**   (Cucurbitaceae)

Si–gua (C), See–gwa (H), Hechima (J), Su–se–mi–o–i (K)

Fruit
Local Drug Name: Si–gua (C), See–gwa (H), Shi–ka (J), Sa–gwa (K).
Method of Administration: Oral (decoction: C, H, J, K).
Folk Medicinal Uses:
        1) Febrile diseases (C, H, K).
        2) Sputum and coughing (C, J, K).
        3) Uterine hemorrhage (C, J, K).
        4) Boils (C).
        5) Lack of milk (C, J).
        6) Hemorrhoid (C).
Side Effects: Impotence, diarrhea.

Leaf
Local Drug Name: Si–gua–ye (C), Sa–gwa–yeop (K).
Processing: Dry under the sun.
Method of Administration: Oral (decoction: C).
Folk Medicinal Uses:
        1) Febrile diseases (C).
        2) Boils (C).
        3) Snake bite (C).
        4) Burns (C).
        5) Scabies (C).
        6) Tinea (C).

Root
Local Drug Name: Si–guo–gen (C); Sa–gwa–geun (K).
Processing: Dry under the sun (C).
Method of Administration: Oral (decoction: C).
Folk Medicinal Uses:
        1) Migraine (C).
        2) Lumbago (C).
        3) Mastitits (C).
        4) Soar throat (C).
        5) Hemorrhoid (C).

Luffa (CP)
Local Drug Name: Si–gua–luo (C), See–gwa–lok (H), Shi–ka–raku (J), Sa–gwa–rak (K).
Processing: Remove the remaining seeds and exocarp, cut into sections.
Method of Administration: Oral (decoction: C).
Folk Medicinal Uses:
        1) Abdominalgia (C).
        2) Lumbago (C, H).
        3) Menoschesis (C).
        4) Lack of milk (C, H).
        5) Hemorrhoid (C, H).
        6) Pyodermas (C).
        7) Arthralgia with muscular contracture (C).

Seed
Local Drug Name: Si–gua–zi (C), Sa–gwa–ja (K).

Processing: Dry under the sun.
Method of Administration: Oral (decoction: C).
Folk Medicinal Uses:
> 1) Edema (C).
> 2) Hemorrhoid (C).
> 3) Ascariasis (C).

Contraindication: Pregnancy, spleen–deficiency.
Side Effects: Diarrhea.

Vine
Local Drug Name: Si–gua–teng (C), Shi–ka–to (J), Sa–gwa–deung (K).
Processing: Dry under the sun.
Method of Administration: Oral (decoction: C).
Folk Medicinal Uses:
> 1) Irregular menses (C).
> 2) Edema (C).
> 3) Numbing of limbs (C).
> 4) Toothache (C).

Stem Sap
Local Drug Name: Hechima–sui (J).
Processing: Cut the stem at *ca.* 30 cm above ground, and collect the sap secreted from the root.
Method of Administration: Topical (fresh juice: J).
Folk Medicinal Uses:
> 1) Skin roughness (J).

Fruit sap
Local Drug Name: Cheon–ra–su (K).
Method of Administration: Oral (fresh: K).
Folk Medicinal Uses:
> 1) Sputum (K).
> 2) Leukorrhea (K).
> 3) Cough (K).

Scientific Researches:
Chemistry
1) Fruit and seed contain cucurbitacin B, lucyosides A–H [4], I–M [5], N and P [3], ginsenosides Re and Rg$_1$ [4], 3–O–β–D–glucopyranosyl hederagenin, 3–O–β–D–glucopyranosyl oleanolic acid [5], bioactive proteins [10], luffin–a, luffin–b [17], ribosome–inactivating protein [19].
2) Leaf contains lucyin A (21β–hydroxy–gypsogenin), lucyoside (3–O–β–D–glucopyranosyl–21–β–hydroxyhederagenin), 3–O–β–D–glucopyranosyl–arjunolic acid [1], machaerinic acid lactone as acetate and apigenin [9].
3) Ribosome–inactivating protein [6].
4) Bryonolic acid [7], malonic acid, malic acid, citric acid [11].
5) Palmitic acid, linoleic acid [11].
6) Trypsin inhibitors [15].
7) β–Sitosterol, apigenin, oleanolic acid (male flower) [18].

Pharmacology
1) Antitussive effects.
2) Fribrinolytic effects (lucyosides) [3, 16].
3) Anti–allergic effects (bryonolic acid) [7].
4) Skin–lightening uses [8] and skin–moisturizing uses [12].
5) Ribosome–inactivating effects [10].
6) Cytotoxic effects [10].

7) Abortifacient effects [10].

8) Antiinflammatory uses [13].

9) Antiperspirant and astringent uses [14].

10) Trypsin inhibitory effects [15].

11) Anti–platelet aggregation effects [16].

Literatures:

[1] Liang, L. et al.: *Yaoxue Xuebao* **1993**, 28, 836.

[2] Liang, L. et al.: *Huaxi Yaoxue Zazhi* **1993**, 8, 63.

[3] Yoshikawa, K. et al.: *Chem. Pharm. Bull.* **1991**, 39, 1185.

[4] Takemoto, T. et al.: *Yakugaku Zasshi* **1984**, 104, 246.

[5] Takemoto, T. et al.: *Yakugaku Zasshi* **1985**, 105, 834.

[6] Li, B.Y. et al.: *Targeted Diagn. Ther.* **1992**, 7, 223.

[7] Tabata, M. et al.: *J. Nat. Prod.* **1993**, 56, 165.

[8] Shimizu, M. et al.: *Jpn. Kokai Tokkyo Koho* JP 04 26,610 [92 26,610] **1992**.

[9] Khan, M.S.Y. et al.: *Indian J. Pharm. Sci.* **1992**, 54(2), 75.

[10] Ng, T.B. et al.: *Biochem. Int.* **1992**, 27, 197.

[11] Chang, K.W. et al.: *Han'guk Nonghwa Hakhoechi* **1991**, 34, 366.

[12] Shimizu, M. et al.: *Jpn. Kokai Tokkyo Koho* JP 04 29,919 [92, 29,919] **1992**.

[13] Shimizu, M. et al.: *Jpn. Kokai Tokkyo Koho* JP 04 36,215 [92, 36,215] **1992**.

[14] Shimizu, M. et al.: *Jpn. Kokai Tokkyo Koho* JP 04 36,216 [92, 36,216] **1992**.

[15] Hatakeyama, T. et al.: *Agric. Biol. Chem.* **1991**, 55, 2641.

[16] Wang, J.D. et al.: *Shoyakugaku Zasshi* **1991**, 45, 215.

[17] Kamenosono, M. et al.: *Agric. Biol. Chem.* **1988**, 52, 1223.

[18] Khan, M.S.Y. et al.: *Indian Drugs* **1990**, 28, 35.

[19] Islam, M.R. et al.: *Agric. Biol. Chem.* **1991**, 55, 1375.

[P.P.H. But]

---

100.   *Trichosanthes kirilowii* Maxim. (Cucurbitaceae)

Gua–lou (C), Kwa–lou (H), Tokarasu–uri (J), Ha–neul–ta–ri (K)

Related plant: *Trichosanthes kirilowii* Maxim. var. *japonicum* Kitamura (= *T. japonica* Regel):
Ri–ben–gua–lou (C), Kikarasu–uri (J), No–rang–ha–neul–ta–ri (K);
T. bracteata Voigt: Okarasu–uri (J);
T. rosthornii Harms (= *T. uniflora* Hao): Shuang–bian–gua–lou (C).

Root   (CP, JP, KP)

Local Drug Name: Tian–hua–fen (C), Tin–fa–fun (H), Ka–ro–kon (J), Gwal–ru–geun (K).

Processing: 1) Remove skin then dry under the sun (J, K). 2) Slice and dry (C).

Method of Administration: Oral or topical (decoction or powder: C, H, J, K).

Folk Medicinal Uses:

         1) Fever (J, K).

         2) Cough (C, J, K).

         3) Congelation (J).

         4) Thirst (C, J).

         5) Diabetes caused by internal heat (C, H, J, K).

         6) Sores and abscess (C). Carbuncle (H). Skin diseases (J).

         7) Jaundice (H).

         8) Hemorrhoid (H).

Contraindication: Incompatible with Radix Aconiti and allied drugs (C).

Fruit (CP)
  Local Drug Name: Gua–lou (C), Kwa–lou (H), Ka–ro–jitsu (J).
  Processing: Hang in cold and shade for drying (C, J). Cut into slivers or pieces (C).
  Method of Administration: Oral (decoction: C, H, J).
  Folk Medicinal Uses:

  1) Cough with thick purulent sputum (C, H).
  2) Angina pectoris and stuffiness sensation in the chest (C). Chest distention (H).
  3) Mastitis, lung abscess, appendicitis (C).
  4) Tuberculosis (H).
  5) Constipation (C, H).
  6) Jaundice (H).

  Contraindication: Incompatible with Radix Aconiti and allied drugs (C).

Pericarp (CP)
  Local Drug Name: Gua–lou–pi (C), Kwa–lou–pay (H), Ka–ro–hi (J).
  Processing: Dry in heat wind. Cut into slivers and dry under the sun.
  Method of Administration: Oral (decoction: C, H, J).
  Folk Medicinal Uses:

  1) Cough with yellowish sticky expectoration (C, H).
  2) Oppressed feeling in the chest and costal pain (C, H).

  Contraindication: Incompatible with Radix Aconiti and allied drugs (C).

Seed (CP)
  Local Drug Name: Gua–lou–zi (C), Kwa–lou–gee (H), Ka–ro–nin (J), Gwal–ru–in (K).
  Processing: Dry under the sun.
  Method of Administration: Oral (decoction: C, H, J, K).
   Folk Medicinal Uses:

  1) Cough (C, H, J, K).
  2) Phlegm (C, H, J).
  3) Constipation (C. H).
  4) Carbuncle (H).

  Contraindication: Incompatible with Radix Aconiti and allied drugs (C).

Scientific Researches:
  Chemistry
  1) Starch
  2) Acids: trichosantic acid.
  3) Amino acids: citrulline, arginine, glutamic acid [1].
  4) Polysaccharides: trichosan A, B, C, D, E [2].
  5) Steroids [3].
  6) Triterpenoids [4].
  Pharmacology
  1) Blood sugar increasing (decoction) [3].
  2) Blood sugar lowering (trichosan A–E) [2].
  3) Inhibition of stress ulcer (water extract) [5].
  4) Alcohol extinction in blood (water extract) [6].
  5) Liver and muscle glycogen increasing [7].

Literatures:
  [1] Murakami, T.:*Shoyakugaku Zasshi* **1965**, 19, 11.
  [2] Hikino, H. et al.:*Planta Med.* **1989**, 55, 349.
  [3] Kanaoka, M. et al.:*Chem. Pharm. Bull.* **1982**, 30, 2570.
  [4] Kitajima, J. et al.:*Yakugaku Zasshi* **1989**, 109, 250, 265.

[5] Yamazaki, M. et al.: *Shoyakugaku Zasshi* **1981**, 35, 96.
[6] Sakai, K., et al. : *Chem. Pharm. Bull.* **1989**, 37, 155.
[7] Watabe, S.: *Gifu Kenritsu Ikadaigaku, Kiyo* **1954**, 1, 256; **1956**, 3, 419.

[T. Kimura]

101.   *Punica granatum* L.   (Punicaceae)

Shi–liu (C), Shek–lou (H), Zakuro (J), Seok–ryu–na–mu (K)

Pericarp (CP)
Local Drug Name: Shi–liu–pi (C), Shek–lou–pay (H), Seki–ryu–ka–hi (J), Seok–ryu–pi (K).
Processing: (1) Cut into pieces and dry (C).
                      (2) Stir–fry the pieces until charred on the outer surface and brown on the inner
                          surface (C).
Method of Administration: Oral (decoction: C, H, J, K).
Folk Medicinal Uses:
                      1) Dysentery (C, H).
                      2) Prolapse of rectum (C).
                      3) Spermatorrhea (C).
                      4) Leukorrhea (C).
                      5) Uterine hemorrhage (C, H).
                      6) Ascariasis (C).
                      7) Tinea (C, K).
                      8) Tonsillitis (K).

Flower
Local Drug Name: Shi–liu–hua (C), Seok–ryu–hwa (K).
Method of Administration: Oral (decoction: C).
Folk Medicinal Uses:
                      1) Epistaxis (C).
                      2) Irregular menses (C).
                      3) Leukorrhea (C).
                      4) Burns (C).

Root
Local Drug Name: Shi–liu–gen (C), Seok–ryu–geun (K).
Method of Administration: Oral (decoction: C).
Folk Medicinal Uses:
                      1) Leukorrhea (C).
                      2) Ascariasis (C).
                      3) Taeniasis (C).
                      4) Renal calculosis (C).
                      5) Dysentery (C).
                      6) Diabetes (C).
Contraindications: Constipation.

Stem bark and Root bark
Local Drug Name: Zaku–ro–hi (J).
Processing: Dry under the sun.
Method of Administration: Oral (decoction: J).
Folk Medicinal Uses:

1) Taeniasis (J).
2) Tonsillitis (J).
3) Sore throat (J).

Scientific Researches:
Chemistry
1) Alkaloids: pelletierine, pseudo–pelletierine, isopelletierine, methylisopelletierine [1, 4, 6, 14, 17].
2) Tannins: punicalagin and punicalin [9], 2–O–galloyl–4,6–(S,S)–gallagyl–D–glucose [10], punicacorteins A–D, punigluconin, casuariin, casuarinin [11], punicafolin, granatins A and B, corilagin, strictinin, 1,2,4,6–tetra–O–galloyl–β–D–glucose, 1,2,3,4,6–penta–O–galloyl–β–D–glucose [12, 13].
3) Sitosterol, ursolic acid, betulic acid, D–mannitol, friedelin, maslinic acid, asiatic acid [1, 8], 2–(2–propenyl)–Δ^1–piperideine [7], chlorogenic acid, p–coumaric acid, neochlorogenic acid, protocatechuic acid [19], elaidic acid, gallic acid [20].
4) Estrone, estradiol [15, 21].
5) Polyphenols: cyanidin–3,5–diglucoside, cyanidin–3–glucoside, delphinidin–3–glucoside [19].
Pharmacology
1) Anthelmintic effects [1, 6].
2) Antibacterial effects [2].
3) Anti–implantation effects [3].
4) Amebicidic effects [5].
5) Estrogenic effects [17].

Literatures:
[1] Fayez, M.B.E. et al.:*Planta Med.* **1963,** 11, 439.
[2] Jimenez Misas, C.A. et al.:*Rev. Cubana Med. Trop.* **1979,** 31, 29.
[3] Prakash, A.O. et al.:*Acta Eur. Fertil.* **1985,** 16, 441.
[4] Ferrara, L. et al.:*Boll. Soc. Ital. Biol. Sper.* **1989,** 65, 385.
[5] Segura, J.J. et al.:*Arch. Invest. Med. (Mex.)* **1990,** 21, 235.
[6] Noordwijk, J.V. et al.:*Rec. Trav. Chim. Pays–Bas* **1963,** 82, 763.
[7] Roberts, M.F. et al.:*Phytochem.* **1967,** 6, 711.
[8] Batta, A.K. et al.:*Phytochem.* **1973,** 12, 214.
[9] Mayer, W. et al.:*Justus Liebigs Ann. Chem.* **1977,** 1976.
[10] Tanaka, T. et al.:*Chem. Pharm. Bull.* **1986,** 34, 650.
[11] Tanaka, T. et al.:*Chem. Pharm. Bull.* **1986,** 34, 656.
[12] Tanaka, T. et al.:*Phytochem.* **1985,** 24, 2075.
[13] Tanaka, T. et al.:*Chem. Pharm. Bull.* **1990,** 38, 2424.
[14] Liebisch, H.W.:*Abh. Deut. Akad. Wiss. Berlin, Kl. Chem., Geol. Biol.* **1966,** 525.
[15] Heftmann, E. et al.:*Phytochem.* **1966,** 5, 1337.
[16] O'Donovan, D.G. et al.:*Tetrahedron Lett.* **1968,** 265.
[17] Sharaf, A.:*Arab Sci. Congr., 5th, Bagdad* **1966,** 281.
[18] Liebisch, H.w. et al.:*Z. Naturforsch., B,* **1968,** 23, 1116.
[19] Markh, A.T. et al.:*Izv. Vyssh. Ucheb. Zaved., Pishch. Tekhnol* **1973,** (2), 36.
[20] Nosacheva, E.P. et al.:*Khim. Prir. Soedin.* **1973,** 9, 108.
[21] Dean, P.D.G. et al.:*Phytochem.* **1971,** 10, 2215.

[P.P.H. But]

102.   *Quisqualis indica* L.,
                    Q. indica L. var. *villosa* Clarke   (Combretaceae)

Shi–jun–zi (C), See–gwun–gee (H), Indoshikunshi, Shikunshi (J), Sa–gun–ja (K)

Fruit (CP)
Local Drug Name: Shi–jun–zi (C), See–gwun–gee (H), Shi–kun–shi (J), Sa–gun–ja (K).
Processing: 1) Eliminate foreign matter, break into pieces before use (C). 2) Remove the pericarp (C).
                3) Stir–fry the seeds to scented (C).
Method of Administration: Oral (decoction: C, H, J, K).
Folk Medicinal Uses:
                1) Ascariasis (C, H, J, K).
                2) Infantile maldigestion (C, H).
                3) Dysentery (C, H).
Contraindications: Avoid drinking strong tea during dosing.
Side Effects: Hiccup, dizziness, nausea, purpurea [4].

Leaf
Local Drug Name: Shi–jun–zi–ye (C), Sa–gun–ja–yeop (K).
Method of Administration: Oral (decoction: C).
Folk Medicinal Uses:
                1) Ascariasis (C).
                2) Infantile maldigestion (C).

Root
Local Drug Name: Shi–jun–zi–gen (C), Sa–gun–ja–geun (K).
Method of Administration: Oral (Water extract, C).
Folk Medicinal Uses:
                1) Ascariasis (C).

Scientific Researches:
Chemistry
    1) Fruit contains potassium quisqualate, trigonelline, pyridine, quisqualic acid, arginineγ –aminobutyric
                acid, aspartic acid, glutamic acid, serine, glycine, proline, leucine, valine, alanine, threonine,
                asparagine, histidine, lysine [7].
    2) Leaf contains trigonelline,*l*–proline, *l*–asparagine, potassium quisqualate [2], rutin [3].
    3) Flower contains rutin and pelargonidin–3–glucoside [3].
Pharmacology
    1) Ascaricidal effects [5].
    2) Antifungal effects against skin fungi (fruit aqueous extract).
    3) Anthelmintic effects [6, 9].

Literatures:
[1] Deng, W.L. In: Chang HM, But PPH. (Eds.): ''*Pharmacology and Applications of Chinese Materia*
    Medica'' World Scientific, Singapore,**1987**, 2, 809.
[2] Fang, S.T. et al.:*Hua Hsueh Hsueh Pao* **1964**, 30, 226.
[3] Nair, G. et al.:*Indian J. Chem.* **1979**, 18B, 291.
[4] Sun, X.X.:*Zhongji Yikan* **1982**, (5), 33.
[5] Chen, J.Y. et al.:*Xinzhongyi* **1982**, (9), 32, 28.
[6] Tuan, Y.C. et al.:*Yao Hsueh Hsueh Pao* **1957**, 5, 87.
[7] Takemoto T. et al.:*Yakugaku Zasshi* **1975**, 95, 176.
[8] Takemoto T. et al.:*Yakugaku Zasshi* **1975**, 95, 326.
[9] Pan, P.C. et al.:*Sci. Sin.* **1976**, 19, 691.   [P.P.H. But]

103.   *Cornus officinalis* **Sieb. et Zucc.** (Cornaceae)

Shan–zhu–yu (C), San–tsue–yue (H), Sanshuyu (J), San–su–yu (K)

Fruits (pseudocarp) (CP, JP, KP)
Local Drug Name: Shan–zhu–yu (C), San–tsue–yue (H), San–shu–yu (J), San–su–yu (K).
Processing: 1) Remove the kernel (the principal fruit) then dry under the sun. 2) Stew or steam the pulp
              with wine until absorbed entirely (C).
Method of Administration: Oral (decoction: C, H, J, K).
Folk Medicinal Uses:
              1) Weakness (C, J).
              2) Bleeding (C, J).
              3) Tinnitus (C, H, K).
              4) Dizziness, tinnitus, soreness in the loins and knees (C, J).
              5) Spermatorrhea, seminal emission, impotence, enuresis, frequency of urination, excessive
                 uterine bleeding and leukorrhea (C, H, J, K).
              6) Nocturia (K).
              7) Collapse with profuse sweating (C).
              8) Diabetes (C, J).
              9) Lumbago (H).

Scientific Research:
  Chemistry
    1) Iridoids: morroniside, loganin, sweroside [1].
    2) Tannins [2].
  Pharmacology
    1) Improvement of experimental diabetes (water suspension of the powder) [3].
    2) Inhibition of anaphylaxis (water extract) [4].
    3) Trypsin like protease increasing (ethanol extract) [5].
    4) Antihistamic (water extract) [6].
    5) Central nervous system depressing (water extract) [6].
Literatures:
[1] Endo, T. et al.: *Yakugaku Zasshi* **1973**, 93, 30.
[2] Okuda, T. et al.: *Chem. Pharm. Bull.* **1984**, 32, 4662.
[3] Yamahara, J.: *Yakugaku Zasshi* **1981**, 101, 86.
[4] Koda, A. et al.: *Nippon Yakurigaku Zasshi* **1973**, 69, 88.
[5] Huang, A. et al.: *Wakan Iyaku Gakkaishi* **1989**, 6, 20, 58.
[6] Ito, T.: *Nippon Yakurigaku Zasshi* **1961**, 57, 15.

[T. Kimura]

104.   *Eleutherococcus senticosus* **Rupr. et Maxim.**   (Araliaceae)
                  (= Acanthopanax senticosus (Rupr. et Maxim.) Harms)

Ci–wu–jia (C), Tzi–ng–gar (H), Ezoukogi (J), Ga–si–o–gal–pi–na–mu (K)

Root and Rhizome (CP)
Local Drug Name: Ci–wu–jia (C), Tzi–ng–gar (H), Shi–go–ka (J), Ga–si–o–ga–pi (K).
Processing: Wash clean, and dry (C, K).
Method of Administration: Oral (extract or tablet: C, H, K).
Folk Medicinal Uses:
              1) Hypofunction of the spleen and the kindey marked by general weakness, lassitude,

anorexia, aching of the loins and knees (C, H, K).

  2) Insomnia and dream–disturbed sleep (C).

  3) Rheumatalgia (H).

  4) Lumbago (H).

  5) Edema (H).

  6) Beriberi (H).

  7) Traumatic injury (H).

  8) Weakness (J).

Scientific Researches:

Chemistry

  1) Steroids: eleutheroside A (β–sitosterol glucoside) [1].

  2) Phenolic glycoside: eleutheroside B (syringin) [2], sinapaldehyde glucodside, coniferaldehyde
         glucoside [3], coniferin [4].

  3) Coumarins: eleutheroside B [1], iso–faxidin [3].

  4) Lignans: eleutheroside D, E (syringaresinol, dl–lirioresinol B) [1], l–sesamin [3, 5].

  5) Saponins: 3β–[O–β–D–glucopyranosyl–(1→3)–O–β–D–galactopyranosyl–(1→4)–[O–α–L–rhamno–
         pyranosyl–(1→2)–O–β–D–glucuronopyranosyl]–16α–hydroxy–13β,28–epoxyoleanane,
         3β–[O–α–L–rhamnopyranosyl–(1→4)–O–α–L–rhamnopyranosyl–(1→4)–[O–α–L–rhamno–
         pyranosyl–(1→2)]–O–β–D–glucopyranosyl–(1→x)–O–β–D–glucuronopyranosyl]–16-α–
         hydroxy–13β,28–epoxyoleanane [6], betulic acid [7].

  6) Cyanogenic glucoside: amygdalin [7].

  7) Stilbenes: $trans$–4,4'–dihydroxy–3,3'–dimethostilbene [3].

  8) Orgnic acids: 1,5–di-O,O–caffeoylquinic acid [3].

  9) Polysaccharides [4].

Pharmacology

  1) Sedative effect on central nervous system [7].

  2) Antifatigue effect [7].

  3) Anti–inflammatory effect [7].

  4) Antitumor effect [7].

  5) Increasing the body's insistance to nonspecific noxious stimulations [8].

  6) Insulinoid effect [9].

  7) Increasing brain's insistance to ischemia [10, 11].

  8) Inhibitory effect on lipid peroxidation (hyperin, chlorogenic acid, dl-α–tocopherol) [12].

  9) Immunomodulatory activities (polysaccharides) [13].

  10) Inducing interferon (polysaccharides) [14].

  11) Inhibitory effect on platelet aggregation (3,4–dihydroxybenzoic acid) [15].

Literatures:

[1] Yu, S. et al.: *Khim. Prir. Soedin* **1967,** 3(1), 63.

[2] Yu, S. et al.: *Izv, Akad. Nauk SSSR, Ser. Khim.* **1969,** (6), 1370.

[3] Zhao, Y.Q. et al.: *Zhongcaoyao* **1991,** 2(11), 516.

[4] "*Zhongyao Zhi*", Vol. 1, **1979,** 459.

[5] Suprunov, N. I. et al.: *Khim. Prir. Soedin.* **1971,** 7(4), 524.

[6] Seqiet–kujawa, et al.: *J. Nat. Prod.* **1991,** 54(4), 1044.

[7] Zhao, Y.Q. et al.: *Yaoxue Xuebao* **1988,** 23(9), 551.

[8] Brekhaman, I. et al.: *Ann. Rev. Pharmacol.*, **1969,** 9, 419.

[9] ДАРЦЫМВ, H. B. et al.: *РАСТИТ РЕСУРСМ,* **1978,** 14, ВМ 2, 186.

[10] Leonava, E. V. et al.: *Vestsi Akad. Navuk BSSR, Ser. Bigal. Navuk* **1979,** (1), 93.

[11] Levonnava, E. V. et al.: *Idravookhr Beloruss,* **1979,** (3), 13.

[12] Takahashi et al.: *Hokkaidoritsu Eisei Kenkynshoho,* **1989,** (39), 94.

[13] Shen, M.L. et al.: *Int. J. Immumopharmacol,* **1991,** 13(5), 549.

[14] Yang, L.C. et al.: *Zhongcaoyao* **1990,** 21(1), 27.

[15] Yun–choi et al.:*J. Nat. Prod.*, **1987**, 50(6), 1059.

[J.X. Guo]

105   *Acanthopanax spinosus* **Miq.**   (Araliaceae)
                          (=*A. gracilistylus* W. W. Smith)

Xi–zhu–wu–jia (C), Ng–gar–pay (H), Yamaukogi (J)

Related plant:*A. sessiliflorus*(Rupr. et Max.) Seem.: Wu–geng–wu–jia (C), O–gal–pi–na–mu (K).

Bark (CP, KP)
   Local Drug Name: Wu–jia–pi (C), Ng–gar–pay (H), Go–ka–hi (J), O–ga–pi (K).
   Processing: soften thoroughly, cut into thick slices and dry under the sun (C, H, J, K).
   Method of Administration: Oral (decoction: C, H, J, K).
   Folk Medicinal Uses:

           1) Lumbago (H, J, K).
           2) Beri–beri (H, J, K).
           3) Neurlagia (J, K).
           4) Arthritis (J, K).
           5) Edema (C, H).
           6) Traumatic injury (C, H).
           7) Weakness (H, K).
           8) Rheumatalgia (C, H).
           9) Gonorrhoea (K).
           10) Sputum (K).
           11) Acute gastritis (K).
           12) Apepsia (K).
           13) Eczema (K).
           14) Urticaria (K).
           15) Impotence (C).
           16) Retarded walking and lack of strength in children (C).

Scientific Researches:
   Chemistry
     1) Diterpenes: kaurenoic acid[1], 16-α–hydroxy–kauran–18–oic acid [2], (–)–ent–kaur–16–en–
                19–oic acid [7].
     2) Lignans: sesamin [2].
     3) Saponins [6,8].
     4) Phenylpropanoids: syringin [1].
     5) Sterols: β–sitosterol, β–sitosterol glucoside [2], cholesterol [5].
     6) Coumarins: eleutheroside B$_1$ [2].
     7) Essential oils: eucarvone, dihydrocarvone,α–copaene, cuparene, myristin.
     8) Fatty acid: stearic acid [2], myristic acid, palmatic acid, oleic acid, linoleic acid, arachidic acid [5].
     9) Amino acids: aspartic acid, threonine, serine, glycine, alanine, cysteine, valine, methionine, leucine,
                tyrosine, arginine [5].
   10) Sugars: glucose [5].
   Pharmacology
     1) Antiedemic and antiinflammatory action (extract) [3].
     2) Decrease of conditioned avoidance behavior (glycoside) [4].
     3) Increase of blood flow in myocardium (saponins) [6].
     4) Lipid lowering effects [8].

Literatures:

[1] Song, X. H. et al.:*Nanjing Yaoxueyuan Xuebao* **1983**, 15.
[2] Xiang, R. D. et al.: *Zhiwu Xuebao* **1983,** 25, 356.
[3] Cherkashin, G. V.: *Stimulyatory Tsentl. Nerv. Sist.* **1966**, 91.
[4] Hong, S. A. et al.:*Soul Uidae Chapchi* **1972**, 13(1), 41.
[5] Takahashi, M. et al.:*Annu. Rep. Tohoku Coll. Pharm.* **1982**, (29), 77.
[6] Yang, S. et al.:*Hunan Yixueyuan Xuebao* **1986**, 11(4), 333.
[7] Song, X. et al.:*Zhongguo Yaoke Daxue Xuebao* **1987**, 18(3), 203.
[8] Yang, Y. et al.:*Hunan Yixueyuan Xuebao* **1987**, 12, 217.

[C.K. Sung]

106. *Aralia cordata* Thunb. (Araliaceae)

Xin–ye–jiu–yan–du–huo (C), Udo (J), Dok–hwal (K)

Root
Local Drug Name: Jiu–yan–du–huo, Tu–dang–gui (C), Wa–dok–katsu, Wa–kyo–katsu (J), Dok–hwal (K).
Processing: Eliminate the up–ground stem and dirt, dry under the sun (C, J, K).
Method of Administration: Oral (water extract)(J, K), bathing (decoction)(J).
Folk Medicinal Uses:

        1) Common cold (J, K).
        2) Headache (J, K).
        3) Migraine (J, K).
        4) Psychoneurosis (J).
        5) Schyzophrenia (J).
        6) Rheumatism (J).
        7) Neuralgia (J).
        8) Hemorrhoid (bath, J).
        9) Rheumatic lumbago and scelalgia (C).
        10) Lumbar muscle strain (C).

Scientific Researches:

Chemistry
1) Diterpenoids: (–)–pimara–8(14),15–diene [1], grandifloric acid, 17–hydroxy–ent–kaur–15–en–19–oic
        acid [3], (ent)–kaur–16–en–19–oic acid, (ent)–pimara–8(14),15–dien–19–oic acid [7].
2) Essential oils: camphene, α–pinene, γ–terpinene, sabinene, myrcene, limonene, humulene [2, 6].
3) Saponins: aralosides A, B, C [4], udosaponins A, B, C, D, E, F [5].
Pharmacology
1) Analgesic action [7].
2) Hypothemia [7].
3) Duration of pentobarbital–induced anesthesia [7].
4) Depression of locomotor activity by methampetamine [7].

Literatures:

[1] Shibata, S. et al.: *Tetrahedron Lett.* **1967**, (51), 5241–3.
[2] Yoshihara, K. and Hirose, Y.:*Phytochemistry* **1973,** 12(2), 468.
[3] Yahara, S. et al.:*Chem. Pharm. Bull.* **1974,** 22(7), 1629.
[4] Orudzheva, K. F. et al.:*Azerb. Med.* **1989,** 66(5), 14.
[5] Kawai, H. et al.: *Chem. Pharm. Bull.* **1989,** 37(9), 2318.
[6] Sawamura, M. et al.:*Kochi Daigaku Gakujutsu Kenkyu Hokuku, Nogaku* **1990,** 38, 49.
[7] Okuyama, E. et al.:*Chem. Pharm. Bull.* **1991,** 39(2), 405.

[C.K. Sung]

107.   *Kalopanax septemlobus* (**Thunb.**) **Nakai**(= *K. pictus* Nakai) (Araliaceae)

Ci–qiu (C), Tzi–tsau (H), Harigiri (J), Eom–na–mu (K)

Bark, Root bark
Local Drug Name: Ci–qiu–shu–pi (C), Shi–shu–kon–pi (J), Hae–dong–pi (K).
Processing: Dry under the sun (J, K).
Method of Administration: Oral (decoction: K).
Folk Medicinal Uses:
        1) Contusion (J, K).
        2) Beri–beri (K).
        3) Lumbago (K).
        4) Neuralgia (K).
        5) Sore shoulder and arms (K).
        6) Acute gastritis (K).
        7) Pleurisy (K).
        8) Hemorrhoids (C, J).
        9) Rheumatism (C, J).
        10) Sputum (J).

Scientific Researches:
Chemistry
  1) Saponins (leaf): kalopanaxsaponin JLa, JLb, kalopanaxsaponin A, B, kizuta saponin K_{11} [1],
        kalopanaxsaponin G, pericarpsaponin Pj3, hederasaponin B [2].
  2) Lignans: syringin, liriodendrin, glucosyringic acid, kalopanaxin A, B, C, D [2].
  3) Phenols: coniferin, protocatechuic acid, chlorogenic acid [2].

Literatures:
[1] Shao, C. et al.: *Chem. Pharm. Bull.* **1990,** 38(4), 1087.
[2] Sano. K. et al.: *Chem. Pharm. Bull.* **1991,** 39(4), 865.

[C.K. Sung]

108.   *Panax ginseng* **C. A. Meyer**   (Araliaceae)

Ren–shen (C), Yan–sum (H), Otaneninjin (J), In–sam (K)

Root (CP)
Local Drug Name: Sheng–shai–shen (sun–dried Ginseng), Hong–shen (red Ginseng), Sheng–shai–shan–
        shen (sun–dried wild Ginseng)(C), Yan–sum, Bak–sum (white), Hung–sum (red)(H),
        Nin–jin (white), Ko–jin (red) (J), Baek–sam (white ginseng), hong–sam (red ginseng) (K).
Processing: 1) Sun–dried Ginseng: Remove rhizomes, soften thoroughly, cut into slices and dry (C).
        2) Red Ginseng: Remove rhizomes, soften thoroughly, cut into slices, and dry. Or break
        into pieces before use (C). 3) Sun–dried wild Ginseng: Remove rhizomes, pulverize or break
        into pieces before use (C). Curing by steam (red ginseng)(K).
Method of Administration: Oral (decoction: C, H, J, K).
Folk Medicinal Uses:
        1) Weakness(C, H, J, K).
        2) Thirsty (C, J, K).
        3) Cough (C, J, K).
        4) Acute gastitis (J, K).
        5) Infant diarrhea (J, K).

6) Convalescens (H, K).
7) Diabetes (J, K).
8) Regurgitation (C, H).
9) Amnesia (C, H).
10) Dizziness (C, H).
11) Dyscrasia (K).
12) Endometritis (K).
13) Nipple–wound, papillitis (K).
14) Suppuration (K).
15) Malaria (K).
16) Hysteria (K).
17) Consumptive cough (H).
18) Gastroatony (J).
19) Gastro intestinal neurosis (J).
20) Dyspepsia (J).
21) Diarrhea (J).
22) Vomiting (J).
23) Hypotonia (J).
24) Prostration with impending collapse maked by cold limbs and faint pulse (C).
25) Diminished function of the "spleen" with loss of appetite (C).
26) General weakness with irritability and insomnia in chronic diseases (C, J).
27) Frigidity (C).
28) Heart failure (C).
29) Cardiogenic shock (C).
30) Alcoholism (K).
31) Impotence (C).
32) Uterine hemorrhage (C).
33) Drunkenness (H).
34) Protecting body heat, chill (K).

Contraindications: Excessive symptom–complex, heat symptom–complex.

Scientific Researches:

Chemistry

1) Saponins: ginsenoside Ro, Ra–Rh$_{1-3}$ [8], malonyl–ginsenoside Rb$_1$, Rb$_2$, Rc, Rd [9].
2) Sesquiterpenes: eremophilene, β–gurjunene, *trans–, cis*–caryophyllene, ε–muurolene, γ–patchoulene, β–eudesmol, β–farnesene, β–bisabolene, aromadendrene, alloaromadendrene, β–guaiene, γ–elemene, mayurone [10].
3) Polyacetylenes: panaxynol, panaxydol, panaxytriol, heptadeca–1–ene–4,6–diyne–3,9–diol [11].
4) Peptide glycans: panaxan A, B, C, D, E [12], F, G, H [13], I, J, K, L [14], Q, R, S, T, U [15].
5) Phenols: maltol, 3–hydroxy–2–methyl–pyran–4–one 3-O–β–D–glucopyranose [16], salicylic acid, vanillic acid, p–hydroxycinnamic acid [32].
6) Flavonoids: kaempferol, trifolin, panasenoside [17].

Pharmacology

1) Increase of RNA, DNA and protein synthesis [18–20].
2) Immunostimulating action [21–22].
3) Decreasing total cholesterol, free cholesterol, LDL cholesterol, triglyceride [23, 24].
4) Increasing HDL cholesterol [25].
5) Stimulation of alcohol dehydrogenase [26].
6) Hypoglycemic action [27].
7) Stimulating pituitary – adrenocortical system [28, 29].
8) Antitumor activity [30].
9) Antioxidant activity [31].

Literatures:

[1] Sanada, S. et al.:*Chem. Pharm. Bull.* **1974,** 22, 421.

[2] Besso, H. et al.: *Chem. Pharm. Bull.* **1982,** 30, 2380.

[3] Koizumi, H. et al.:*Chem. Pharm. Bull.* **1982,** 30,2393.

[4] Matsuura, H. et al.: *Chem. Pharm. Bull.* **1984,** 32, 1188.

[5] Kasai, R. et al.: *Chem. Pharm. Bull.* **1983,** 31, 2120.

[6] Sanada, S. et al.:*Chem. Pharm. Bull.* **1978,** 26, 1694.

[7] Luo, S. D. et al.:*Chem. Pharm. Bull.* **1983,** 18, 468.

[8] Kitagawa, I. et al.: *Yakugaku Zasshi* **1983,** 103, 612.

[9] Kitagawa, I. et al.: *Chem. Pharm. Bull.* **1983,** 31, 3353.

[10] Zhang, H. X. et al.:*Kexue Tongbao* **1985,** 30, 195.

[11] Dabrowski, Z. et al.:*Phytochemistry* **1980,** 19, 2464.

[12] Konno, C. et al.:*Planta Med.* **1984,** 50, 434.

[13] Hikino, H. et al.:*Shoyakugaku Zasshi* **1985,** 39, 331.

[14] Oshima, Y. et al.:*J. Ethnopharmacol,* **1985,** 14, 255.

[15] Konno, C, et al.:*J. Ethnopharmacol.* **1985,** 14, 69.

[16] Xu, S. X. et al.:*Yaoxue Xuebao* **1986,** 21, 71.

[17] Wang, Z. X. et al.:*Shenyang Yaoxueyuan Xuebao* **1985,** 2, 284.

[18] Wang, B. X. et al.:*Yaoxue Xuebaoin.* **1982,** 17, 899.

[19] Nagasawa, T. et al.:*Chem. Pharm. Bull.* **1977,** 25, 1665.

[20] Zhang, B. F. et al.:*Shenyang Yaoxueyuan Xuebao.* **1985,** 2, 121.

[21] Jie, Y. H. et al.:*Agents Actions* **1984,** 15, 386.

[22] Cui, J. C. et al.:*Zhongcaoyao* **1982,** 13, 29.

[23] Lim, C. J. et al.:*Hanguk Saenghwa Hakhoe Chi* **1981,** 14, 188.

[24] Moon, C. K. et al.:*Arch. Pharmaco.l Res.* **1984,** 7, 41.

[25] Yokozawa, T. et al.:*Chem. Pharm. Bull.* **1985,** 33, 722.

[26] Joo, C. N. et al.:*Hanguk Saenghwa Hakhoe Chi* **1977,** 10, 109.

[27] Yokozawa, T. et al.:*Chem. Pharm. Bull.* **1985,** 33, 869.

[28] Zong, R. Y. et al.:*Bethune Yike Daxue Xuebao.* **1985,** 11, 254.

[29] Hiai, S. et al.: *Planta Med.* **1985,** 37, 15.

[30] Tahara, M. et al.: *Wakan Iyaku Gakkaishi* **1985,** 2, 170.

[31] Han, B. H. et al.:*Kor. J. Biochem.* **1979,** 12, 33.

[32] Han, B. H. et al.:*Seoul Taehakkyo Saengyak Yonguso Opjukjip,* **1981,** 20, 14.

[C.K. Sung]

109.   *Panax japonicus* **C. A. Meyer**   (Araliaceae)

(= *P. pseudo-ginseng* Wall. *var. japonicus* (C. A. Meyer) Hoo et Tseng)

Zhu–jie–shen (C), Tsue–gee–sum (H), Tochiba–ninjin (J), Juk–jeol–in–sam (K)

Related plants: *P. japonicus* C. A. Meyer *var. major* (Burk.) C. Y. Wu et K. M. Feng (=*P. pseudo-*
ginseng Wall. *var. japonicus (C. A. Meyer) Hoo et Tseng)* Zhu–jie–shen (C);
P. japonicus C. A. Meyer *var. bipinnatifidus* (Seem.) C. Y. Wu et K. M. Feng (=*P.*
pseudo–ginseng Wall. *var. bipinnatifidus* (Seem.) Li): Yu–ye–san–qi (C).

Rhizome (CP, JP)

Local Drug Name: Zhu–jie–shen (C), Tsue–gee–sum (H), Chiku–setsu–nin–jin (J), Juk–jeol–in–sam (K).

Processing: Boil for a short time then dry under the sun (J).

Method of Administration: Oral (decoction: C, J, K).

Folk Medicinal Uses:

114

1) Dyspepsia (J).
2) Anorexia (J).
3) Cough (C, H, J).
4) Phlegm (C, J).
5) Fever (J).
6) Bleeding (C, J).
7) Weakness after disease (C, H).
8) Traumatic injuries (C).

Scientific Researches:
Chemistry
1) Saponins: Chikusetsusaponin Ia, Ib, III, IV, V [1].
2) Polysaccharides: Tochibanan A, B [2].
Pharmacology
1) Central nervous system depressing (methanol extr., butanol extr., chikusetsusaponin III, IV, V) [2].
2) Cholinergic, anti-cholin esterase activity (water extr., methanol extr., butanol extr., chikusetsusaponin III) [2].
3) Histamic and antihistamic (methanol extr., butanol extr., chikusetsusaponin III, IV) [2].
4) Muscle relaxation (methanol extr., butanol extr., chikusetsusaponin III) [2].
5) Anti nicotine-like activity (methanol extr., butanol extr., chikusetsusaponin III) [2].
6) Antipyretic (methanol extr., butanol extr., chikusetsusaponin III, V) [2].
7) Analgesic (methanol extr., chikusetsusaponin V) [2].
8) Antiinflammatory (methanol extr., chikusetsusaponin III, IV, V) [2].
9) Local irritant (methanol extr., butanol exr., chikusetsusaponin III, IV) [2].
10) Antitussive (methanol extr., butanol extr., chikusetsusaponin III) [2].
11) Gastric secretion decreasing (methanol extr., butanol extr.) [2].
12) Bowel movement (methanol extr., water extr., chikusetsusaponin III, IV) [2].
13) Anti-stress ulcer (butanol extr., chikusetsusaponin III, IV, V) [2].
14) Blood pressure raising and lowering (water extr., chikusetsusaponin III, IV, V) [2].
15) Diuretic (water extr.) [2].
16) Antiallergic (ethanol extr.) [3].
17) Hair growing (50% ethanol extr.) [4].
18) Corticosterone secretion increasing (saponins) [5].
19) Fibrinolytic stimulation (chikusetsusaponin III, IV, V) [6].
20) Anti-gastric ulcer (chikusetsusaponin III) [7].
21) Reticulo-endothelial system stimulation (tochibanan-A, B) [8].
22) Inhibition of cyclic AMP phosphodiesterase activity [9].

Literatures:
[1] Shoji, J. et al.: *Yakugaku Zasshi* **1968**, 88, 325; **1969**, 89, 846; *Chem. Pharm. Bull.* **1970**, 18, 1558; **1971**, 19, 1103; **1976**, 24, 253; Morita, M. et al.: *Chem. Pharm. Bull.* **1983**, 31, 3205; **1985**, 33, 3852.
[2] Saito, H. et al.: *Chem. Pharm. Bull.* **1977**, 25, 1017; Lee, Y.-M. et al.: *ibid.* **1977**, 25, 1391.
[3] Goda, A. et al.: *Nippon Yakurigaku Zasshi* **1973**, 69, 88.
[4] Kubo, M. et al.: *Yakugaku Zasshi* **1988**, 108, 971.
[5] Yokoyama, H. et al.: *Yakugaku Zasshi* **1982**, 102, 555.
[6] Matsuda, H. et al.: *Planta Med.* **1989**, 55, 18.
[7] Yamahara, J. et al.: *Yakugaku Zasshi* **1987**, 107, 135.
[8] Ohtani, K. et al.: *Chem. Pharm. Bull.* **1989**, 37, 2587.
[9] Nikaido, T. et al.: *Chem. Pharm. Bull.* **1984**, 32, 1477.

[T. Kimura]

110.   *Angelica acutiloba* Kitagawa (Umbelliferae)

Dong–dang–gui (C), Toki (J), Il–dang–gwi (K)

Related plant: *Angelica sinensis* Diels; Dang–gui (C), Karatoki (J), Dang–gwi (K).
A. *gigas* Nakai: Tu–dang–gui (C), Cham–dang–gwi (K).

Root (JP, KP)
 Local Drug Name: To–ki (J), Dang–gwi (K).
 Processing: Steam for short time then air dry.
 Method of Administration: Oral or topical (decoction, powder or ointment: J, K).
 Folk Medicinal Uses:
             1) Menstrual disorder (J, K).
             2) Hysteria (J).
             3) Feeling of cold (J, K).
             4) Pain (J, K).
             5) Hypotonia (J).
             6) Sterilitas (J, K).
             7) Weakness (K).
             8) Anemia (K).
             9) Hemiplegia (K).
             10) Woman's diseases (J, K).

Leaf
 Local Drug Name: To–ki–yo (J), Dang–gwi–yeop (K).
 Processing: Dry under the sun (J).
 Method of Administration: Bath (J).
 Folk Medicinal Uses:
             1) Menstrual disorder (J).
             2) Congelation (J).
             3) Feeling of cold (J).

Scientific Researches:
 Chemistry
  1) Essential Oil: safrole, isosafrole, *p*–cymene [1, 2].
  2) Phthalides: ligustilide, butylidenephthalide, butylphthalide, sedaonnic acid lactone, bergaptene [2, 3].
  3) Cumarins: scopoletin, umbelliferone [4].
  4) Polyacetylenes: falcarinol, falcarindiol, falcarinolone [4].
  5) Polysaccharides: AGⅡ a, AGⅡ b–1, AR2Ⅱ a, AR2Ⅱ b, AR2Ⅱ c, AR2Ⅱ d, AR4E–2 [5, 6].
  6) β–Carbolines [7]
 Pharmacology
  1) Analgesic (decoction) [4, 8].
  2) Antiinflammatory (decoction) [4, 8]
  3) Antiallergic (water extract, ethanol extract) [5, 6, 9, 10, 17].
  4) Antihypertensive (decoction) [11].
  5) Blood sugar lowering (water extract) [12].
  6) Cholilytic (ligustilide, butylidenephthalide) [13].
  7) Sedative [11].
  8) Blood or platelet coagulation inhibition (adenosine) [14]
  9) Antispasmodic (ligustilide) [15].
  10) Antitumor (AR–4E–2) [5].
  11) Anti–tumor–promoter (methanol extract) [16].
  12) Others [18].

Literatures

[1] Takahashi, S. et al.:*Yakugaku Zasshi* **1958**, 78, 1156 (1958).

[2] Noguchi, K. et al.:*Yakugaku Zasshi* **1932**, 52, 769; **1937**, 57, 783.

[3] Mitsuhashi, H. et al.:*Chem. Pharm. Bull.* **1961**, 9, 115; **1963**, 11, 1317; **1967**, 15, 1606; *Tetrahedron* **1963**, 19, 1277; **1964**, 20, 1971.

[4] Tanaka, S. et al.: *Yakugaku Zasshi* **1977**, 97, 14; Idem.:*Arzneim. Forsch.* **1977**, 27, 2039.

[5] Yamada, H. et al.:*Shoyakugaku Zasshi* **1984**, 38, 111; *Planta Med.* **1984**, 50, 163; *Phytochemistry* **1984**, 23, 587; Kiyohara, H., et al.:*Carbohydr. Res.* **1988**, 182, 259.

[6] Yamada, H. et al.:*Planta Med.* **1990**, 56, 182.

[7] Nagai, M. et al.: *109th Ann. Meeting Jap. Soc. Pharm., Abstr.***1988**, Ⅲ, 226.

[8] Tanaka, S. et al.: *Yakugaku Zasshi* **1971**, 91, 1098.

[9] Cho, S. et al.:*Shoyakugaku Zasshi* **1982**, 36, 78.

[10] Koda, A. et al.:*Nippon Yakurigaku Zasshi***1973**, 69, 88.

[11] Okada, N.:*Rinsho Ganka* **1965**, 19, 279; Saeki, T.:*ibid.* **1965**, 19, 647.

[12] Bin, H.: *Nippon Yakubutsugaku Zasshi***1930**, 11, 22.

[13] Mitsuhashi, H., et al.:*Chem. Pharm. Bull.* **1960**, 8, 243.

[14] Kosuge, T.:*Yakugaku Zasshi* **1984**, 104, 1050; Toriizuka, K. et al.:*Chem. Pharm. Bull.* **1986**, 34, 5011.

[15] Tao, J.–Y. et al.:*Yaoxue Xuebao* **1984**, 19, 561.

[16] Konoshima, T. et al.:*Yakugaku Zasshi* **1989**, 109, 843.

[17] Yamada, H. et al.:*Mol. Immunol.* **1985**, 22, 295; Kiyohara, H. et al.:*J. Pharm. Dyn.* **1986**, 9, 339; Kumazawa, Y. et al.:*Immunolgy* **1982**, 47, 75; *J. Pharm. Dyn.* **1985**, 8, 417; Ohno, N. et al.:*ibid.* **1983**, 6, 903.

[18] Matsumoto, S.: *Gifu Daigaku Igakubu Kiyo***1958**, 6, 554; Hayashi, M.:*Nippon Yakurigaku Zasshi***1977**, 73, 177, 205; Harada, M. et al.:*J. Pharm. Dyn.* **1984**, 7, 304.

[T. Kimura]

111.　　*Angelica dahurica* (Fisch. ex Hoffm.) Benth. et Hook. f. (Umbelliferae)

Bai–zhi (C), Bak–gee (H), Yoroigusa (J), Gu–rit–dae (K)

Related plant:　　*Angelica dahurica* (Fisch. ex Hoffm.) Benth. et Hook. f. var.*formosana* (Boiss.) Shan et Yuan (= *A. taiwaniana* Boiss.): Hang–bai–zhi (C).

Root (CP, JP, KP)
Local Drug Name: Bai–zhi (C), Bak–gee (H), Byaku–shi (J), Baek–ji (K).
Processing: Dry under the sun.
Method of Administration: Oral (decoction: C, H, J, K).
Folk Medicinal Uses:
　　　　　　1) Women's diseases (C, J).
　　　　　　2) Menstrual disorder (J).
　　　　　　3) Pain (C, J, K). Abdominal pain (H).
　　　　　　4) Hysteria (J).
　　　　　　5) Bleeding (J).
　　　　　　6) Headache (C, H, J, K).
　　　　　　7) Stuffed nose due to colds, sinusitis (C).
　　　　　　8) Toothache (C, H, K).
　　　　　　9) Excessive leukorrhea (C, H).
　　　　　　10) Swelling and pain of sores and wounds (C).
　　　　　　11) Tinea (H).

12) Pruritus (H).

Scientific Researches:
Chemistry
  1) Cumarins: byak−angelicin, byak−angelicol [1], imperatorin, phellopterin, oxypeucedanin [2], xanthotoxin, marmesin, scopoletin, anhydrobyakangelicin, neobyakangelicol [3].
Pharmacology
  1) Inhibition of heat and Cu ion induced denaturation of human gamma−globulin (methanol extr.) [4].
  2) Stimulation of adrenalin or ACTH induced degradation of lipid (furocumarins) [5].
  3) Inhibition of insulin indused lipid genaration (furocumarins) [5].
  4) Inhibition of phosphorus acceptance in HeLa cell [6].

Literatures:
[1] Noguchi, K. et al.:*Yakugaku Zasshi* **1938**, 58, 370, 578, 1052; **1941**, 61, 77; Fujiwara, H. et al.: *Yakugaku Zasshi* **1980**, 100, 1258; Kozawa, M. et al.:*Shoyakugaku Zasshi* **1981**, 35, 90.
[2] Hata, K. et al.:*Yakugaku Zasshi* **1963**, 83, 606; Shlvun' Ko E. K. et al.:*Khim. Prir. Soedin.* **1977**, 280; Zhou, J. et al.:*Zhongcaoyao* **1987**, 18, 242.
[3] Saiki, Y.:*Yakugaku Zasshi* **1971**, 91, 1313; Baba, K. et al.:*Planta Med.* **1985**, 64.
[4] Yamahara, J. et al.:*Shoyakugaku Zasshi* **1981**, 35, 103.
[5] Kimura, Y., et al. :*Planta Med.* **1982**, 45, 183.
[6] Okuyama, T., et al. :*Chem. Pharm. Bull.* **1990**, 38, 1084.

[T. Kimura]

112.   *Angelica decursiva* **Fr. et Sav.**   (Umbellliferae)
                          (= *Peucedanum decursivum* (Miq.) Maxim.)

Zi−hua−qian−hu (C), Nodake (J), Ba−di−na−mul (K)

Related plant: *Peucedanum praeruptorum* Dunn: Bai−hua−qian−hu (C).

Root
Local Drug Name: Qian−hu (C), Zen−ko (J), Jeon−ho (K).
Processing: Dry under the sun (J, K).
Method of Administration: Oral (decoction: C, J, K).
Folk Medicinal Uses:
          1) Cough (J, K).
          2) Asthma (J).
          3) Pneumonia (J).

Scientific Researches:
Chemistry
  1) Polyacetylenes [1].
  2) Coumarins: decursin, decursidin, 3'(*S*)−angeloyloxy−4'(*R* and *S*)−isovaleroyl−oxy−3',4'−dihydro xanthyletin, 3'(*S*)−angeloyloxy−4'(*R*)−senecioyloxy−3',4'−di−hydroxanthyletin [2, 3].

Literatures:
[1] Park, D. S. et al.:*Seoul Taehakkyo Yakhak Nonmunjip* **1976**, 1, 132.
[2] Sano, K. et al.:*Chem. Pharm. Bull.* **1975**, 23(1), 20.
[3] Sano, K. et al.:*Chem. Pharm. Bull.* **1973**, 21(9), 2095.

[C.K. Sung]

113.   **Angelica pubescens Maxim.**(= *A. polyclada* Franch.) (Umbelliferae)

Mao–dang–gui (C), Duk–wood (H), Shishiudo (J)

Related plant: *Angelica pubescens* Maxim. f. *bisserrata* Shau et Yuan: Chong–chi–mao–dang–gui (C); *A. koreana*: Gang–hwal (K).

Root
Local Drug Name: Du–huo(C), Duk–wood (H), Dok–katsu (J), Gang–hwal (K).
Processing: Eliminate fibrous root and mud, dry under the sun or in the shade (C, H, J, K).
Method of Administration: Oral (decoction: C, H, J, K); bathing (decoction, J).
Folk Medicinal Uses:
   1) Headache and body pain (C, H, J, K).
   2) Common cold (C, J, K).
   3) Rheumatism (C, H, J).
   4) Wind expulsion (C, H, K).
   5) Perspiration (J, K).
   6) Apoplexy (J, K).
   7) Toothache (H, J).
   8) Lumbago (C, H).
   9) Laryngitis (K).
   10) Edema (J).
   11) Feeling of cold (J).
   12) Chronic bronchitis (H).
   13) Gonalgia (C).

Scientific Researches:
Chemistry
   1) Coumarins: osthol, glabralactone, isopimpinellin, coumurrayin, angelol A–H [1, 3, 6], bergapten, psoralen, xanthotoxin, byakangelicin, osthenol coumurrayin, 7–methoxy–8–senecioylcoumarin, scopoletin, angelin, 8–(3–hydroxy–isovaleroyl)–5,7–dimethoxycoumarin [2,4,5], isoangelol, anpubesol, columbianetin [8].
Pharmacology
   1) Antiinflammatory effects (osthol) [7].
   2) Analgesic effect (osthol) [7].
   3) Blood platelet aggregation inhibition (osthol, columbianetin) [8].
   4) Inhibition of platelet thromboxane formation (osthol) [10].

Literatures:
[1] Hata, K. et al.: *Yakugaku Zasshi* **1968,** 88(3), 283.
[2] Kozawa, M. et al.: *Chem. Pharm. Bull.* **1980,** 28(6), 1782.
[3] Hata, K. et al.: *Yakugaku Zasshi* **1981,** 101(1), 67.
[4] Chen, S. et al.: *Yaoxue Tongbao* **1982,** 17(2), 120.
[5] Chen, S. et al.: *Yaoxue Tongbao* **1982,** 17(5), 392.
[6] Baba, K. et al.: *Chem. Pharm. Bull.* **1982,** 30(6), 2025.
[7] Kosuge, T. et al.: *Chem. Pharm. Bull.* **1985,** 33(12), 5351.
[8] Pan, J. et al.: *Yaoxue Xuebao* **1987,** 22(5), 380.
[9] Wang, Z. et al.: *Shenyang Yaoxueyuan Xuebao* **1988,** 5(3), 183.
[10] Ko, F. N. et al.: *Thromb. Haemostasis* **1989,** 62(3), 996.

[C.K. Sung]

114.   *Angelica sinensis* (Oliv.) **Diels**   (Umbelliferae)

Dang–gui (C), Dong–gwai (H), Karatoki (J)

Relative Plants:*Anglica gigas* Nakai: Tu–dang–gui (C), Cham–dang–gwi (K);
           A. acutiloba Kitagawa: Dong–dang–gui (C), Toki (J).

Root (CP)
Local Drug Name: Dang–gui (C), Dong–gwai (H), To–ki, Kara–to–ki (J), Dang–gwi (K).
Processing: 1) Eliminate foreign matter, wash, soften thoroughly, cut into slices, and dry under the sun
           or at a low temperature (C, J, K).
Method of Administration: Oral (decoction: C, H, J, K).
Folk Medicinal Uses:
           1) Anemia with dizziness and palpitation (C, H, J, K).
           2) Menstrual disorders (C, H, J, K).
           3) Amenorrhea (C, H, J).
           4) Dysmenorrhea, constipation (C, H, J).
           5) Rheumatic arthralgia, traumatic injuries, carbuncles, boils and sore (C, H, J).
           6) Soft stool (H).
           7) Hemiplegia (K).
Side Effects: Pain, fever, aversion to cold, headache, nause, thirsty (volatile oil) (C).

Scientific Researches:
Chemistry
     1) Volatile oil: ligustilide [1], *n*–butylidene phthalide, *n*–valerophenon–*O*–carboxylic acid, $\Delta^{2,4}$–
           dihydrophthalic anhydride [2], angelicone, carvacrol [3], angelicide [4], etc.
     2) Water–soluble substances: ferulic acid, butanediolic acid, uracil, nicotinic acid, adenine [5],
           polysaccharide [6], amino acids.
Pharmacology
     1) Excitory or inhibitory effect on uterine smooth muscle [7, 8].
     2) Effects on the cardiovascular system[9–14]:
           a. Antiarrhythmic effect.
           b. Effect of dilating coronary artery and decreasing oxygen consumption of myocardium.
           c. Antihypertensive effect.
           d. Inhibitory effect on platelet aggregation.
           e. Effect of decreasing blood–lipid.
     3) Inhibitory effect on antibody formation [15].
     4) Effct of increasing the macrophage phagocytic function.
     5) Anti–inflammatory effct, analgesic effect (ferulic acid) [16].
     6) Avitaminous E–resistant effect,antianemic effect [17, 18].
     7) Antibacterial effect [19].
     8) Sedative effect on cerebrum (ligustilide) [20].
     9) Radiation–resistant effect [6].

Literatures:
[1] Fang, H. J.: *Yaoxue Xuebao* **1979**, (10), 617.
[2] Hikino, H.: *Shoyakugaku Zasshi* **1962**, 16, 12.
[3] Liu, G. S.: *Yaoxue Xuebao* **1979**, (8), 375.
[4] Chen, Y.Z.: *Kexue Tongbao* **1983**, 28(19), 1206.
[5] Lin, M. et al.: *Yaoxue Xuebao* **1979**, (9), 529.
[6] Ma, L.F. et al.: *Lanzhou Yixueyuan Xuebao* **1988**, (2), 44.
[7] Lu, F.H.: *Zhonghua Yixue Zazhi* **1954**, 40(9), 670.
[8] Pi, X.P.: *ibid*, **1955**, 41(10), 967.

[9] Mei, Q. B. et al.:*Zhongcaoyao* **1983**, 14(8), 43.

[10] Wang, Y.S. et al.: "*Zhongyao Yaoli Yu Yingyong*", **1983**, 424.

[11] Peng, R. Q. et al.:*Zhongcaoyao 1981*, 12(7), 33.

[12] Cha, L.:*Yaoxue Xuebao* **1981**, 16(5), 3.

[13] Zhang, Y. Y. et al.:*Shengwu Yixue Gongcheng Xuebao***1984**, 3(2), 90.

[14] Ying, Z. Z. et al.:*Yaoxue Xuebao* **1980**, 15(6), 321.

[15] Goda, S.:*Nippon Yakurigaku–ho,* **1973**, 69, 88.

[16] Ozaki, Y. et al.:*Chem. Pharm. Bull.* **1992**, 40(4), 954.

[17] Schimidt, C. F. et al.:*Chin. J. Physiol.* **1941**, 16(3), 397.

[18] Goto, M.: *Yakugaku Zasshi* **1955,** 75(10), 1180.

[19] Liu, G. S.: *Chinese J. of Modern Med. Sci.***1950**, 1(2), 95.

[20] Xi, F. X.: *Shanxi Xinyiyao* **1985**, 14(8), 59.

[J.X. Guo]

115.　　　　　*Bupleurum chinense* DC.　　(Umbelliferae)

Bei–chaihu (C)

Related plant:　*B. scorzonerifolium* Willd.: Xiaye–chaihu (C);

B. scorzonerifolium Willd. var. *stenophyllum* Nakai (= *B. falcatum* L.): Mishimasaiko (J), Cham–si–ho (K).

Root　(CP, JP, KP)

Local Drug Name: Chai–hu (C), Chai–woo (H), Sai–ko (J), Si–ho.

Processing: Dry under the sun (J).

Method of Administration: Oral (decoction or powder: C, H, J, K).

Folk Medicinal Uses:

　　　　　1) Fever (C, H, J, K).

　　　　　2) Hepatitis (C, J, K).

　　　　　3) Pain (C, J). Headache (C, H).

　　　　　4) Dyspepsia (J).

　　　　　5) Nephritis (J).

　　　　　6) Alternating chills and fever (C, J). Malarial disease (H).

　　　　　7) Stuffiness sensation in thorax (J). Chest distention (H).

　　　　　8) Menstrual disorder (C, H).

　　　　　9) Prolapse of the uterus and the rectum (C, H).

　　　　　10) Apoplexy (K).

Scientific Researches:

Chemistry

　1) Saponins: saikosaponin a, b, c, d, e, f, saikoside Ia, Ib–1 Ib–2,II [1, 2, 5, 6].

　2) Steroids: α–spinasterol.

　3) Adonitol.

Pharmacology

　1) Antipyretic effect (decoction [3, 4]), crude saponin [18]).

　2) Hepatotonic activity (decoction) [4, 5, 6], (saikosaponins [14]).

　3) Weight increasing of adrenal glands and relative weight decreasing of thymus glands (decoction)[7].

　4) Serum corticosterone increasing (extract)[8].

　5) Blood urea nitrogen (BUN) decreasing and serum total cholesterol increasing [9].

　6) Blood cyclic AMP increasing [10].

　7) Passive cutaneous anaphylaxis (PCA) inhibition (water or 50% methanol extract)[11].

8) Central sedative, analgesic, antipyretic, and antitussive (crude saponin fraction) [12].

9) Local irritant activity and anti–inflammatory effects (crude saponin) [12].

10) Serum ALP lowering on experimental liver disorder (crude saponins) [12].

11) Stress ulcer inhibition [12].

12) Anti–inflammatory effect (saikosaponin a, d) [13, 21, 22].

13) Others [15–23].

Literatures:

[1] Shibata, S. et al.: *Chem. Pharm. Bull.* **1966**, 14, 1023; **1968**, 16, 641; Yamasaki, K. et al.:*Tetrahedron Letters* **1977**, 1231.

[2] Shimaoka, A. et al.:*J. Chem. Soc. Perkin I* **1975**, 2043; Takeda, K.: *Taisha* **1973**, 10, 676; Ishii, H. et al.: *Chem. Pharm. Bull.* **1980**, 28, 2367; Shimizu, K. et al.:*Chem. Pharm. Bull.* **1985**, 33, 3349; Akabori, A.: *Gendai Toyo Igaku* **1980**, 1(1), 45.

[3] Kondo, T. et al.:*Nippon Yakubutsugaku Zasshi* **1928**, 7, 296.

[4] Haginiwa, T. et al.: *Yakugaku Zasshi* **1960**, 80, 617.

[5] Mizoguchi, Y. et al.:*Wakan Iyaku Gakkaishi* **1985**, 2, 27.

[6] Yang, L. et al.:*Wakan Iyaku Gakkaishi* **1990**, 7, 28.

[7] Abe, H. et al.:*Yakugaku Zasshi* **1980**, 100, 602.

[8] Hattori, T. et al.:*Japan. J. Pharmacol.* **1989**, 51, 117.

[9] Nagasawa, T. et al.:*Yakugaku Zasshi* **1979**, 99, 71.

[10] Tei, M. et al.: *Wakan Iyaku Gakkaishi* **1985**, 2, 272.

[11] Goda, A. et al.:*Nippon Yakurigaku Zasshi* **1982**, 80, 31.

[12] Takagi, K. et al.:*Yakugaku Zasshi* **1969**, 89, 1367; Shibata, M. et al.:*ibid.* **1970**, 90, 398; **1973**, 93, 1660;*Shoyakugaku Zasshi* **1976**, 30, 62.

[13] Yamamoto, M. et al.:*Arzneim. Forsch.* **1975**, 25, 1021, 1240.

[14] Arichi, S. et al.:*Kanzo* **1978**, 19, 430, 1053, 1058; Abe, H., et al.:*Planta Med.* **1980**, 40, 366 (1980); Abe, H., et al.:*Naunyn–Schmiedeberg's Arch. Pharmacol.* **1982**, 320, 266; Abe, H., et al.:*J. Pharm. Pharmacol.* **1985**, 37, 555.

[15] Abe, H., et al.:*Eur. J. Pharmacol.* **1986**, 120, 171.

[16] Hiai, S., et al.: *Chem. Pharm. Bull.* **1981**, 29, 495; Yokoyama, H., et al.:*ibid.* **1981**, 29, 500; **1984**, 32, 1244;*Yakugaku Zasshi* **1982**, 102, 555; Hiai, S. et al.:*Chem. Pharm. Bull.* **1986**, 34, 1195; **1987**, 35, 2900.

[17] Kita, T. et al.:*J. Pharm. Dyn.* **1980**, 3, 269.

[18] Kimura, Y. et al.:*Chem. Pharm. Bull.* **1980**, 28, 1788.

[19] Abe, H. et al.:*Planta Med.* **1978**, 34, 160, 287; **1981**, 42, 356;*Naunyn–Schmiedeberg's Arch. Pharmacol.* **1981**, 316, 262.

[20] Nose, M.,:*Chem. Pharm. Bull.* **1989**, 37, 2736.

[21] Cheng, J.-T., et al.:*Biochem. Pharmacol.* **1986**, 35, 2483.

[22] Chou, C. C. et al.:*Yaoxue Xuebao* **1985**, 20,   257.

[23] Yamada, H. et al.:*Phytochemistry* **1988**, 27, 3163;*Carbohydr. Res.* **1989**, 189, 209.

[T. Kimura]

116.   *Cnidium officinale* Makino   (Umbelliferae)

Yang–chuan–xiong (C), Senkyu (J), Cheon–gung (K)

Related plant: *Ligusticum chuanxiong* Hort. (= *L. wallichii Franch.*): Chuan–xiong (C); *Cnidium monnieri* (L.) Cussor: She–chuang (C).

Rhizome (JP, KP)

Local Drug Name: Sen–kyu (J), Cheon–Gung (K).

Processing: Steam for a short time then dry under the sun (J, K).
Method of Administration: Oral (decoction or powder: J, K).
  Folk Medicinal Uses:
                    1) Anemia (J).
                    2) Weakness (J, K).
                    3) Women's diseases (J, K).
                    4) Pain (J, K).
                    5) Feeling of cold (J, K).

Scientific Researches:
  Chemistry
    1) Phthalides: cnidilide, neocnidilide, ligustilide, senkyunolide, butylphthalide, butylidenephthalide,
                    senkyunolide B~J [1, 2].
    2) Steroids: pregnenolone.
    3) Aromatic compounds: vanillin, coniferyl ferulate, ferulic acid [2].
  Pharmacology
    1) Vasodilator effect (ether extract) [3].
    2) Sedative activity (ethanol extract) [4].
    3) Intestinal blood flow increasing (ether extract)[5].
    4) Analgesic, anti–inflammatory and antifebrile activity (water and 50% ethanol extract) [6, 7].
    5) Central muscle relaxation effect (cnidilide, ligustilide, senkyunolide) [8].
    6) Antispasmodic (butylidenephthalide) [9].
    7) Others [10–16].

Literatures:
  [1] Mitsuhashi, H. et al.:*Tetrahedron* **1964**, 20, 1971; *Chem. Pharm. Bull.* **1967**, 15, 1606.
  [2] Kobayashi, M. et al.:*Chem. Pharm. Bull.* **1984**, 32, 3770.
  [3] Matsumoto, S.: *Gifu Ikadaigaku Kiyo* **1958**, 6, 554.
  [4] Kanashima, H. et al.:*Hokkaido Eisei Kenkyusho* **1975**, 25, 12; **1976**, 26, 22.
  [5] Ohmoto, T., et al. :*Shoyakugaku Zasshi* **1985**, 39, 28.
  [6] Ka, B. et al.:*Nippon Yakurigaku Zasshi* **1979**, 75, 135.
  [7] Yamahara, J. et al.:*Yakugaku Zasshi* **1980**, 100, 713.
  [8] Ozaki, Y. et al.:*Yakugaku Zasshi* **1989**, 109, 402.
  [9] Ka, B. et al.:*Nippon Yakurigaku Zasshi* **1978**, 74, 171.
  [10] Yamagishi, T. et al.:*Yakugaku Zasshi* **1977**, 97, 237.
  [11] Kano, Y. et al.:*Shoyakugaku Zasshi* **1985**, 39, 88.
  [12] Pushan, W. et al.:*Phytochemistry* **1984**, 23, 2033; Baronnat, M. P. et al.:*Planta Med.* **1984**, 50, 105;
    Wang, P. et al.:*Zhongcaoyao* **1985**, 16, 137, 227; Huang, Y. Z. et al.:*Yaoxue Xuepao* **1988**, 23,
    426.
  [13] Suzuki, Y. et al.:*Nippon Yakurigaku Zasshi* **1983**, 82, 164.
  [14] Nakazawa, K. et al.:*Yakugaku Zasshi* **1989**, 109, 662.
  [15] Ohta, S. et al.:*Yakugaku Zasshi* **1985**, 105, 874; **1990**, 110, 746.
  [16] Kimura, K. et al.:*Shoyakygaku Zasshi* **1961**, 15, 5.

[T. Kimura]

117.   *Foeniculum vulgare* **Miller**   (Umbelliferae)

                Hui–xiang (C), Wui–heung (H), Uikyo (J), Hoe–hyang (K)

Fruit (CP, JP, KP)
  Local Drug Name: Xiao–hui–xiang (C), Wui–heung (H), Ui–kyo (J), Hoe–hyang (K).

Processing: 1) Dry under the sun. 2) Stir–fry with Salt water until yellow (C).
Method of Administration: Oral (decoction: C, H, J, K) or powder: H, J, K).
Folk Medicinal Uses:

   1) Dyspepsia (C, J, K).
   2) Carminative (C, H, J, K).
   3) Colic (K).
   4) Lumbago (H).
   5) Abdominal pain (H).
   6) Stomachache (H).
   7) Vomiting (H).
   8) Distending pain in the epigastrium with anorexia, vomiting and diarrhea (C).
   9) Scrotal hernia with pain and cold extremities (C).
   10) Dysmenorrhea with lower abdominal pain and cold sensation (C).
   11) Hydrocele of tunica vaginalis (C).

Scientific Researches:
Chemistry
   1) Phenylpropanoids: anethole, estragol.
   2) Monoterpenes: d–fenchone, dl–limonene, α–, β–pinene, camphene, γ–terpinene, p–cymene,
         camphor [1, 2].
Pharmacology
   1) Gastrointestinal movement stimulation (powder, essential oil) [3,4,5]
   2) Antispasmodic (31% ethanol extract) [4].
   3) Pancreas protease precursor activation [5].

Literatures:
[1] Betts, T. J.:*J. Pharm. Pharmacol.* **1968**, 20, suppl. 61; Toth, L.:*Planta Med.* **1967**, 15, 157;
   Karlsen, J. et al.:*ibid.* **1969**, 17, 281.
[2] Ravid, U. et al.:*J. Nat. Prod.* **1983**, 46, 848.
[3] Takagi, K. et al.:*Nippon Yakurigaku Zasshi* **1977**, 73, 45.
[4] Sone, Y. et al.:*Tohoku J. Exptl. Med.* **1937**, 30, 540; Imazeki, I. et al.:*Yakugaku Zasshi* **1962**, 82,
   1326.
[5] Forster, H. B. et al.:*Planta Med.* **1980**, 40, 309.
[6] Uchiyama, T. et al.:*Wakan Iyaku Gakkaishi* **1989**, 6, 201.

[T. Kimura]

118.   *Glehnia littoralis* **Fr. Schmidt ex Miquel** (Umbelliferae)

Shan–hu–cai (C), Sha–sum (H), Hamabofu (J), Gaet–bang–pung (K)

Root and Rhizome (CP, JP, KP)
Local Drug Name: Bei–sha–shen (C), Sha–sum (H), Hama–bo–fu (J), Bin–bang–pung (K).
Processing: Dry under the sun.
Method of Administration: Oral (decoction: C, H, J, K).
Folk Medicinal Uses:

   1) Common cold (J, K).
   2) Cough (C, H, J, K).
   3) Phlegm (C, H, J, K).
   4) Thirst in febrile diseases (C).
   5) Chronic bronchitis (H).

Scientific Researches:
Chemistry
  1) Cumarins: osthenol–7–*O*–β–gentiobioside [1,2].
Pharmacology
  1) Antipyretic (ethanol extract) [3].
  2) Analgesic (ethanol extract) [3].
  3) Immunosuppressive (polysacchalide) [4].

Literatures:
[1] Sasaki, H. et al.: *Chem. Pharm. Bull.* **1980**, 28, 1847.
[2] Wang, J.: *Zhongyao Tongbao* **1987**, 12, 742.
[3] Taki, K.: *Gifu Daigaku Igakubu Kiyo* **1960**, 8, 464, 471.
[4] Fang, X. D. et al.: *Yaoxue Xuebao* **1986**, 21, 931.

[T. Kimura]

119.　　　*Saposhnikovia divaricata* (**Turcz.**) **Schischkin**　(Umbelliferae)
(= *Ledebouriella divaricata* Hiroe)

Fang–feng (C), Fong–fung (H), Bofu (J), Bang–pung (K)

Root　(CP, JP, KP)
Local Drug Name: Fang–feng (C), Bo–fu (J), Bang–pung (K).
Processing: Dry under the sun.
Method of Administration: Oral (decoction: C, H, J, K).
Folk Medicinal Uses:
　　　　　　1) Common cold (C, H, J, K).
　　　　　　2) Pain (C, J, K).
　　　　　　3) Headache (H).
　　　　　　4) Suppuration (J).
　　　　　　5) Urticaria (C).
　　　　　　6) Rheumatic arthralgia (C, H).
　　　　　　7) Tetanus (C, H).
　　　　　　8) Eczema (H).
　　　　　　9) Apoplexy (K).

Scientific Researches:
Chemistry
  1) Cumarins [1].
  2) Chromones [1].
  3) Polyacetylenes: falcarinol, falcarindiol [2].
  4) Polysaccharides: saposhinkovan A, B, C [3].
  5) Essential oil [4].
Pharmacology
  1) Adjuvant arthritis inhibition (decoction) [5,6].
  2) Analgesic (30% ethanol extract) [6].
  3) Anti–stress ulcer (30% ethanol extract) [6].
  4) Cyclooxygenase inhibition (falcarindiol) [7].
  5) Reticulo–endothelinal system activation (polysaccharides) [3].

Literatures:
[1] Sasaki, H. et al.: *Chem. Pharm. Bull.* **1982**, 30, 3555; Kobayashi, H.: *Shoyakugaku Zasshi* **1983**, 37,

276; Ding, A. et al.:*Zhongcaoyao* **1987**, 18, 247.

[2] Baba, K. et al.:*Shoyakugaku Zasshi* **1987**, 41, 189.

[3] Shimizu, N. et al.:*Chem. Pharm. Bull.* **1989**, 37, 1329, 3054.

[4] Wang, J. et al. :*Yaoxue Tongbao* **1987**, 22, 335.

[5] Cho, S. et al.:*Shoyakugaku Zasshi* **1982**, 36, 78.

[6] Kinoshita, T. et al.: *Wakan Iyaku Gakkaishi* **1987**, 4, 130.

[7] Baba, K. et al. :*Shoyakugaku Zasshi* **1987**, 41, 189.

[T. Kimura]

120. *Rhododendron dahuricum* L. (Ericaeae)

Xing–an–du–juan (C), Ezomurasakitsutsuji (J), San–jin–dal–rae (K)

Leaf (CP)

Local Drug Name: Man–shan–hong (C), Moon–san–hung (H), Man–zan–ko (J), Man–san–hong (K).

Processing: Dry in the shade (C, J, K).

Method of Administration: Oral (Water or alcohol extract: C, H, J, K).

Folk Medicinal Uses:

1) Acute and chronic bronchitis (C, H).

2) Cough (H, J, K).

3) Sputum (H).

Side Effects: Dizziness, headache, perspiration, palpitation, hepatic dysfunction when used in a long term.

Scientific Researches:

Chemistry

1) Flavonoids: farrerol, hyperin, avicularin, azaleatin, farrerol B, myricetin, dihydroquercetin [1, 2].

2) Triterpenes: daurichromenic acid, ursolic acid [2, 3].

3) Volatile oils: germacrone, cineole, caryophyllene, guaiazulene, selinane, humulane, vanillic acid, anisic acid, *p*–hydroxybenzoic acid, syringic acid, rhododendrol [1, 2].

4) Others: andromedotoxin, gallic acid 3–monomethyl ether, protocatechuic acid, hydroquinone [2, 4].

Pharmacology [1].

1) Antitussive effect (water–soluble matter, volatile extract, germacrone).

2) Expectorant effect (water–soluble matter, volatile extract, farrerol).

3) Preventing bronchospasm (water–soluble matter, volatile extract, farrerol).

4) Antibacterial effect (water or alcohol extract).

Literatures:

[1] Nanjing College of Pharmacy: "*Zhongcaoyao Xue*" Vol. 2, **1975**, 793.

[2] "*Zhongyao Dacidian*", **1977**, 2507.

[3] Suntory, Ltd.:*Jpn. Kokai Tokkyo Koho* JP 82 28, 080 (CL. CO7D311/58). 15 Feb.**1982**, Appl. 80/102, 700, 25 Jul. 1980.

[4] Liu, Y.L. et al.:*Zhongcaoyao* **1980**, 11(4), 152.

[J.X. Guo]

121.   *Forsythia suspensa* (Thunb.) Vahl   (Oleaceae)

Lian–qiao (C), Lin–kiu (H), Rengyo (J), Dang–gae–na–ri (K)

Related plants: *Forsythia viridissima* Lindley: Shinarengyo (J), Eui–seong–gae–na–ri (K);
F. koreana Nakai: Chosenrengyo (J), Gae–na–ri.

Fruit (CP, JP, KP)
   Local Drug Name: Lin–qiao (C), Lin–kiu (H), Ren–gyo (J), Yeon–gyo (K).
   Processing: Dry under the sun.
   Method of Administration: Oral (decoction: C, H, J, K).
   Folk Medicinal Uses:
                    1) Carbuncles, boils, lymphadenitis, mastitis, erysipelas (C). Suppuration (J, K).
                    2) Inflammation (H, J, K).
                    3) Erysipelas (H).
                    4) Fever (C, H).
                    5) Erythemas (H).
                    6) Scrofula (H).
                    7) Upper respiratory infection (C).
                    8) Acute urinary infection with oliguria (C).

Scientific Researches:
   Chemistry
      1) Triterpenoids: oleanolic acid, betulinic acid, ursolic acid [1].
      2) Lignans: phillygenin, (+)–pinoresinol, (+)–pinoresinol glucoside, phillyrin [2–6].
      3) Flavonoids: rutin [2–6].
   Pharmacology
      1) Choleretic (methanol extract) [7].
      2) Inhibition of cyclic AMP phosphodiesterase activity ((+)–pinoresinol, (–)–matairesinol) [8].
      3) Antibacterial and 5–lipoxygenase inhibition (forsythiaside, suspensaside) [9, 10].

Literatures:
   [1] Murakami, S.: *Yakugaku Zasshi* **1957**, 77, 437.
   [2] Nishibe, S. et al.: *Yakugaku Zasshi* **1977**, 97, 1134; *Shoyakugaku Zasshi* **1977**, 31, 131.
   [3] Chiba, M. et al.: *Chem. Pharm. Bull.* **1977**, 25, 3435; *Shoyakugaku Zasshi* **1978**, 32, 194; **1979**, 33, 150.
   [4] Nishibe, S. et al.: *Chem. Pharm. Bull.* **1982**, 30, 1048, 4548; **1984**, 32, 1209; *Yakugaku Zasshi* **1987**, 107, 274.
   [5] Endo, K. et al.: *Tetrahedron* **1987**, 43, 2681.
   [6] Kuang, H. X. et al.: *Zhongyao Tongbao* **1988**, 13, 416.
   [7] Miura, M. et al.: *Yakugaku Zasshi* **1987**, 107, 992.
   [8] Nikaido, T. et al.: *Chem. Pharm. Bull.* **1981**, 29, 3586.
   [9] Nishibe, S. et al.: *Chem. Pharm. Bull.* **1972**, 30, 4548; Kitagawa, S. et al.: *Yakugaku Zasshi* **1987**, 107, 274.
   [10] Kimura, Y. et al.: *Planta Med.* **1987**, 53, 148.

[T. Kimura]

122.   *Fraxinus japonica* Blume   (Oleaceae)

Toneriko (J)

Related plant: *Fraxinus rhynchophylla* Hance: Ku–li–bai–la–shu (C), Mul–pu–re–na–mu (K).

Bark
  Local Drug Name: Qin–pi (C), Shin–pi (J), Jin–pi (K).
  Processing: Dry under the sun (J, K).
  Method of Administration: Oral (decoction: J, K) or topical (J).
  Folk Medicinal Uses:
                1) Eye diseases (J, K).
                2) Pyrexia (J).
                3) Weakness (J).
                4) Apoplexy (K).
                5) Diarrhea (J).
Scientific Researches:
  Chemistry
    1) Lignans: (+)–fraxiresinol[(1*S*,2*R*,5*R*,6*S*)–1–hydroxy–2–(3,5–dimethoxy–4–hydroxy–phenyl)–6–
                (4–hydroxy–3–methoxyphenyl)–3,7–dioxabicyclo[3,3,0]octane], (+)–1–hydroxysyringaresinol
                (+)–1–hydroxypinoresinol–4'–β–D–glucoside, (+)–pinoresinol, (+)–1–hydroxypinoresinol,
                (–)–olivil, (+)–cyclo–olivil, (+)–pinoresinol–β–D–glucoside [2, 4].
    2) Coumarins: scopoletin, isofraxidin, esculetin, fraxetin, esculin, fraxin [3], fraxidin, fraxinol [4].
  Pharmacology
    1) Anti–platelet aggregation (coumarin).
    2) Antibacterial [5].
    3) Inhibition of lipooxygenase (esculin, esculetin) [6].

Literatures:
  [1] Kodaira, H. et al.:*Chem. Pharm. Bull.* **1983,** 31(7), 2262.
  [2] Tsukamoto, H. et al.:*Chem. Pharm. Bull.* **1984,** 32(11), 4482.
  [3] Tsukamoto, H. et al.:*Chem. Pharm. Bull.* **1985,** 33(9), 4069.
  [4] Miyachi, H. et al.: *Yakugaku Zasshi* **1987,** 107(6), 435.
  [5] Mei, P. F. et al.:*Acta Chim. Sin.* **1962,** 28, 25.
  [6] Sekiya, K. et al.:*Biochim. Biophys. Acta* **1982,** 713, 68.

[C.K. Sung]

123.   *Ligustrum lucidum* **Ait.**   (Oleaceae)

Nu–zhen (C), Lui–jing (H), Tonezumimochi (J), Je–ju–gwang–na–mu (K)

Related Plants: *Ligustrum japonicum* Thunb.: Nezumimochi (J).

Fruit (CP)
  Local Drug Name: Nu–zhen–zi (C), Lui–jing–gee (H), Jo–tei–shi (J), Yeo–jeong–sil (K).
  Processing: 1) Eliminate foreign matter, wash clean and dry (C, K).
                2) Stew or steam with wine (C).
  Method of Administration: Oral (decoction: C, H).
  Folk Medicinal Uses:
                1) Vertigo (C, H).
                2) Tinnitus (C, H).

3) Weakness in the loins and knees (C, H, J, K).
4) Pemature whitening of hair (C, H).
5) Impaired eyesight due to deficiency of yin of the liver and kidney (C, H, J).

Leaf
Local Drug Name: Nezumimochi (J).
Processing: Fresh leaves (J).
Method of Administration: Oral (Warer extrat or external, J).
Folk Medicinal Uses:
1) Gastric ulcer (J).
2) Sore, swelling (J).

Scientific Researches:
Chemistry
1) Triterpenes: oleanolic acid, acetyloleanolic acid, ursolic acid, betulin, lupeol [1, 2].
2) Volatile oils [3].
3) Others: ligustroside, nuzhenide, oleuropein, salidroside, linoleic acid, oleic acid, palmatic acid [1].
Pharmacology
1) Leukogennic effect (Alc. extract,C) [2].
2) Immunoregulation (water extract) [4].
3) Antibiosis (water extract) [1].
4) Decreasing the intraocular pressure of rabbit (Water extract) [5].
5) Recovering fatigue (salidroside) [2].
6) Anticancer effect (water ectract) [2].

Literatures:
[1] "*Zhongyao Zhi*", Vol. 3, **1984**, 172.
[2] Wang, Y. S. et al.: "*Zhongyao Yaoli Yu Yingyong*", **1983**, 131.
[3] Li, K. H. et al.: *Zhongchengyao* **1990**, 12(12), 32.
[4] Dai, Y. et al.: *Zhongguo Yaoke Daxue Xuebao* **1987**, 18(4), 301.
[5] Li, W.M. et al.: *Yuannan Zhongyi Zazhi* **1990**, 11(4), 27.

[J.X. Guo]

124.   *Gentiana scabra* Bunge.   (Gentianaceae)

Long–dan (C), Lung–darm (H), To–rindo (J)

Related plants: *Gentiana scabra* Bunge var. *buergeri* Maxim.: Rindo (J), Yong–dam (K).

Root and Rhizome (CP, JP, KP)
Local Drug Name: Long–dan (C), Long–darm (H), Ryu–tan (J), Yong–dam (K).
Processing: Dry under the sun.
Method of Administration: Oral (decoction or powder: C, H, J, K).
Folk Medicinal Uses:
1) Anorexia (J, K).
2) Dyspepsia (J, K).
3) Inflammation (H, J, K).
4) Fever (H, J).
5) Hepatitis, jaundice (H, J). Jaundice caused by damp–heat (C).
6) Sputum (K).
7) Encephalitis (H).

8) Epilepsy (H).
9) Dysentery (H).
10) Swelling and itching of the vulva with excessive leuckorrhea (C).
11) Eczema accompanied by itchung (C).
12) Prolonged erection of penis with spontaneous emission (C).

Scientific Researches:
Chemistry
  1) Secoiridoid glycosides: gentiopicroside [1].
  2) Xanthones: gentisin [1].
Pharmacology
  1) Stimulation of stomach movement (water extract, decoction) [2, 3].
  2) Gastric secretion increasing (extract, gentiopicroside) [4, 5, 6].
  3) Stimulation of isolated bowel movement (water extract) [7].
  4) Choleretic effect (methanol extract) [8].
  5) Inhibition of skin sensitizing antibody (reagin) production (water, ethanol extract) [9].

Literatures:
[1] Hayashi, T.: *Yakugaku Zasshi* **1976**, 96, 356, 366, 679; Akada, Y. et al.:*ibid.* **1979**, 99, 1047.
[2] Sone, Y.: *Tohoku J. Exptl. Med.* **1936**, 29, 321.
[3] Suga, S.: *Osaka Igakkai Zasshi* **1942**, 41, 649.
[4] Uchida, S.: *Tokyo Igakkai Zasshi* **1938**, 52, 779; Saeki, T.: *Nippon Yakubutsugaku Zasshi* **1943**, 38, 405.
[5] Ikuta, M.: *Osaka Igakkai Zasshi* **1940**, 39, 2072; **1941**, 40, 711, 727.
[6] Haginiwa, T. et al.: *Yakugaku Zasshi* **1961**, 81, 1387.
[7] Ito, T.: *Nippon Yakurigaku Zasshi* **1960**, 56, 63.
[8] Miura, M. et al.: *Yakugaku Zasshi* **1987**, 107, 992.
[9] Koda, A. et al.: *Nippon Yakurigaku Zasshi* **1973**, 69, 88.

[T. Kimura]

125.   *Swertia japonica* Makino (= *Ophelia japonica* Griseb.) (Gentianaceae)

Ri–ben–dang–yao (C), Senburi (J), Sseun–pul (K)

Whole plant (JP)
Local drug name: Dang–yao (C), Senburi, To–yaku (J), Dang–yak (K).
Processing: Air dry (J, K).
Administration: Oral (decoction: J, K).
Folk Medicinal Uses:
  1) Dyspepsia (J, K).
  2) Anorexia (J, K).
  3) Diarrhea (J).
  4) Alopecia pitirodes (J).
  5) Water eczema (J).
  6) Abdominal Pain (K).
  7) Stomach ache (J, K).
  8) Psoriasis (K).

Scientific Researches:
Chemistry
  1) Secoiridoid glycosides: swertiamarin(2~ 10 %), sweroside, gentiopicroside, amarogentin,

amaroswerin [1, 2, 3].
2) Xanthones: swertianin, swertianolin, bellidifolin [4].
3) Triterpene and its glycoside [5].
4) Flavonoids [6].
5) Volatile compounds [7].

Pharmacology
1) Secretion of gastric juice (water extract) [8–12].
2) Choleretic (methanol extract) [13].
3) Lowering death rate on carbon tetrachloride (ethanol extract) [14].
4) Bowel movement stimulation in low and depression in high concentration (ethanol extract) [14].
5) Pancreas protease activity stimulation (water extract) [15].
6) Secretion of saliva, bile and pancreatic juice (swertiamarin) [16].
7) Central nervous system depressing (swertiamarin)[17].
8) Inhibiting experimental disorder of liver function (amarogentin, swertiajaponin, bellidifolin) [18].
9) Mutagenicity (bellidifolin) [19].

Literatures:

[1] Inouye, H. et al.:*Chem. Pharm. Bull.* **1970**, 18, 1856, 2043; *Tetrahedron* **1971**, 27, 1951; Ikeshiro, Y. et al.: *Planta Medica* **1984**, 50, 485; **1985**, 51, 390.

[2] Hayashi, H. et al.:*Yakugaku Zasshi* **1976**, 96, 366, 498; Takino, Y. et al.:*Planta Medica* **1980**, 38, 351; Akada, Y. et al.:*Yakugaku Zasshi* **1980**, 100, 770; Sakamoto, I. et al.:*Chem. Pharm. Bull.* **1983**, 31, 25.

[3] D. Teshima et al.: *Shoyakugaku Zasshi* **1980**, 34, 251.

[4] Komatsu, K. et al.:*Chem. Pharm. Bull.* **1969**, 17, 155; *Yakugaku Zasshi* **1969**, 89, 410; Sakamoto, I. et al.: *Chem. Pharm. Bull.* **1982**, 30, 4088.

[5] Ikeshiro, Y. et al.:*Planta Med.* **1983**, 47, 26; Kanamori, H. et al.:*Chem. Pharm. Bull.* **1984**, 32, 4942.

[6] Komatsu, K. et al.:*Yakugaku Zasshi* **1968**, 88, 832.

[7] Sakai, T. et al.:*Bull. Chem. Soc. Japan* **1983**, 56, 3477.

[8] M. Ikuta: *Osaka Igakkai Zasshi* **1940**, 39, 2072; **1941**, 40, 711, 727.

[9] Saeki, T.:*Nippon Yakubutsugaku Zasshi* **1943**, 38, 405.

[10] Esaki, T.:*Nippon Yakurigaku Zasshi* **1954**, 50, 103; **1955**, 51, 62.

[11] Suga, S.: *Osaka Igakkai Zasshi* **1942**, 41, 649.

[12] Haginiwa, T. et al.:*Yakugaku Zasshi* **1961**, 81, 1387.

[13] Miura, M. et al.: *Yakugaku Zasshi* **1987**, 107, 992.

[14] Hasegawa, S. et al.:*Nippon Shokakibyo Zasshi* **1964**, 61, 976.

[15] Uchiyama, T., et al.:*Wakan Iyaku Gakkaishi* **1989**, 6, 201.

[16] Yamahara, J. et al.:*Yakugaku Zasshi* **1978**, 98, 1446; Hoshino, K.:*Hokuetsu Igakkaishi* **1939**, 54, 1221.

[17] Bhattacharya, S. K., et al.:*J. Pharm. Sci.* **1976**, 65, 1547.

[18] Hikino, H. et al.:*Shoyakugaku Zasshi* **1984**, 38, 359.

[19] Kanamori, H. et al.:*Chem. Pharm. Bull.* **1984**, 32, 2290; Nozaka, T. et al.:*Shoyakugaku Zasshi* **1984**, 38, 96.

[T. Kimura]

126.   *Gardenia jasminoides* Ellis   (Rubiaceae)

Zhi–zi (C), Gee–gee (H), Korin–kuchinashi (J), Chi–ja–na–mu (K)

Fruit (CP, JP, KP)
Local Drug Name: Zhi–zi (C), Gee–gee (H), San–shi–shi (J), Chi–ja.
Processing: 1) Dry under the sun. 2) Stir–fry until the outer part turned to yellowish brown (C).

3) Stir–fry until the outer part charred (C).

Method of Administration: Oral or topical (decoction, powder or plaster: C, H, J, K).

Folk Medicinal Uses:

    1) Suppurative inflammation, abscess (J, K).

    2) Dermatitis (J, K).

    3) Jaundice (C, H, J, K). Jaundice with dark urine (C).

    4) Febrile diseases with restlessness (C).

    5) Dysuria (H, K).

    6) Hematuria with difficult painful urination (C).

    7) Hemoptysis and epistaxis caused by heat in the blood (C). Hematemesis, epistaxis (H).

    8) Inflammation of the eyes (C). Conjunctivitis, pharyngitis (H).

    9) Twist (H).

Scientific Researches:

Chemistry

  1) Iridoid glycosides: geniposide (genipin β–D–glucoside), geniposidic acid, 10–acetylgeniposide, genipin 1–β–gentiobioside, gardenoside, shanzhiside, methyl deacetylasperulosidate, gardoside, scandoside methyl ester [1, 4].

  2) Carotenoids: crocin [2].

  3) Phenylpropanoids:p–hydroxycinnamic acid [3].

Pharmacology

  1) Inhibition of blood bilirubin ascending (methanol extr.) [5].

  2) Choleretic effect (methanol extr., genipin) [6, 12].

  3) Inhibition of ethanol gastritis occurrence (hot water extr.) [7].

  4) Inhibition of serum cholesterol ascending (hot water extr.) [8].

  5) Lowering blood pressure (decoction or ethanol extr.) [9].

  6) Stimulating growth in aortic endotherium culture (decoction) [10].

  7) Moderate laxative (decoction, methanol extr. or genipin) [11].

  8) Anticholinergic decreasing of gastric secretion and total acidity, ascending pH value of gastric juice, anti–acetylcholine and antihistamic activity (genipin) [12].

  9) Decreasing of stomach movement and tension (geniposide, genipin) [12].

  10) Decreasing of lipids in blood serum and liver (geniposide) [13].

  11) Inhibition of liver parenchymal disorder (geniposide) [14].

  12) Preventive effect for decreasing sexual and learning behaviors caused by stress (iridoids) [15].

  13) Inhibition of 5–lipoxygenase (chlorogenic acid and 4 other ingredients) [16].

  14) Prevention of experimental arteriosclerosis (crocetin) [17].

  15) Stimulation of oxigen supplement in lung and brain (crocetin) [18].

  16) Toxicity [19].

Literatures:

[1] Inouye, H., et al.:*Tetrahedron Letters* **1969**, 2347, **1970**, 3581; Endo, T. et al.:*Chem. Pharm. Bull.* **1970**, 18, 1066; **1973**, 21, 2684; Inouye, H. et al.:*Yakugaku Zasshi*, **1974**, 94, 577; Inouye, H. et al.: *Phytochemistry* **1974**, 13, 2219; Takeda, Y. et al.:*Chem. Pharm. Bull.* **1976**, 24, 2644; Inouye, H.: *Gendai Toyo Igaku*, **1983**, 4, 48.

[2] Munesada, T.:*Yakugaku Zasshi*, **1922**, 42, 666; Kuhn, R. et al.:*Helv. Chim. Acta* **1928**, 11, 716.

[3] Nishizawa, M. et al., *Chem. Pharm. Bull.* **1988**, 36, 87.

[4] Yamauchi, K., et al.:*Planta Med.* **1974**, 25, 219; Hayakawa, J. et al.:*Yakugaku Zasshi* **1985**, 105, 966; Harada, M. et al.: *"Hanyo Shoyaku no Seibun Teiryo",* **1989**, 170, Hirokawa Publ. Co.

[5] Li, K. et al.:*Nippon Yakurigaku Zasshi,* **1944**, 41, 207; Miwa, T.:*Japan. J. Pharmacol.* **1953**, 2, 139; **1953**, 3, 1; Che, C.T., et al.:*Planta Med.* **1977**, 18.

[6] Miura, M. et al.:*Yakugaku Zasshi,* **1987**, 107, 992; Miyagoshi, M. et al.:*J. Pharmacobio–Dyn.* **1988**, 11, 186.

[7] Takase, H., et al.:*Japan. J. Pharmacol.* **1989**, 49, 301.

[8] Maemura, S. et al.:*Wakan Iyakugaku Zasshi,* **1987**, 4, 300.

[9] Zhang, S. F. et al.:*Yaoxue Xuepao,* **1965**, 12, 636.

[10] Kaji, T., et al.:*Planta Med.* **1990**, 56, 353.

[11] Yamauchi, K., et al.:*Planta Med.* **1974**, 25, 219, 285; **1976**, 30, 39.

[12] Harada, M. et al.:*Yakugaku Zasshi,* **1974**, 94, 157; Aburada, M., et al.:*J. Pharm. Dyn.* **1978**, 1, 81; **1980,** 3, 423; Takeda, S., et al.:*Ibid.* **1981,** 4, 612.

[13] Kimura, Y. et al.:*Chem. Pharm. Bull.* **1982**, 30, 4444.

[14] Yang, L. L., et al.:*Wakan Iyakugaku Zasshi,* **1990**, 7, 28.

[15] Imai, T. et al.:*Yakugaku Zasshi,* **1988**, 108, 572.

[16] Nishizawa, M., et al.:*Chem. Pharm. Bull.* **1986**, 34, 1419; **1987**, 35, 2133; **1988**, 36, 87.

[17] Gainer, J. L., et al.:*Experientia* **1975**, 31, 548; Pool, J. D., et al.:*Adv. Exp. Med. Biol.* **1976**, 67, 205; Kuwano, S.: *Gendai Toyo Igaku,* **1983**, 4, 57.

[18] Seyde, W. C., et al.:*J. Cereb. Blood Flow Metab.* **1986**, 6, 703; Holloway, G. M. et al.:*J. Appl. Physiol.* **1988**, 65, 683.

[19] Aburada, M. et al.:*Oyoyakuri,* **1980**, 19, 259.

[T. Kimura]

127.   *Paederia scandens* (Lour.) Merr.,
P. scandens (Lour.) Merr. var. *mairei* (Leveille) Hara   (Rubiaceae)

Ji–shi–teng (C), Gait–see–teng (H), Hekusokazura (J)

Seed

Local Drug Name: Ji–shi–teng (C), Gait–see–teng (H), Kei–shi–to (J), Gye–ngo–deung (K).

Processing: Dry under the sun or use when fresh.

Method of Administration: Oral (decoction: C, H, J). Topical (juice: C, H).

Folk Medicinal Uses:

1) Biliary and gastrointestinal pain (C, H).

2) Rheumatalgia (C, H).

3) Infantile maldigestion (C, H).

4) Icteric hepatitis (C, H).

5) Enteritis, dysentery, diarrhea (H, J).

6) Bronchitis, whooping cough (H).

7) Pulmonary tuberculosis (H).

8) Traumatic injury (C, H).

9) Leukopenia (H).

10) Poisoning by organic phosphorus (H).

11) Furunculus (C).

12) Beriberi (J).

Scientific Researches:

Chemistry

1) Paederoside, paederosidic acid, asperuloside, scandoside, deacetylasperuloside, sitosterol, oleanolic acid, abutin, volatile oil [1–2, 4–6], paederinin [7].

Pharmacology

1) Antibacterial effects.

2) Analgesic and sedative1 effects.

3) Expectorant effects.

4) Hypotensive effects.

5) Anti–imflammatory effects.

6) Paederoside ingested by aphid functions as a defence against ladybird beetles [8].

Literatures:

[1] Inouye, H. et al.: *Chem. Pharm. Bull.* **1969**, 17, 1942.

[2] Inouye, H. et al.: *Tetrahedron Lett.* **1968**, 6; 683–8.

[3] Nishida, R. et al.: *J. Chem. Ecol.* **1989**, 15, 1837.

[4] Hui, W.H. et al.: *Australian J. Chem.* **1964**, 17, 493.

[5] Inonye, H. et al.: *Tetrahedron Lett.* **1990**, (38), 3351.

[6] Inonye, H. et al.: *J. Chromatogr.* **1976**, 118, 4201.

[7] Ishikura, N. et al.: *Z. Naturforsch., C: Biosci.* **1990**, 45, 1081.

[P.P.H. But]

128.   *Uncaria rhynchophylla* **Miq.**   (Rubiaceae)

Gou–teng (C), Ngou–teng (H), Kagikazura (J)

Related plants: *Uncaria sinensis* (Oliv.) Havil.; *U. macrophylla* Wall.; *U. sessilifructus* Roxb.

Stem with hooks (CP)

Local Drug Name: Gou–teng (C); Ngou–teng (H); Cho–to–ko (J).

Processing: Remove leaf, cut into section, and dry under the sun.

Method of Administration: Oral (decoction: C, H, J).

Folk Medicinal Uses:

       1) Hypertension (C, H, J).

       2) Dizziness, blurred vision (C, H, J).

       3) Infantile convulsion, high fever, night screaming (C, H, J).

       4) Colds, headache, neural headache (C, H).

       5) Hemiplegia (C).

       6) Potential miscarriage, abortion (C).

       7) Arteriosclerosis (J).

Contraindications: Debility, fire–deficiency.

Side Effects: LD_{50} of water extract 29.0 ± 0.8 g/kg IP in mice.

Root

Local Drug Name: Gou–teng–gen (C), Ngou–teng–gun (H).

Processing: Dry under the sun.

Method of Administration: Oral (decoction: C, H).

Folk Medicinal Uses:

       1) Rheumatalgia (C, H).

       2) Hemiplegia (C).

       3) Infantile fever (C).

       4) Edema in pregnancy (C).

       5) Traumatic injury (C).

       6) Schizophrenia (C).

Scientific Researches:

Chemistry

   1) Alkaloids: Akuammigine, cadambine, 3a–dihydrocadambine, 3b–isodihydrocadambine, corynantheine, dihydrocorynantheine, corynoxeine, isocorynoxeine, corynoxine, isocorynoxine, isoformosanine, geissoschizine methyl ether, hirsuteine, hirsutine, mitraphylline,

134

pteropodine, isopteropodine, rhynchophine, rhynchophylline, isorhynchophylline,
isorhynchophyllic acid, strictosamide, tetrahydroalstonine, vallesiachotamine,
vincosamide, vincoside lactam, [9–11, 13–16, 21–22].

2) Hyperin, trifolin, mitraphyllic acid, isomitraphyllic acid, mitraphyllic acid [16–1]–β–D–glucopyranosyl
ester, isomitraphyllic acid [16–1]–β–D–glucopyranosyl ester [10, 12].

Pharmacology

1) Sedative action.

2) Hypotensive effects (3 α–dihydrocadambine, 3 β–isodihydrocadambine) [1, 5, 11].

3) Inhibitory effects on contraction of guinea pig urinary bladder induced by electrical stimulation of the
pelvic nerves (hirsutine) [2].

4) Anesthetic effects on isolated frog sciatic nerve preparation (hirsutine) [2].

5) Stimulatory effects on tone and amplitude of the spontaneous movement of guinea pig urinary bladder
(hirsutine, isorhynchophylline) [2].

6) Blocking effects on rat superior cervical ganglionic preparation (hirsutine) [3].

7) Vasodilation effects (hirsutine, hirsuteine) [4].

8) Central nervous system depressant effects (hirsutine, hirsuteine, rhynchophylline, isorhynchophylline,
dihydrocorynantheine) [5].

9) Anti–spasmodic effects (hirsutine, hirsuteine, rhynchophylline, isorhynchophylline, dihydrocorynantheine) [5].

10) Antioxidant and antiepileptic effects [7].

11) Ca^{2+} channel blocking effects (hirsutine) [6, 8].

12) Partial agonistic effects on 5–hydroxytryptamine receptors [20].

13) Inhibitory effects on adenylate cyclase [23].

Literatures:

[1] Wu, C. C. et al.: *Taiwan I Hsueh Hui Tsa Chih* **1980**, 79, 749.

[2] Harada, M. et al.: *Chem. Pharm. Bull.* **1979**, 27, 1069.

[3] Harada, M. et al.: *Chem. Pharm. Bull.* **1974**, 22, 1372.

[4] Ozaki, Y.: *Nippon Yakurigaku Zasshi* **1990**, 95, 47.

[5] Ozaki, Y.: *Nippon Yakurigaku Zasshi* **1989**, 94, 17.

[6] Horie, S. et al.: *Life Sci.* **1992**, 50, 491.

[7] Liu, J., Mori, A.: *Neuropharmacology* **1992**, 31, 1287.

[8] Yano, S. et al.: *Planta Medica* **1991**, 57, 403.

[9] Aimi, N. et al.: *Chem. Pharm. Bull.* **1982**, 30, 4046.

[10] Aimi, N. et al.: *Chem. Pharm. Bull.* **1982**, 30, 4046.

[11] Endo, K. et al.: *Planta Medica* **1983**, 49, 188.

[12] Liu H.M. et al.: *Yaoxue Xuebao* **1993**; 28, 849.

[13] Liu, H.M. et al.: *Chin. Chem. Lett.* **1992**, 3(6), 425.

[14] Liu, H.M. et al.: *Zhongcaoyao* **1993**, 24(2), 61.

[15] Kawazoe, S. et al.: *Shoyakugaku Zasshi* **1991**, 45, 281.

[16] Aimi, N. et al.: *Chem. Pharm. Bull.* **1977**, 25, 2067.

[17] Haginiwa, J. et al.: *Yakugaka Zasshi* **1971**, 91, 575.

[18] Haginiwa, J. et al.: *Yakugaka Zasshi* **1973**, 93, 448.

[19] Nozoye, T. et al.: *Yakugaku Zasshi* **1975**, 95, 758.

[20] Kanatani, H. et al.: *J. Pharm. Pharmacol.* **1985**, 37, 401.

[21] Liu, G. et al.: *Zhongguo Yaoxue Zazhi* **1991**, 26, 583.

[22] Phillipson, J.D. et al.: *Phytochem.* **1973**, 12, 2795.

[23] Kanatani, H. et al. *Planta Med.* **1985**, (2), 182.

[P.P.H. But]

129. *Cuscuta chinensis* **Lam.**   (Convolvulaceae)
C. japonica Lam., *C. australis* R. Br.

Tu–si–zi (C), To–see–gee (H), Nenashikazura (J), Sae–sam (K)

Seed (CP)

Local Drug Name: Tu–si–zi (C), To–see–gee (H), To–shi–shi (J), To–sa–ja (K).

Processing: a) Eliminate foreign matter, wash clean, dry under the sun. b) Stir–fry cleaned seeds with salt–water until the seeds become slightly bulged.

Method of Administration: Oral (decoction: C, H, J, K).

Folk Medicinal Uses:

    1) Lumbago (C, H, J, K).
    2) Diabetes (C, J).
    3) Miscarriage (C, J).
    4) Spermatorrhea (C, H, J, K).
    5) Blurred vision, tinnitus (C).
    6) Diarrhea due to hypofunction of spleen and kidney (C).
    7) External use for vitiligo (C).
    8) Impotence (J).

Contraindications: Constipation, hemorrhagia, fire in 'kidney', pregnancy.

Whole plant

Local Drug Name: Tu–si (C), To–shi (J), To–sa (K).

Method of Administration: Oral (decoction: C, J).

Folk Medicinal Uses:

    1) Hematuria (C, J).
    2) Hemorrhinia (C, J).
    3) Jaundice (C, J).
    4) Dysentery (C).
    5) Leukorrhea (C).
    6) Pyroderma (C).

Scientific Researches:

Chemistry

  1) Carotenoids; carotene, taraxanthin, lutein [1].
  2) Pentacosane, β–sitosterol, stearic acid, arachidic acid [2].
  3) Polysaccharides [3].

Pharmacology

  1) Immunopotentiating effects [1].

Literatures:

[1] Kim, M.S. et al.:*Korean J. Pharmacog.* **1988**, 19, 193–200.
[2] Wen, D.X. et al.:*Huaxi Yaoxue Zazhi.* **1992**, 7, 11–3.
[3] Ye, P.: *Zhong Chengyao* **1992**, 14(3), 36–7.

[P.P.H. But]

130.   *Pharbitis nil* **Choisy**   (Convolvulaceae)

Lie–ye–qian–niu (C), Hin–ngau (H), Asagao (J), Na–pal–ggot (K)

Seed (CP, JP, KP)
  Local Drug Name: Qian–niu–zi, Hei–chou, Bai–chou (C), Hin–ngau–gee (H), Ken–go–shi (J),
        Heuk–chuk (K)
  Processing: 1) Dry under the sun. 2) Stir–fry to be slightly inflated (C).
  Method of Administration: Oral (powder: C, H, J, K).
  Folk Medicinal Uses:
        1) Constipation (C, H, J, K).
        2) Anasarca with oliguria (C).
        3) Dyspnea and cough caused by retained fluid (C).
        4) Abdominal pain due to intestinal parasitosis (C).
        5) Ascariasis, taeniasis (C).
        6) Edema (H).
        7) Phlegm (H).
        8) Beriberi (H).
  Contraindications: Pregnancy.

Scientific Researches:
  Chemistry
   1) Resin glycosides: pharbitin [1].
  Pharmacology
   1) Purgative [2].

Literatures:
  1) Okabe, H. et al.: *Tetrahedron Letters* **1970**, 3123.
  2) Ito, H. : *Mie Med. J.* **1964**, 14, 47.

[T. Kimura]

131.   *Lithospermum erythrorhizon* **Sieb. et Zucc.**   (Boraginaceae)

Zi–cao (C), Gee–cho (H), Murasaki (J), Ji–chi (K)

Related plant: *Arnebia euchroma* Johnst. (=*Macrotomia euchroma* Pauls.): Xin–zang–ge–zi–cao.

Root (CP, JP, KP)
  Local Drug Name: Zi–cao (C), Gee–cho (H), Shi–kon (J), Ja–cho (K).
  Processing: Dry under the sun.
  Method of Administration: Oral or topical (decoction or ointment: C, H, J, K).
  Folk Medicinal Uses:
        1) Skin diseases, dermatitis (C, J, K).
        2) Burn, congelation, scald (C, H, J, K).
        3) Hemorrhoid (J, K).
        4) Eczema, erysepalis, furunculosis (H).
        5) Dysentery (H).
        6) Hematuria, dysuria (H).
        7) Purpura (H).
        8) Jaundice (H).
        9) Cough (K).
        10) Measles (K).

Scientific Researches:
  Chemistry
   1) Naphthoquinones: acetylshikonin, isobutylshikonin, β,β–dimethylacrylshikonin, shikonin [1].

2) Lithospermic acid [2], lithospermoside [3].

3) Purin base: alantoin [4].

4) Polysaccharide: lithosperman A, B, C [4].

Pharmacology

1) Anti–inflammatory effects [5].

2) Stimulation of granulation tissue growth and acceleration of wound healing (acetylshikonin and shikonin) [6].

3) Bacteriocidal effect (shikonin) [7].

4) Anti–tumor–promoter activity (methnol extract) [8].

5) Antitumor activities on Sarcoma 180 and Ehrlich's ascites carcinoma in mice (shikonin and its derivertives) [9].

6) Blood sugar lowering (water extract, lithosperman A, B, C) [10].

Literatures:

[1] Hirata, Y. et al.: *Tetrahedron Letters* **1965**, 4737; **1966**, 3677; Kyogoku, K. et al.: *Shoyakugaku Zasshi* **1973**, 27, 24; Kudo, S. et al.: *Ibid.* **1982**, 36, 154, 170; Honda, G., et al.: *J. Nat. Prod.* **1988**, 51, 152.

[2] Wagner, H., et al.: *Tetrahedron Letters* **1975**, 547 ; *J. Org. Chem.* **1975**, 33, 105.

[3] Sosa, A., et al.: *Phytochemistry* **1977**, 16, 707.

[4] Yoshizaki, F., et al.: *Chem. Pharm. Bull.* **1982**, 30, 4407.

[5] Hayashi, M.: *Nippon Yakurigaku Zasshi* **1977**, 73, 177, 205.

[6] Hayashi, M.: *Nippon Yakurigaku Zasshi* **1977**, 73, 193.

[7] Tanaka, Y. et al.: *Yakugaku Zasshi* **1972**, 92, 525; Kyogoku, K. et al.: *Shoyakugaku Zasshi* **1973**, 27, 31.

[8] Konoshima, T. et al.: *Yakugaku Zasshi* **1989**, 109, 843.

[9] Sankawa, U., et al.: *Chem. Pharm. Bull.* **1977**, 25, 2392; **1981**, 29, 116; Kosuge, T. et al.: *Yakugaku Zasshi* **1985**, 105, 791.

[10] Konno, C., Mizuno, T., Hikino, H.: *Planta Med.* **1985**, 51, 157.

[T. Kimura]

132   *Clerodendron cyrtophyllum* **Turcz**   (Verbenaceae)

Lu–bian–qing (C), Die–ching–yip (H), Makibakusagi (J)

Root and Leaf

Local Drug Name: Da–qing–ye (C), Die–ching–yip (H), Tai–sei–yo (J).

Processing: 1) Root: Cut into slices, and dry under the sun (C).

               2) Leaf: Wash clean, and dry in the shade or use in fresh (C).

Method of Administration: Oral (decoction: C, H).

Folk Medicinal Uses:

         1) Preventing epidemic encephalomyelitis and epidemic encephalitis B (C, H).

         2) Common cold and headache (C, H).

         3) Measles complicated with pneumonia (C, H).

         4) Tonsillitis (C, H).

         5) Dysentery (C, H).

         6) Epidemic parotitis (H).

         7) Infectious hepatitis (H).

         8) Urinary tract infection (H).

Side Effects: Nausea and vomiting.

Scientific Researches:

Chemistry

1) Indoles: indican, indoxyl, indirubin [1].
2) Flavonoids: cytophyllin [2].
Pharmacology
1) Antibacterial effect (Water extract of leaf,C)

Literatures:

[1] Wang, Y.S. et al.: *"Zhongyao Yaoli Yu Yingyonga"*, **1983**, 88.
[2] *"Zhiwuyao Youxiaochengfen Shouce'*, **1983**, 298.

[J.X. Guo]

133.   *Clerodendron trichotomum* **Thunb.**   (Verbenaceae)

Hai–zhou–chang–shan (C), Kusagi (J), Nu–ri–jang–na–mu (K)

Leaf
Local Drug Name: Chou–wu–tong (C), Shu–go–to (J), Chwi–o–dong (K).
Processing: Wash clean and dry (C).
Method of Administration: Oral (decoction: C).
Folk Medicinal Uses:
1) Rheumatalgia (C, K).
2) Hypertension (C).
3) Hematochezia (C).
4) Arthritis (K).
Side Effects: Nausea, vomiting, anasarca when large dosage is used.

Scientific Researches:
Chemistry
1) Flavonoids: clerodendrin, acacetin–7–di–β–glucuronide [1].
2) Indoles: indolizino indole–5–carboxylic acid [2].
3) Others: kusasginin, clerodendrin A, B, clerodendronin A, B, clerodolone, clerodone, clerosterol, N–acetyl–D–galactosamine, mesoinositol [3, 4, 5].
Pharmacology
1) Antihypertensive effect (water extract) [6].
2) Sedative effect (clerodendronin) [6].
3) Analgesia (clerodendronin B) [6].
4) Anti–inflammatory effect [6].
5) Anthelmintic effect [6].
6) Anti–complementary effect (polysaccharides) [7].

Literatures:

[1] Nanjing College of Pharmacy: *"Zhongcaoyao Xue"* Vol. 3, **1980, **904.
[2] Irikawa, H. et al.: *Bull. Chem. Soc. Jpn.,* **1989**, 62(3), 880.
[3] Sakurai, A. et al.: *ibid*, **1983**, 56(5), 1573.
[4] Jiansu Xinyi–xueyuang (ed.): *"Zhongyao Dacidian"*, Shanghai Renmin Chuban, Shanghai, **1977,** 1891; 1893.
[5] Kitagaki, H. et al.: *J. Biochem.* (Tokyo), **1985**, 97(3), 791.
[6] Wang, Y.S. et al.: *"Zhongyao Yaoli Yu Yingyong"*, **1983, **907.
[7] Hashi, M.: *Shinrin Sogo Kenkyusho Kenkyo Hokoku*, **1991,** 360, 121.

[J.X. Guo]

134.   *Verbena officinalis* L.   (Verbenaceae)

Ma–bian–cao (C), Ma–bin–cho (H), Kumatsuzura (J), Ma–pyeon–cho (K)

Herb (CP)
Local Drug Name: Ma–bian–cao (C), Ma–bin–cho (H), Ba–ben–so (J), Ma–pyeon–cho (K).
Processing: Eliminate the remained roots, soften briefly, cut into sections and dry under the sun (C, J, K).
Method of Administration: Oral (decoction: C, H, J, K).
Folk Medicinal Uses:
       1) Edema (C, H).
       2) Menstrual disorder (J, K).
       3) Amenorrhea and dysmenorrhea(C, H).
       4) Diarrhea (J).
       5) Dermatitis (J).
       6) Masses in the abdomen (C).
       7) Jaundice (J).
       8) Malaria (C, H).
       9) Inflammation of the throat (C).
       10) Carbuncles (C).
       11) Boils (C).
       12) Acute infection of the urinary tract (C).
       13) Metropathy (K).
       14) Filariasis (H).
       15) Schistosomiasis (H).
       16) Common cold, fever (H).
       17) Soar throat (H).
       18) Pertusis (H).
       19) Pyorrhea (H).
       20) Acute gastroenteritis (H).
       21) Bacillary dysentery (H).
       22) Hepatitis (H).
       23) Cirrhosis (H).
       24) Ascites (H).
       25) Nephritis (H).
       26) Urethrites (H).
       27) Sore scrotum (H).
       28) Traumatic injury (topical; H).
       29) Pyodermas (topical; H).
Contraindications: In pregnancy, "spleen" deficiency.

Scientific Researches:
Chemistry
    1) Iridoids: cornin (= verbenalin) [1, 2], hastatoside [3, 4, 5].
    2) Flavonoids: artemetin.
    3) Phenyl propanoids: verbascoside, eukovoside [7, 8].
    4) Triterpenes: lupeol, ursolic acid, β–sitosterol [5, 6].
Pharmacology
    1) Antiphlogistic activity (EtOH ext.) [9].
    2) Antiphlogistic activity on conjunctivitis (EtOH ext.) [9].
    3) Antitussive action (cornin, β–sitosterol) [6].
    4) Synergistic action on the action of PG (cornin) [10].
    5) Stimulation of the phagocytic activity (EtOH ext.) [11].

Literatures:

[1] Jensen, S. R. et al.:*Acta Chem. Scand.* **1973,** 27, 2581.

[2] B chi, G., Manning, R. E.:*Tetrahedron Lett.* **1960,** 5–12.

[3] Rimpler, H. et al.:*Tetrahedron Lett.* **1973,** 1463–4.

[4] Rimpler, H. et al.:*Z. Naturforsch.* **1979,** 34, 311.

[5] Makboul, A. M.:*Fitoterapia* **1986,** 57, 50.

[6] Kui, C. H. et al.:*Bull. Chin. Mater. Med.* **1985,** 10, 467.

[7] Bianco, A. et al.:*J. Nat. Prod.* **1984,** 47, 901.

[8] Haensel, R. et al.:*Arch. Pharm.(Weinheim)* **1986,** 319, 227.

[9] Sakai, S. et al.: *Gifu Ika Daigaku Kiyo* **1963,** 11, 6.

[10] Research group on reproductive physiology:*Dongwu Xuebao* **1974,** 20, 340.

[11] Delavequ, P et al.:*Planta Med.* **1980,** 40(1), 49.

[C.K. Sung]

135. *Vitex rotundifolia* **L.f.** (Verbenaceae)

Dan–ye–man–jing (C), Man–ging (H), Hamago (J), Sun–bi–gi–na–mu (K)

Seed
Local Drug Name: Man–jing–zi (C), Man–ging–gee (H), Man–kei–shi (J), Man–hyung–ja (K).
Processing: Stir–fry until charred yellow.
Method of Administration: Oral (decoction or powder: C, H, J).
Folk Medicinal Uses:
    1) Colds, headache, migraine (C, H, J).
    2) Sore eyes, night blindness (C, H, J).
    3) Myalgia, neuralgia (C, H, J).
Contraindications: Headache of blood–deficiency with fire, stomach–deficiency.

Leaf
Local Drug Name: Man–jing–zi–ye (C), Man–kei–shi–yo (J), Man–hyung–ja–yeop (K).
Method of Administration: Oral or topical (decoction: C, J).
Folk Medicinal Uses:
    1) Headache (C, J).
    2) Traumatic injury (C, J).
    3) Rheumatalgia (C).
Contraindications: Headache of blood–deficiency with fire, stomach–deficiency.

Scientific Researches:
Chemistry
  1) Monoterpenes: camphene, pinene.
  2) Diterpenes: rotundifuran, prerotundifuran, vitexilactone, previtexilactone [1].
  3) Flavones: vitexicarpin (casticin), luteolin, artemetin [1].
  4) *p*–Hydroxybenzoic acid, vanillic acid [1].
  5) Alkaloids: vitricine.
  6) Glucosides: agnuside, eurostoside, 10-*O*-*cis*-*p*-hydroxycinnamoyl aucubin, 3'4'–dihydroxy–
          phenyl–butanone glucoside [2].
Pharmacology
  1) Antibacterial effect.

Literatures:

[1] Kondo, Y. et al.:*Chem. Pharm. Bull.* **1986**, 34, 4829–32.

[2] Kouno, I. et al.:*Phytochem.* **1988**, 27, 611–2.

[3] Haensel, R. et al.:*Phytochem.* **1965**, 4, 19.

[4] Asaka, Y. et al.:*Chem. Lett.* **1973**, 9, 937.

[P.P.H. But]

136   *Agastache rugosa* (Fisch. et Mey.) O. Ktze. (Labiatae)

Huo–xiang (C), Kawamidori (J), Bae–cho–hyang (K)

Aerial Part

Local Drug Name: Huo–xiang (C), Kak–ko (J), Gwak–hyang (K).

Processing: 1) Eliminate foreign matter, wash clean, and dry in the shade (C, K).

            2) Use in fresh (C, K).

Method of Administration: Oral (decoction: C, J, K).

Folk Medicinal Uses:

            1) Rhinitis and chronic nasosinusitis (C).

            2) Pain of the stomach–qi (C).

            3) Abdominal pain due to cold (C, J).

            4) Vomiting and diarrhea (J, K).

            5) Dyspepsia (J).

            6) Common cold (J).

            7) Head ache (J).

            8) Acute gastritis (K)

Contraindications: Hyperactivity of fire due to yin deficiency.

Scientific Researches:

Chemistry

     1) Essential oils: methyl chavicol, limonene, α–, β–pinene, p–cymene, linalool, l–caryophyllene, β–humulene, γ–cadinene, β–elemene, α–ylangene, β–farnesene, calamene, anisaldehyde, anethole [1].

     2) Flavonoids: acacetin, tilianic, isoagastachoside, gastachin, linarin, agastachoside, daucosterol [2,3].

     3) Terpenes: oleanolic acid, 3–O–acetyloleanolic acid, erythrodiol–3–O–acetate, 3–O–acetyloleanolic aldehyde, dehydroagastol [4–6].

     4) Others: maslinic acid, rosmarinnic acid, β–sitosterol [7].

Pharmacology

         1) Antifungal effect[1].

         2) Antispirochetic effect (Water extract)[8].

Literatures:

[1] Nanjing College of Pharmacy:*"Zhongcaoyao Xue"* Vol. 3, **1980**, 915.

[2] Itokawa, H. et al.:*Chem. Pharm. Bull.* **1981**, 29(6), 1777.

[3] Zakharova, D.I. et al.:*Khim. Prir. Soedin.* **1979**, 5, 642.

[4] Han, D.S. et al.:*Saengyak Hakhoechi,* **1988,** 19(2), 97.

[5] Han, D.S. et al.:*ibid.,* **1987,** 18(1), 50.

[6] Zhou, Z.H. et al.:*Yaoxue Xuebao,* **1991**, 26(12), 906.

[7] Okuda, T. et al.:*Yakugaku Zasshi,* **1986**, 106(12), 1108.

[8] *"Zhongyao Dacidian"*, **1977**, 2711.

[J.X. Guo]

137.   *Ajuga decumbens* Thunb.   (Labiatae)

Jin–gu–cao, Bai–mao–xia–ku–cao (C), Gun–gwut–cho (H), Kiranso (J), Geum–chang–cho (K)

Herb
Local Drug Name: Jin–gu–cao (C), Gun–gwut–cho (H), Ki–ran–so (J), Baek–mo–ha–go–cho (K).
Processing: Eliminate the seeds, dry under the sun (C, H, J).
Method of Administration: Oral (decoction: C, H, J); topical (paste: C).
Folk Medicinal Uses:

    1) Cough (H, J).
    2) Upper respiratory infection (C, H).
    3) Tonsilitis (C, H).
    4) Hepatitis (C, H).
    5) Bronchitis (H, J).
    6) Pneumonitis (H).
    7) Lung abscess (H).
    8) Gastroenteritis (H).
    9) Mastitis (H).
    10) Appendicitis (H).
    11) Hemoptysis (H).
    12) Sputum (J).
    13) Diarrhea (J).
    14) Sore throat (J).
    15) Carbuncle (J).
    16) Hypertension (C).
    17) Boils (C).
    18) Burns (C).
    19) Venomous snake bite (C).
    20) Traumatic hemorrhage (C).

Scientific Researches:
Chemistry
    1) Steroids: ajugalactone [1, 4], ajugasterone C, ecdysterone [2, 3].
    2) Iridoids: decumbeside A, B, C, D [5], 8-acetyl–harpagide [9].
    3) Diterpenoids: ajugamarin A2, B2, F4, G1, H1 [6], ajugacumbin A, B, C, D [7], E, F [9],
                    ajugamarin [9].
Pharmacology
    1) Insect molting inhibition effects (ajugalactone) [1, 2].
    2) Wound healing and skin regeneration (ecdysteroid–rich ext.) [8].

Literatures:
[1] Nakanishi, K. et al.:*J. Amer. Chem. Soc.* **1970,** 92(25), 7512.
[2] Imai, S. et al.:*Japan.* 71 14,665, 20 Apr. 1971.
[3] Imai, S. et al.:*Japan.* 71 28,038, 14 Aug. 1971.
[4] Imai, S. et al.:*Japan.* 73 08,640, 16 Mar. 1973.
[5] Takeda, Y. et al.:*Phytochemistry* **1987,** 26(8), 2303.
[6] Shimomura, H. et al.:*Chem. Pharm. Bull.* **1989,** 37(4), 996.
[7] Min, Z. et al.:*Chem. Pharm. Bull.* **1989,** 37(9), 2505.
[8] Meybeck, A. et al.:*Fr. Demande FR* 2,637,182, 06 Apr. 1990.
[9] Min, Z. et al.:*Chem. Pharm. Bull.* **1990,** 38(11), 3167.

                                              [C.K. Sung]

138.   *Leonurus artemisia*(Lour.) S. Y. Hu (= *L. heterophylla* Sweet) (Labiatae)

Yi–mu–cao (C), Yik–mo–cho (H), Ik–mo–cho (K)

Related plant: *Leonurus sibiricus* L. (= *L. japonicus Houtt.*): Mehajiki (J).

Whole plant (CP)
Local Drug Name: Yi–mu–cao (C), Yik–mo–cho (H), Yaku–mo–so (J); Ik–mo–cho (K).
Processing: Eliminate foreign matter, clean, cut into sections, and dry.
Method of Administration: Oral (decoction: C, H, J, K).
Folk Medicinal Uses:
>   1) Menstrual irregularities, amenorrhea, post–partum, hematoma (C, H, J, K).
>   2) Hypogastric pain (C, H, J, K).
>   3) Nephritis, edema, oliguria, hematuria (C, H, J, K).
>   4) Abscess (C).
>   5) Malarial disease (K).

Contraindications: Yin–deficiency and blood–deficiency.

Fruit (CP)
Local Drug Name: Chong–wei–zi (C), Tsung–wai–gee (H), Ju–i–shi (J); Chung–ul–ja (K).
Processing: (1) Eliminate foreign matter, wash and dry. (2) Stir–fry until the fruits crack open.
Method of Administration: Oral (decoction: C, H, J).
Folk Medicinal Uses:
>   1) Menstrual irregularities, amenorrhea, post–partum. hematoma (C, H, K).
>   2) Conjunctivitis (C, H).
>   3) Prolapse of uterus (C).
>   4) Edema (C).
>   5) Dizziness and headache (C).

Scientific Researches:
Chemistry
>   1) Alkaloids: leuronurine, stachydrine, leonuridine, leonurinine.
>   2) Diterpenes: prehispanolone [1].
>   3) Peptide: cycloleonurinin [4]

Pharmacology
>   1) Uteronic effects [3].
>   2) Inhibitory effects on precancerous mammary nodule formation [2].
>   3) Antagonistic effects on platelet activating factor (prehispanolone) [5].

Literatures:
[1] Hon, P.M. et al.:*Phytochem.* **1991**, 30, 354–6.
[2] Nagasawa, H. et al.:*Shoyakugaku Zasshi* **1990**, 44, 176–8.
[3] Teng, J.M. et al.:*Acta Univ. Med. Tongji* **1992**, 21, 103–5.
[4] Kinoshita, K. et al.:*Chem. Pharm. Bull.* **1991**, 39, 712–5.
[5] Lee, C.M. et al.:*Br. J. Pharmacol.* **1991**, 103, 1719–24.

[P.P.H. But]

139.   *Mentha arvensis* **Linn. var.** *piperascens* **Malinv.**
          (= *M. haplocalyx* Briq.)   (Labiatae)

Bo–he (C), Bok–hor (H), Hakka (J), Bak–ha (K)

Related plant: *Mentha piperita* L.; Seiyo–hakka (J), Yang–bak–ha (K).

Herb   (CP, JP, KP)
Local Drug Name: Bo–he (C), Bok–hor (H), Hak–ka (J), Bak–ha (K).
Processing: Air dry.
Method of Administration: Oral (decoction, powder or ointment: C, H, J, K).
Folk Medicinal Uses:

1) Nausea (H, J, K).
2) Dyspepsia (J, K).
3) Toothache, boils (H, J).
4) Trauma, insect bite (C, J).
5) Common cold, headache (C, H, J).
6) Pharyngitis (C, H, J, K).
7) Chest distention (H).

Scientific Researches:
Chemistry
1) Essential oil: *l*–menthol, methyl acetate, *l*–menthone, 1,8–cineole, β–caryophyllene, *l*–limonene, iso–menthone, germacrene–D, piperitone, pulegone [1].
Pharmacology
1) Analgesic (50% methanol extract) [2].
2) Inhibition of heat and Cu ion induced denaturation of human γ–globulin (methanol extract) [3].
3) Local vasodilation (essential oil) [4].
4) Skin irritant (essential oil) [4].
5) Antispasmodic (essential oil) [5].
6) Cholagogue (*l*–menthol) [6].

Literatures:

[1] Bicchi, C. et al.: *J. High. Resolut. Chromatogr.* **1989**, 12, 316.
[2] Yamahara, J. et al.: *Yakugaku Zasshi* **1980**, 100, 713.
[3] Yamahara, J. et al.: *Shoyakugaku Zasshi* **1981**, 35, 103.
[4] Masaki, Y. et al.: *Nippon Yakurigaku Zasshi*, **1948**, 43, 80.
[5] Giachetti, D. et al.: *Planta Med.* **1988**, 54, 389.
[6] Yamahara, J. et al.: *Shoyakugaku Zasshi* **1985**, 39, 93.

[T. Kimura]

140.   *Perilla frutescens* (**L.**) **Britton var.** *acuta* **Kudo**   (Labiatae)

Zi–su (C), Gee–so (H), Shiso (J), So–yeop (K)

Leaf and Upper stem   (CP, JP, KP)
Local Drug Name: Zisu–ye (C), Gee–so (H), So–yo (J), So–yep (K).
Processing: Air dry (J).
Method of Administration: Oral (decoction: C, H, J, K).
Folk Medicinal Uses:

1) Cough and wheezing (C, H, J, K).
2) Fever (H, J, K).
3) Fish and crab poisoning (C, H, J, K).
4) Dyspnea (C).
5) Phlegm (C).
6) Constipation (C).

7) Common cold with cough and nausea (C).

8) Vomiting in pregnancy (C).

9) Chest distention (H).

Seed

Local Drug Name: Gee–so–gee (H), Shi–so–shi (J), Ja–so–ja (K).

Processing: Air dry.

Method of Administration: Oral (decoction: H, J, K).

Folk Medicinal Uses:

1) Cough (H, J, K).

2) Fever (H, J, K).

3) Phlegm (H).

4) Constipation (K).

Scientific Researches:

Chemistry

1) Essential oil: (–)–perillaldehyde, (+)–limonene, α–, β–pinene, 3–octanol, 1–octen–3–ol, linalool, caryophyllene, α–farnesene, 8–p–menthen–7–ol, ℓ–perillylalcohol [1–3].

2) Anthocyans: cyanin, cyanin–p–cumarate, shisonin [4, 5].

3) Flavonoids: apigenin, luteolin and their glycosides [4, 6, 7].

Pharmacology

1) Antipyretic (decoction) [8].

2) Extension of sleeping (water extract, methanol extract and perillaldehyde) [9, 10].

3) Sedative (water extract) [9, 11].

4) Antiulcer (50% methanol extract) [12].

5) Antifungal (perillaldehyde and citral) [13].

Literatures:

[1] Ito, H.: *Yakugaku Zasshi* **1964**, 84, 1123; **1970**, 90, 883; *Shoyakugaku Zasshi* **1964**, 18, 24, 58; **1966**, 20, 73; **1968**, 22, 151; Nagao, Y. et al.: *Takeda Kenkyusho hokoku* **1974**, 33, 111.

[2] Fujita, Y. et al.: *Nogeikagaku Zasshi* **1970**, 44, 428.

[3] Honda, G. et al.: *Shoyakugaku Zasshi* **1984**, 38, 238; *Phytochemistry* **1986**, 25, 859.

[4] Ishikura, N.: *Agric. Biol. Chem.* **1981**, 45, 1855.

[5] Tamura, H. et al.: *Agric. Biol. Chem.* **1989**, 53, 1971.

[6] Aritomi, M. et al.: *Phytochemistry* **1985**, 24, 2438.

[7] Okuda, T. et al.: *Yakugaku Zasshi* **1986**, 106, 1108.

[8] Kondo, T. : *Nippon Yakubutsugaku Zasshi* **1928**, 7, 296.

[9] Sugaya, A. et al.: *Yakugaku Zasshi* **1981**, 101, 642; Sugaya, A. et al.: *Planta Med.* **1983**, 47, 59.

[10] Honda, G. et al.: *Chem. Pharm. Bull.* **1986**, 34, 1672; **1988**, 36, 3153.

[11] Honda, G. et al.: *Chem. Pharm. Bull.* **1986**, 34, 1672.

[12] Yamahara, J. et al.: *Wakan Iyaku Gakkaishi* **1987**, 4, 100.

[13] Honda, G. et al.: *Shoyakugaku Zasshi* **1984**, 38, 127.

[T. Kimura]

141.   *Prunella vulgaris* **Linn.**   (Labiatae)

(= *P. vulgaris* var. *asiatica* Hara, *P. vulgaris* var. *lilacina* Nakai)

Xia–ku–cao (C), Har–fu–cho (H), Utsubogusa (J), Ggul–pul (K).

Inflorescence   (CP, JP, KP)

Local Drug Name: Xia–ku–cao (C), Har–fu–cho (H), Ka–go–so (J), Ha–go–cho (K).
Processing: Dry under the sun.
Method of Administration: Oral (decoction: C, H, J, K).
Folk Medicinal Uses:

         1) Edema (C, J, K).
         2) Nephritis (J, K).
         3) Eyediseases, eye pain at night (C, H).
         4) Headache and dizziness (C).
         5) Scropfula, goitre, mastitis with swelling and pain, hyperplasia of breast (C, H, K).
         6) Hypertension (C).
         7) Hepatitis (H).
         8) Leukorrhea (H).
         9) Tuberculosis (H).
         10) Mammary cancer (H).

Scientific Researches:
  Chemistry
   1) Triterpenoids: ursolic acid [1].
  Pharmacology
   1) Diuretic [2].
   2) Antileukemia, antitumor [3].

Literatures:
[1] Kojima, H. et al.: *Phytochem.* **1986**, 25, 729.
[2] Haginiwa, T. et al.: *Shoyakugaku Zasshi* **1963**, 17, 6.
[3] Lee, K. H., et al.: *Planta Med.* **1988**, 54, 308.

                                        [T. Kimura]

142.   *Schizonepeta tenuifolia* **Briquet**   (Labiatae)

Jing–jie (C), Ging–gie (H), Keigai (J), Hyung–gae (K)

Inflorescence   (CP, JP, KP)

Local Drug Name: Jing–jie (C), Ging–gie (H), Kei–gai (J), Hyung–gae (K).
Processing: 1) Dry under the sun. 2) Cut and carbonize until the surface turned dark brown (C).
            3) Cut and carbonize the fruit spike until the surface turned charred black (C).
Method of Administration: Oral (decoction: C, H, J, K).
Folk Medicinal Uses:

             1) Pharyngitis (H, J, K).
             2) Rhinitis (J).
             3) Suppurative inflammation (J).
             4) Common cold, fever, headache (C, H).
             5) Measles rubella (C).
             6) Sores at early stage (C).
             7) Hematochezia, abnormal uterine bleeding, fainting after delivery due to excessive

bleeding (C, H).
8) Hematemesis (H).
9) Epistaxis (H).
10) Tinea, scrofula (H).
11) Palsy (K).
12) Vertigo (K).

Scientific Researches:
Chemistry
1) Monoterpenoids:l–pulegone, d–menthone, l–isomenthone, d–limonene, isopulegone, α–, β–pinene, camphene, piperitone, piperitenone [1], schizo–nepetosides A, B, C, D, E [2].
2) Sesquiterpenoids: caryophyllene, β–elemene, β–humulene [1].
3) Aliphatic compounds: 3–octanone, 3–octanol, 1–octen–3–ol [1].
4) Flavonoids: diosmetin, hesperetin, luteolin [2].
Pharmacology
1) Antiinflammatory [4].

Literatures:
[1] Murayama, Y. et al.:*Yakugaku Zasshi* **1921**, 41, 869; Fujita, S. et al:*ibid.* **1973**, 93, 1622.
[2] Sasaki, H. et al.:*Chem. Pharm. Bull.* **1981**, 29, 1636, **1986**, 34, 3097; Oshima, Y. et al.:*Planta Med.* **1989**, 55, 179.
[3] Fujita, S. et al.:*Yakugaku Zasshi* **1987**, 107, 959.
[4] Yamahara, J. et al.:*Yakugaku Zasshi* **1980**, 100, 713.

[T. Kimura]

143.   *Scutellaria baicalensis* **Georgi**   (Labiatae)

Huang–qin (C), Wong–sum (H), Koganebana (J), Hwang–geum (K).

Root   (CP, JP, KP)
Local Drug Name: Huang–qin(C), Wong–sum (H), O–gon(J), Hwang–geum.
Processing: 1) Boil for 10 min. or steam for 30 min. and dry in the shade. (C).
                 2) Stir–fry with wine until dryness (C).
Method of Administration: Oral (decoction: C, H, J, K).
Folk Medicinal Uses:
1) Anorexia (C, J).
2) Diarrhea (C, H, J).
3) Fever (C, H, J, K).
4) Hypertension (J).
5) Discomfort in the chest, nausea and vomiting in epidemic febric diseases caused by damp–heat or summer heat (C).
6) Feeling of stuffness in the abdomen (C).
7) Jaundice (C, H, J, K).
8) Pleurisy (K).
9) Common cold (J, K), Bronchitis (J), Cough due to heat in the lung (C).
10) Inflammation (K).
11) Hematemesis, epistaxis, uterine hemorrhage (H). Spitting of blood and epistaxis due to heat in blood (C).
12) Conjunctivitis (H).
13) Furunculosis (H).
14) Carbuncles and sores (C).

15) Threatend abortion (C).

Scientific Researches:
Chemistry
  1) Flavonoids: wogonin, baicalin, baicalein, scutellarin, skullcapflavone I , II [1].
Pharmacology
  1) Choleretic (methanol extract) [2].
  2) Laxative (ethanol extract) [3].
  3) Against arteriosclerosis [4].
  4) Antiallergic (water or ethanol extract) [5].
  5) Antiinflammation (70% methanol or water extract, baicalin, baicalein) [6].
  6) Antibacterial (ether extract) [7].
  7) Antidotes (baicalin, baicalein) [8].
  8) Hyperlipemia lowering (flavonoids) [9].

Literatures:
  [1] Popova, T. P. et al.:*Khim. Prir. Soedin.* **1973**, 729; *Farm. Zh. (Kiev)* **1974**, 29, 91; Takido, M. et al.:
     Yakugaku Zasshi **1975**, 95, 108, **1979**, 99, 443; Horie, T. et al.:*Bull. Chim. Soc. Japan* **1979**, 52,
     2950; Takagi, S. et al.:*Yakugaku Zasshi* **1980**, 100, 1220; **1981**, 101, 899; Tomimori, T. et al.:*ibid.*
     1982, 102, 388; **1983**, 103, 607, **1984**, 104, 524, 529; *Shoyakugaku Zasshi* **1988**, 42, 216.
  [2] Miura, M. et al.:*Yakugaku Zasshi* **1987**, 107, 992.
  [3] Kumasaki, H.: *Gifu Ikadaigaku Kiyo* **1958**, 6, 372.
  [4] Aonuma, S.:*Yakugaku Zasshi* **1957**, 77, 1303.
  [5] Koda, A. et al.:*Arerugii* **1972**, 21, 346: *Nippon Yakurigaku Zasshi* **1982**, 80, 31; **1970**, 66, 194, 237;
     1970, 66, 471; Nagai, H. et al.:*Japan. J. Pharmacol.* **1975**, 25, 763.
  [6] Kubo, M. et al.:*Chem. Pharm. Bull.* **1984**, 32, 2724.
  [7] Kubo, M., et al.:*Planta Med.* **1981**, 43, 194.
  [8] Kuboki, N. et al.:*Yakkyoku* **1962**, 13, 1011, **1963**, 14, 968.
  [9] Kimura, Y. et al.:*Chem. Pharm. Bull.* **1981**, 29, 2308; **1982**, 30, 219.

[T. Kimura]

144.   *Stachys sieboldii* **Miq.**   (Labiatae)

Gan–lu–zi (C), Chorogi (J), Mong–ul–su–so (K)

Related plant: *Stachys geobombycis* (H).

Rhyzome
  Local Drug Name: Gan–lu–zi (C), So–seki–san, Kan–ro–shi (J), Gwang–yeop–su–so (K).
  Processing: Dry under the sun (J, K).
  Method of Administration: Oral (decoction: C, J, K).
  Folk Medicinal Uses:
                1) Pain (J, K).
                2) Blood stasis (J, K).
                3) Jaundice (C).
                4) Urethritis (C).
                5) Cold caused by wind and heat (C).
                6) Snake and insect bite (C).

Scientific Researches:
Chemistry

1) Phenethyl alcohol glycosides: stachysoside B, C [1].
2) Flavonoid glycosides: isoscutellarein 4'-methylester 7-O-β-(6"-O-acetyl-2"-allosyl) glucoside [2], acteoside.
3) Iridoids: stachsoside A [3].
Pharmacology
1) Inhibition of hyaluronidase (flavonoid glycosides) [2].

Literatures:
[1] Nishimura, H. et al.:*Phytochem.* **1991,** 30(3), 965.
[2] Takeda, Y. et al.:*Yakugaku Zasshi* **1985,** 105(10), 955.
[3] Miyase, T. et al.: *Yakugaku Zasshi* **1990,** 110(9), 652.

[C.K. Sung]

145.　　　　　*Datura metel* **L.** (= *D. alba* Nees)　　(Solanaceae)

Bai–man–tuo–luo (C), Lou–yeung–fa (H), Chosen–asagao (J), Hin–dok–mal–pul (K)

Flower (CP)
Local Drug Name: Yang–jin–hua (C), Lou–yeung–fa (H), Yo–kin–ka (J), Yang–geum–hwa (K).
Processing: Dry under the sun.
Method of Administration: Oral (decoction or smoking: C, H).
Folk Medicinal Uses:
　　　　1) Bronchial asthma (C, H, J).
　　　　2) Chronic bronchitis (C, J).
　　　　3) Epigastric pain, toothache, rheumatalgia (C, J).
　　　　4) Traumatic injury (C).
　　　　5) Epilepsy (C).
　　　　6) Cough (C).
　　　　7) Chronic infantile convulsion (C).
　　　　8) Anaesthesia for surgical operation (C).
Contraindications: Debility.
Side Effects: Dizziness, drowsiness, respiratory failure, death.

Fruit
Local Drug Name: Man–tuo–luo (C), Man–da–ra (K).
Method of Administration: Oral or topical (decoction or tincture: C, K).
Folk Medicinal Uses:
　　　　1) Asthma (C).
　　　　2) Epilepsy (C, K).
　　　　3) Rheumatalgia (C).
　　　　4) Traumatic injury (C).
　　　　5) Prolapse of rectum (C).
　　　　6) Diarrhea (C).
　　　　7) Schizophrenia (K).
Contraindications: Debility.
Side Effects: Dizziness, drowsiness, respiratory failure, death.

Seed
Local Drug Name: Man–da–ra–shi (J).
Method of Administration: Oral or topical (decoction or tincture: J).
Folk Medicinal Uses: 1) Asthma (J).

Root

Local Drug Name: Man–tuo–luo–gen (C), Man–da–ra–geun (K).
Method of Administration: Topical (decoction: C).
Folk Medicinal Uses:
        1) Scabies (C).
        2) Tinea (C).
        3) Traumatic injury (C).
Contraindications: Cold disease.
Side Effects: Dizziness, drowsiness, respiratory failure, death.

Scientific Researches:
Chemistry
  1) Alkaloids: *l*–hyoscyamine, scopolamine [11].
  2) Withametelin B, 12–deoxywithastramonolide, physalindicanol A (leaf) [2], withanolides A, B, C [12].
  3) Daturametelin [4,8,9], daturilin [8].
  4) Daturilinol [5], secowithametelin [6].
  5) Glucose esters [7], *p*–hydroxycinnamic acid amide of tyramine, lycium susbstance B [12].
Pharmacology
  1) Mutagenicity [1].
  2) Spasmogenic effect (root) [3].

Literatures:

[1] Yin, X.J. et at.:*Mutation Res.* **1991**, 260, 73–82.
[2] Gupta, M. et al.:*J. Nat. Prod.* **1991**, 54, 599–602.
[3] Nanda Kumar, N.V. et al.:*Phytother. Res.* **1991**, 5, 41–2.
[4] Shingu, K. et al.:*Chem. Pharm. Bull.* **1990**, 38, 2866–7.
[5] Mahmood, T. et al.:*Heterocycles* **1988**, 27, 101–3.
[6] Kundu, S. et al.:*Phytochem.* **1989**, 28, 1769–70.
[7] King, R.R. et al.:*Phytochem.* **1988**, 27, 3761–3.
[8] Mahmood, T. et al.:*Planta Med.* **1988**, 54, 468.
[9] Mahmood, T. et al.:*J. Indian Chem. Soc.* **1988**, 65, 526–7.
[10] Shingu, K. et al.:*Chem. Pharm. Bull.* **1987**, 35, 4352–61.
[11] Kundu, D. et al.:*Indian J. Pharmacol.* **1991**, 23(3), 177–8.
[12] Gupta, M. et al.:*Phytochem.* **1992**, 31, 2423–5.

                                              [P.P.H. But]

146.   *Lycium chinense* Mill., *L. barbarum* L.   (Solanaceae)

                Gou–qi (C), Gou–gay (H), Kuko (J), Gu–gi–ja–na–mu (K)

Fruit (CP)

Local Drug Name: Gou–qi–zi (C), Gou–gay–gee (H), Ku–ko–shi (J), Gu–gi–ja (K).
Processing: Collect the mature fruit and dry.
Method of Administration: Oral (decoction, spirit or fresh: C, H, J, K).
Folk Medicinal Uses:
        1) Lumbago (C, H, J).
        2) Dizziness (C).
        3) Diabetes (C, J).
        4) Spermatorrhea (C, H, J).
        5) Exhaustive coughing (C, K).
        6) Debility (K).

Contraindications: Spleen–deficiency, diarrhea.

Leaf
Local Drug Name: Gou–qi–ye (C), Gou–gay–yip (H), Ku–ko–yo (J), Gu–gi–yeop (K).
Method of Administration: Oral (decoction or tea: C, J).
Folk Medicinal Uses:
          1) Consumptive fever (C, H).
          2) Conjunctivitis (C, H).
          3) Abscess (C).
          4) Leukorrhea (C).
          5) Night–blindness (C, H).
          6) Hemorrhoid (C).
          7) Hypertension (J).
Contraindications: Milk.

Root bark (CP)
Local Drug Name: Di–gu–pi (C), Day–gwut–pay (H), Ji–kop–pi (J), Ji–gol–pi (K).
Processing: Eliminate foreign matter, wash clean, dry under the sun.
Method of Administration: Oral (decoction: C, H, J).
Folk Medicinal Uses:
          1) Consumptive fever (C, H, J).
          2) Hemorrhinia (C).
          3) Diabetes (C, J).
          4) Hypertension (C, H, J).
          5) Abscess (C, H).
          6) Hematuria (C, H).
          7) Edema, oliguria (C, H, J).
          8) Rheumatalgia (C, H).
          9) Cough, hemoptysis and epistaxis due to lung–heat (C).
Contraindications: Spleen– and Stomach–deficiency.

Scientific Researches:
Chemistry
  1) Betaine, zeaxanthine, physalein, carotene, thiamine, riboflavine, nicotinic acid, ascorbic acid,
          cholesterol, campesterol, stigmasterol, sitosterol, tricosane, tritriacontane [16].
  2) Hyoscyamine, atropine [3].
  3) Scopoletin, aurantiamide acetate, (S)–9–hydroxy–E–10, Z–12–octa–decadienoic acid (=α–dimorphecolic
          acid), (S)–9–hydroxy–E–10,Z–12–Z–15–octadecatrienoic acid [5].
  4) Vanillic acid, salicylic acid [6].
  5) Polysacchrides [7, 18].
  6) Peptides: lyciumins A–D [11, 20].
  7) Glycosides: lyciumosdies I–III, and others [11].
  8) Amino acids: proline, taurine, γ–aminobutanoic acid [23].
Pharmacology
  1) Immunopotentiating effect [1, 2, 7, 8, 10, 13, 18].
  2) Hematopoietic effect [1].
  3) Antilipemic, liver–protective and lipotropic effects [1].
  4) Hypoglycemic effect [1].
  5) Stimulate neurite outgrowth of brain cells and increased pyruvate dehydrogenase complex in chicken
          embryo brain cells [4].
  6) Inhibitory effects on rennin and angiotensin converting enzyme [5, 20, 21].
  7) LD50 of methanol–water extract of stem >1 g/kg in mice [9].
  8) Anti–peroxidation and antioxidant effects [12, 19].

9) Glucosidase inhibitory effects [14].
10) Enhancing cytotoxic effects [22].

Literatures:

[1] Ye, S.B. In: Chang HM, But PPH (Eds.): *Pharmacology and Applications of Chinese Materia Medica*
   World Scientific, Singapore, Vol 2, **1987,** 852.

[2] Kim, M.S. et al.: *Korean J. Pharmacog.* **1988**, 19, 193–200.

[3] Harsh, M.L.: *Curr. Sci.* **1989**, 58, 817–8.

[4] Park, M.J. et al.: *Korean J. Pharmacog.* **1989**, 20, 32–6.

[5] Morota, T. et al.: *Shoyakugaku Zasshi* **1987**, 41, 169–73.

[6] Zhao, Q.C. et al.: *Zhongcaoyao* **1987**, 18, 104,133.

[7] Geng, C.S. et al.: *Zhongcaoyao* **1988**, 19, 313–5.

[8] Zhang, Y.X. et al.: *Zhongguo Yaolixue Yu Dulixue Zazhi* **1989**, 3, 169–74.

[9] Nakanishi, K.: *Chem. Pharm. Bull.* **1965**, 13, 882–90.

[10] Qian, Y.K. et al.: *Beijing Yike Daxue Xuebao* **1989**, 21, 31–2.

[11] Yahara, S. et al.: *Chem. Pharm. Bull.* **1993**, 41, 703–9.

[12] Zhang, X. et al.: *Zhongyuo Zhongyao Zazhi* **1993**, 18(2), 110–2.

[13] Cao, G.W. et al.: *Zhonghua Weishengwuxue He Mianyixue Zazhi* **1992**, 12(6), 390–2.

[14] Yamada, H. et al.: *Jpn. Kokai Tokkyo Koho JP 04, 208,264 [92, 208,264]* **1992**.

[15] Harsh, M.L. et al.: *Geobios* **1988**, 15, 32–5.

[16] MAldoni, B.E. et al.: *Rev. Latinoam. Quim.* **1988**, 19, 15–7.

[17] Baghdadi, H.H. et al.: *Alexandria J. Pharm. Sci.* **1988**, 2, 73–6.

[18] Geng, C.S. et al.: *Zhongguo Yaolixue Yu Dulixue Zazhi* **1989**, 3, 175–9.

[19] Zhan, H. et al.: *Zhongguo Yaolixue Yu Dulixue Zazhi* **1989**, 3, 163–8.

[20] Yahara, S. et al.: *Tetrahedron Lett.* **1989**, 30, 6041–2.

[21] Yahara, S. et al.: *Tennen Yuki Kagobutsu Toronkai Koen Yoshishu* **1989**, 31, 633–40.

[22] Wang, B.K. et al.: *Zhongguo Yaolixue Yu Dulixue Zazhi* **1990**, 4, 39–43.

[23] Chen, S.Q. et al.: *Zhongguo Yaoke Daxue Xuebao* **1991**, 22, 53–5.

[P.P.H. But]

147.   *Solanum nigrum* **L.**   (Solanaceae)

Long–kui (C), Lung–kwai (H), Inuhozuki (J), Gga–ma–jung (K)

Herb
Local Drug Name: Long–kui (C), Lung–kwai (H), Ryu–ki (J), Yong–gyu (K).
Processing: 1) Wash clean, and dry (C, K). 2) Use in fresh (C, K).
Method of Administration: Oral (decoction: C, H) or topical (fresh herb: C, H, J).
Folk Medicinal Uses:
        1) Chronic tracheitis (C, J).
        2) Carcinomatosis (C, H).
        3) Eczematoid dermatitis (C, H, J, K).
        4) Urticaria (C, H).
        5) Snake–bite (C, H).
        6) Chronic bronchitis (H).
        7) Colds, fever, sore throat (H).
        8) Urinary tract infection (H).
        9) Acute nephritis (H, J).
        10) Mastitis (H).
        11) Bruise (J).
        12) Abcess (J).

13) Uterus cancer (K).
14) Tonsillitis (K).
15) Erysipelas (K).
16) Acute gastritis (K).
Side Effects: Fatigue, thirsty, laryngoxerosis, dizziness, dim eyesight and even to coma.

Scientific Researches:
Chemistry
1) Alkaloids: solanine, solasomine, solamargine, solavilline, solasodamine, solamaviol, solasodine, 23–O–acetyl–12 β–hydroxysolasodine, 12 β,27–dihydroxysolasodine.
2) Saponins: uttronin B, 26–O–(β–D–glucopyranosyl)–22–methoxy–25–D–5 α–furost–3β, 26–diol–3–O–β–lycotetraoside [1–3,8]. Dopsgenin, tigogenin, desgalactotigonin [4].
3) Flavonoids: quercetin 3–O–(2–α–rhamnosyl)–β–glucosyl–(1⁻6)–β–glactoside, quercetin–3–O–α–rhamnosyl–(1⁻2)–β–galactoside, quercetin 3–glucosyl–(1⁻6)–galactoside, quercetin 3–gentiobioside, querectin 3–galasctoside, querectin 3–glucoside [5].
Pharmacology
1) Antihypertensive effect (Water or alcohol extract) [6].
2) Increasing activities of some liver drug metabolizeing enzymes [7].
3) Anti–inflammatory effect and antishock (solasodine) [8].
4) Antiallergic effect (solanine) [8].
5) Antipyretic analgesic effect (solasodine) [8].
6) Expectorant and antitussive effect (alcohol extract) [8].
7) Antibiosis (Water extract, mixture of solasonine and solamargine) [8].
8) Anticancer effect (solanine) [8].
9) Antivenene effect (water ectract) [8].
10) Anticholinesterase effect (solanine) [8].
11) Leuogenic effect (solanine) [8].
12) Increasing blood surgar (solanine) [8].
13) Cordial effect (solanine) [8].

Literatures:

[1] Sharna, S.C. et al.:*Pharmazie* **1982**, 37(12), 870.
[2] Doepke, W. et al.:*Z. Chem.* **1988**, 28(5), 185.
[3] Yoshida, K. et al.:*Chem. Pharm. Bull.* **1987**, 35(4), 1645.
[4] Saijo, R. et al.: *Yakugaku Zasshi* **1982**,102(3), 300.
[5] Nawwar, M.A.M. et al.:*Phytochem.* **1989**, 28(6), 1755.
[6] Ye, J.R. et al.: *Zhongyao Tongbao,* **1984**, 9(1), 35.
[7] Moundipa, P. F. et al.:*Br. J. Nutr.* **1991**, 65(1), 81.
[8] Wnag, Y.S. et al.: *"Zhongyao Yaoli Yu Yingyang",* **1983**, 299.

[J.X. Guo]

148.   *Rehmannia glutinosa* **Libosch.**   (Scrophulariaceae)
(= *R. glutinosa* Libosch. var.*purpurea* Makino)

Di–huang (C), Day–wong (H), Akayajio (J), Ji–hwang

Related plant: *Rehmannia glutinosa* Libosch. f. *huichingensis* Hsiao: Kaikei–jio (J)

Root (CP, JP, KP)
Local Drug Name: Di–huang (C), Day–wong (H), Ji–o (J), Ji–hwang (K).
Processing: 1) Dry under the sun (Sound–day–wong; H, Sho–jio; J).

2) Boil or steam with wine then dry under the sun (Suk–day–wong; H, Juku–jio; J).
Method of Administration: Oral (decoction: C, H, J, K).
  Folk Medicinal Uses (Process 1):
            1) Impairment of yin in febrile diseases marked by deep red tongue and thirst (C).
            2) Spitting of blood (C).
            3) Bleeding, spitting of blood, hematemesis, epistaxis (C, H, J, K).
            4) Anorexia (H, J)
            5) Menstrual disorder (C, H, J).
            6) Skin eruption and maculation (C).
            7) Constipation (H).
            8) Traumatic injury. Apply fresh juice for trauma (H, J, K).
  Folk Medicinal Uses (Process 2):
            1) Anemia, weakness (J, K).
            2) Irregular menses (C, H).
            3) Diabetes caused by internal heat (C).
            4) Cough, sore throat (C, H).
            5) Lumbago (H).
            6) Spermatorrhea (C, H, J).
            7) Deafness, dizzines, tinnitus (C, H).
            8) Deficiency of yin of the liver and the kidney marked by aching and limpness of the
            loins and knees, night sweating and seminal emission (C).
            9) Cardiac palpitation (C).
            10) Premature greying of beard and hair (C).

Scientific Researches:
  Chemistry
    1) Iridoids: Catalpol, rehmanoside A, B, C, D, cerebroside, acteoside, purpureaside, jionoside A, B.
    2) Sugars: stachyose, mannitol [1,2].
  Pharmacology
    1) Blood sugar lowering (water, ethanol and methanol extract) [1,3].
    2) Coagulation inhibiting (70% methanol extract) [4].
    3) Protease activity acceleration (ethanol extract) [5].
    4) Laxative and diuretic (catalpol) [6].
    5) Immunosupressing (acteoside, purpureaside, jionoside A, B) [7].

Literatures:
[1] Kitagawa, I. et al.:*Yakugaku Zasshi* **1971**, 91, 593; Oshio, H. et al.:*Phytochem.* **1982**, 21, 133;
   Kitagawa, I. et al.:*Chem. Pharm. Bull.* **1986**, 34, 1399, 1403, 2294; Oshio, H. et al.:*Shoyakugaku
   Zasshi* **1981**, 35, 291.
[2] Tomoda, M. et al.:*Chem. Pharm. Bull.* **1971**, 19, 1455, 2411.
[3] Kim, K.: *Chosen Igakkai Zasshi***1932**, 22, 131; Bin, H.:*Nippon Yakubutsugaku Zasshi***1930,** 11, 22,
   181.
[4] Matsuda, H. et al.:*Shoyakugaku Zasshi* **1986**, 40, 182.
[5] Huang, A. et al.:*Wakan Iyaku Gakkaishi***1988**, 5, 191; **1989**, 6, 20, 58.
[6] Suzuki, Y.:*Nippon Yakurigaku Zasshi***1964**, 60, 550.
[7] Sasaki, H. et al.:*Planta Med.* **1989**, 55, 458.

                                                                            [T. Kimura]

149.   *Catalpa ovata* **G. Don**   (Bignoniaceae)

Zi (C), Gee–sue (H), Kisasage (J), Gae–o–dong (K).

Related plant: *Catalpa bungei* C. A. Mey.: Qiu–shu (C), To–kisasage (J).

Fruit   (JP, KP)
  Local Drug Name: Zi–shi (C), Gee–bak–pay (H), Kisasage (J), Ja–sil (K).
  Processing: Air dry.
  Method of Administration: Oral or topical (decoction: C, H, J, K).
  Folk Medicinal Uses:
                    1) Edema (C, J, K).
                    2) Nephritis (C, J, K).
                    3) Cystitis (C).
                    4) Ascites due to cirrhosis (C).
                    5) Eczema (C).
                    6) Jaundice (H).
                    7) Nausea (H).
                    8) Pruritus (H).
                    9) Boils (H).
                    10) Leprosy (K).
                    11) Gastric cancer (K).
                    12) Acute gastritis (K).

Scientific Researches:
  Chemistry
    1) Iridoids: catalposide, catalpa lactone [1].
  Pharmacology
    1) Diuretic (catalposide) [2].

Literatures:
  [1] Lunn, W. H., et al.: *Canad. J. Chem.* **1962**, 40, 104; Bobbitt, J. B. et al.: *Tetrahedron Letters* **1962**,
      321; *J. Org. Chem.* **1967**, 32, 1459; Kimura, K. et al.: *Yakugaku Zasshi* **1963**, 83, 635; Inouye,
      H. et al.: *Chem. Pharm. Bull.* **1967**, 15, 786.
  [2] Suzuki, Y.: *Nippon Yakurigaku Zasshi* **1964**, 60, 544, 550; **1968**, 64, 93; Tsurumi, S. et al.: *Gifu*
      Daigaku Igakubu Kiyo **1963**, 11, 129; Haginiwa, T. et al.: *Shoyakugaku Zasshi* **1963**, 17, 6.

[T. Kimura]

150.   *Sesamum indicum* **L.**   (Pedaliaceae)

Hei–zhi–ma (C), Gee–ma (H), Goma (J), Cham–ggae (K)

Seed (CP)
  Local Drug Name: Hei–zhi–ma (C), Hak–gee–ma (H), Go–ma–shi, Koku–shi–ma (J), Ho–ma (K).
  Method of Administration: Oral (decoction or whole: C, H, J, K).
  Folk Medicinal Uses:
                    1) Rheumatalgia (C).
                    2) Constipation (C, H, J, K).
                    3) Premature white hair (C, H).
                    4) Paralysis (C).
                    5) Weakness (J).

6) Hyperacidity (K).

7) Pneumonia (K).

Seed oil (JP)

Local Drug Name: Goma–abura (J), Cham–gi–reum (K).

Method of Administration: Base for ointment (J). Oral (fresh: K).

Folk Medicinal Uses:

  1) Poisoning (K).

  2) Scabies (K).

  3) Eczema (K).

Leaf

Local Drug Name: Hu–ma–ye (C), Ho–ma–yeop (K).

Method of Administration: Oral (decoction: C).

Folk Medicinal Uses:

  1) Constipation (C).

  2) Hematuria (C).

  3) Rheumatalgia (C).

Stem

Local Drug Name: Ma–jie (C), Ma–gal (K).

Method of Administration: Oral (decoction: C).

Folk Medicinal Uses:

  1) Infantile asthma (C).

  2) Edema (C).

Scientific Researches

Chemistry

  1) Lignanes: sesamin, sesamolin, sesamol (seed) [1].

  2) Pedaliin (leaf) [3].

  3) Octanal, 2,4–undecadienal, 3–methylbutanal, 2,3–dimethylpyrazine, 2,5–dimethylpyrazine, 2–ethyl–
      pyrazine, 2,5–diethylpyrazine, 2–furfuryl alcohol [4].

Pharmacology

  1) Antioxidants [1].

  2) Anticancer [2].

Literatures:

[1] Larson, R.A.: *Phytochem.* **1988**, 27, 969–78.

[2] Jain, S.C. et al.: *J. Res. Ayurveda Siddha.* **1987**, 8, 70–3.

[3] Morita, N.: *Chem. Pharm. Bull.* **1960**, 8, 59–65.

[4] El–Sawy, A.A.: *Grasas Aceites (Seville)* **1988**, 39, 160–2.

[P.P.H. But]

151.   *Plantago asiatica* **Linn.**   (Plantaginaceae)

Che–qian (C), Che–chin (H), Obako (J), Jil–gyung–i (K)

Related plants: *Plantago depressa* Willd.; *P. major* L.

Seed (CP, JP, KP)

Local Drug Name: Che–qian–zi (C), Che–chin–gee (H), Sha–zen–shi (J), Cha–jeon–ja (K).

Processing: 1) Dry ander the sun. 2) Stir–fry with salt water (C).

Method of Administration: Oral (decoction: C, H, J, K).
Folk Medicinal Uses:

1) Cough (C, H, J, K). Cough caused by phlegm–heat (C).
2) Phlegm (H).
3) Diarrhea (C, H, J, K). Diarrhea caused by summer–damp (C).
4) Cystitis (C, J).
5) Oliguria, dysuria, hematuria (H, J).
6) Leukorrhea (H), menstrual disorder (K).
7) Jaundice (H).
8) Edema (C).
9) Inflammation of eyes (C). Conjunctivitis (H), trachoma, stye (K).

Whole herb (CP, JP)
Local Drug Name: Che–qian–cao (C), Che–chin–cho (H), Sha–zen–so (J), Cha–jeon–cho (K).
Processing: Dry under the sun.
Method of Administration: Oral (decoction: C, H, J, K).
Folk Medicinal Uses:

1) Cystitis (C, J).
2) Asthma (J).
3) Articular pain (J, K).
4) Eye congestion (J, K).
5) Gastritis (J, K).
6) Diarrhea (C, K), dysentery (H).
7) Gonorrhea (K).
8) Edema with oliguria, dysuria (C, H).
9) Cough, pharyngitis (C, H).
10) Spitting of blood, epistaxis (C, H).
11) Carbuncles and sores (C).
12) Jaundice, hepatitis (H).
13) Hematuria (H).
14) Urinary tract calculus (H).
15) Leukorrhea (H).

Scientific Researches:
Chemistry
1) Polysaccharide: Plantasan, plantago–mucilage A [1].
2) Flavonoids: plantagoside [2], plantaginin, homoplantaginin [3].
3) Iridoids: aucubin [4].
4) Triterpenes [11].
Pharmacology
1) Choleretic (methanol extract) [5].
2) Intestine blood flow increasing (decoction) [6].
3) Inhibition of heat and Cu ion induced denaturation of humanγ–globulin (50% methanol extract) [7].
4) Blood sugar lowering (plantago–mucilage A) [8].
5) Complement activation inhibition (plantago–mucilage A) [9].
6) Antitussive and expectorant (plantagin) [10].

Literatures:
[1] Tomoda, M., et al.: *Chem. Pharm. Bull.* **1973**, **21**, 989; **1984**, 32, 2182.
[2] Endo, T., et al.: *Chem. Pharm. Bull.* **1981**, 29, 1000.
[3] Nakaoki, T., et al.: *Yakugaku Zasshi* **1961**, 81, 1697; Aritomi, M.: *Chem. Pharm. Bull.* **1967**, 15, 432.
[4] Nishibe, S., et al.: *Yakugaku Zasshi* **1990**, 110, 453; Oshio, H., et al.: *Planta Med.* **1981**, 43, 204.
[5] Miura, M., et al.: *Yakugaku Zasshi* **1987**, 107, 992.

[6] Ohmoto, T., et al.:*Shoyakugaku Zasshi* **1985**, 39, 28.

[7] Yamahara, J., et al.:*Shoyakugaku Zasshi* **1981**, 35, 103.

[8] Tomoda, M., et al.: *Planta Med.* **1987**, 53, 8.

[9] Yamada, H., et al.: *Carbohydr. Res.* **1986**, 156, 137.

[10] Takahashi, T.: *Okayama Igakkai Zasshi* **1922**, 34, 59.

[11] Torigoe, Y.: *Yakugaku Zasshi* **1965**, 85, 176.

[T. Kimura]

152.   *Sambucus sieboldiana* **Blume**   (Caprifoliaceae)

Mao–jie–gu–mu (C), Niwatoko (J), Deot–na–mu (K)

Related plant: *Sambucus williamsii* Hance: Jie–gu–mu (C).

Stem
Local Drug Name: Jie–gu–mu (C), Sek–kotsu–boku (J), Jeop–gol–mok (K).
Processing: Dry under the sun (J, K).
Method of Administration: Oral (decoction: C, J, K); topical (decoction or powder: C); or bathing (J).
Folk Medicinal Uses:
    1) Dropsy caused by nephritis (C, J, K).
    2) Hypoacidity (K).
    3) Fever (K).
    4) Gastrectasis (K).
    5) Nocturia (J).
    6) Articular pain (J).
    7) Fracture, sprain (J).
    8) Rheumatic pain (C).
    9) Injury due to fall (C).
    10) Traumatic bleeding (C).
Contraindications: In pregnancy.
Side Effects: Vomitting.

Flower
Local Drug Name: Sek–kotsu–boku–ka (J), Jeop–gol–mok–hwa (K).
Processing: Dry under the sun (J, K).
Method of Administration: Oral (decoction: J, K).
Folk Medicinal Uses:
    1) Rheumatism (K).
    2) Comon cold (J).

Leaf
Local drug name: Sek–kotsu–boku–yo (J).
Processing: Dry under the sun (J).
Method of Administration: Oral(decoction: J).
Folk Medicinal Uses:
    1) Constipation (J).
    2) Nocturia (J).

Scientific Researches:
Chemistry
 1) Essential oils: pyranoid, furanoid, linalool oxides, hotrienol, hexenol, hexanol, benzaldehyde,

citronellol, geraniol [1].
2) Lectins: S. sieboldiana agglutinin (SSA) [2].

Literatures:
[1] Eberhardt, R., Pfannhauser, W.:*Mikrochim. Acta* **1985,** 1(1–2), 55.
[2] Tazaki, K., Shibuya, N.:*Plant Cell Physiol.* **1989,** 30(6), 899.

[C.K. Sung]

153.   *Adenophora triphylla* var. *japonica* Hara   (Campanulaceae)

Tsuriganeninjin (J), Jan–dae (K)

Related plant:*Adenophora tetraphylla*(Thunb) Fisch.: Lun–ye–shashen (C), Sha–sum (H).

Root
 Local Drug Name: Sha–shen (C), Sha–sum (H), Sha–jin (J), Sa–sam (K).
 Processing: Dry under the sun (C, H, J, K).
 Method of Administration: Oral (deccoction: C, H, J, K).
 Folk Medicinal Uses:
              1) Sputum (C, H, J, K).
              2) Cough (C, H, J, K).
              3) Sore throat (C, H).
              4) Bronchial catarrh (J, K).
              5) Tinea (C).
              6) Weakness (K).
 Contraindications: Coughing in "wind–cold" disease.

Scientific Researches:
 Chemistry
  1) Triterpenoids: methyl adenophorate, triphyllol [1].

Literature:
 [1] Konno, C., et al.:*Planta Med.* **1981,** 42(3), 268.

[C.K. Sung]

154.   *Codonopsis lanceolata* **(Sieb. et Zucc.) Benth. et Hook.f.** (Campanulaceae)

Yang–ru (C), Say–yip–sum (H), Tsuruninjin (J), Deo–deok (K)

Root
 Local Drug Name: Yang–ru (C), Say–yip–sum (H), San–kai–ra (J), Sa–sam (K).
 Processing: 1) Eliminate foreign matter, wash clean, dry, cut into slices, and dry (C, K).
              2) Steam thoroughly, cut into slices, and dry (C).
 Method of Adminiatration: Oral (decoction: C, H, K).
 Folk Medicinal Uses:
              1) Valetudinarianism (C, K).
              2) Postpartum hypogalactia (C, H, K).
              3) Pulmonary abscess (C, H, J).
              4) Mastadenitis (C).

5) Mastitis (H).

6) Boils, pyoderma (H).

Scientific Researches:

Chemistry

1) Alkaloids: *N*-9-formulharman, 1-carbomethoxycarboline, perlolyrine, norgharman [1].

2) Triterpenes: echinocystic acid, codonoside A, B, C, cycloartenol [2-5].

3) Volatile oils: hexanal, 7,3-*trans*-2-hexanal, 1-hexanol, *cis*-3-hexen-1-ol, *trans*-2-hexen-1-ol [6].

4) Others: phospholipid, triglycerides, monoglycerides, sterol ester, linoleic acid, palmitic acid, lauric acid [7].

Pharmacology

1) Hematopoietic system effect (water extract) [8].

2) Accumalate activity and stimulate spiration (Water extract) [8].

3) Antifatigue effect (water extract) [9].

Literatures:

[1] Chang, Y.K. et al.: *Yakhak Hoechi* **1986**, 30(1).

[2] Aladyina, N. G. et al.: *F. E. C. S. Int. Conf. Chem. Biotechnol. Biol. Act. Nat. Prod* **1985**(pub.1987), 5, 446.

[3] Aladyina, N. G. et al.: *Khim. Prir. Soedin.* **1989**, 3, 368.

[4] Aladyina, N. G. et al.: *ibid*, **1988**, (1), 137.

[5] Chung, B. S. et al.: *Saengyak Hakhoe Chi (Hanguk Saengyak Hakhoe)* **1977**, 8(2), 49.

[6] Park, J. Y. et al.: *Honghuk Nonghwa Hakhoechi,* **1989**, 32(4), 338.

[7] Park, B. D. et al.: *Hanguk Yongyang Silklyong Hakhoechi* **1985**, 14(3), 280.

[8] Nanjing College of Pharmacy: "*Chinese Traditional and Herbal Medicines*", Vol. 3, **1980**, 1110.

[9] "*Zhongyao Zhi*", Vol. 1, **1979**, 375.

[J.X. Guo]

155.   *Lobelia sessilifolia* **Lamb.** (Campanulaceae)

Shan-geng-cai (C), Sawagikyo (J), Sut-jan-dae (K)

Root, Leaf or Herb

Local Drug Name: Shan Geng Cai (C), San-ko-sai (J), San-gyung-chae (K).

Processing: 1) Eliminate foreign matter, wash clean and dry (C). 2) Use in fresh (C).

Method of Administration: Oral (decoction: C) or topical (fresh leaf, C).

Folk Medicinal Uses:

       1) Bronchitis (C).

       2) Ascites due to cirrhosis (C).

       3) Carbuncle and furuncle (C).

       4) Snake-bite (C).

Scientific Researches:

Chemistry

1) Alkaloids: lobeline [1].

2) Triterpenes: ursolic acid [2].

3) Others: melissic acid, nonacosane, sessilifolan [1].

Pharmacology

1) Selective exciting effect on spiraion centre (lobeline) [1].

2) Expectorant (water extract) [1].

161

Literatures:

[1] "*Quanguo Zhongcaoyao Huibian*', Vol. 1, **1975**, 114.

[2] "*Zhongyao Dicidian*" **1977,** 196.

[J.X. Guo]

156.   *Platycodon grandiflorum* A. DC.   (Campanulaceae)

Jie–geng (C), Gut–geng (H), Kikyo (J), Do–ra–ji (K).

Root   (CP, JP, KP)

Local Drug Name: Jie–geng (C), Gut–geng (H), Ki–kyo (J), Gil–gyung (K).

Processing: Dry under the sun.

Method of Administration: Oral (decoction or powder: C, H, J, K).

Folk Medicinal Uses:

      1) Common cold (C, H, J, K).

      2) Pharyngitis (C, H, J, K).

      3) Bronchitis (C, H, J, K).

      4) Cough with much phlegm (C, H, J, K).

      5) Hoarseness of voice (C).

      6) Suppuration (C, J).

      7) Lung abscess with purulent sputum (H).

      5) Stomach ache (J).

Scientific Researches:

Chemistry

      1) Saponins: platycodin A, C, D, D2, polygalacin D, D2 [1].

      2) Sugars: inulin [2].

Pharmacology:

      1) Saliva secretion, blood pressure increasing, respiration depressing (water extract) [3].

      2) Tracheal secretion increasing (hot water infusion, water extract) [4].

      3) Weak antitussive (water extract) [5].

      4) Blood sugar lowering (water extract) [6].

      5) Against gastric ulcer (50 % methanol exract, platycodin) [7].

      6) Inhibition of congestive edema, and diuretic (50 % methanol extract) [8].

      7) Hemolytic, local irritant activities. Central nervous system depressing such as sedative, analgesic and antifebrile effects. Antiallergic, antitussive and expectorant (platycodin mixture) [9].

      8) Vasodilation (platycodin mixture) [10].

      9) Corticosterone secretion (total saponin) [11].

      10) Antitumor (crude inulin) [12].

      11) Others [13].

Literatures:

[1] Tada, A., et al.: *Chem. Pharm. Bull.* **1975**, 23, 2965; Konishi, T., et al :*ibid.* **1978**, 26, 668; Ishii, H., et al.: *ibid.* **1978**, 26, 674; *J. Chem. Soc., Perkin* I, **1984**, 661 ; Shoji, J.: *Gendai Toyo Igaku,* **1983**, 4, 47.

[2] Mino, Y., et al.: *Shoyakugaku Zasshi* **1985**, 39, 63, 154; *Chem. Pharm. Bull.* **1985**, 33, 3503.

[3] Kobayashi, Y.: *Jikken Yakubutugaku Zasshi* **1936**, 11, 153.

[4] Igarashi, K.: *Sogo Igaku* **1951**, 8, 526; Akiba, K., et al.: *Oyo Yakuri* **1981**, 22, 339.

[5] Shoji, T. et al.,: *Oyo Yakuri* **1975**, 10, 407.

[6] Koda, A. et al.,: *Nippon Yakurigaku Zasshi* **1971**, 67, 223.

[7] Yamahara, J., et al.: *Shoyakugaku Zasshi* **1974**, 28, 33; Kawashima, K., et al.: *Chem. Pharm. Bull.*

1972, 20, 755.

[8] Yamahara, J., et al.:*Chem. Pharm. Bull.* **1979**, 27, 1464.

[9] Takagi, K., et al.: *Yakugaku Zasshi* **1972**, 92, 951, 961, 969; **1973**, 93, 1188.

[10] Kato, H., et al. :*Japan. J. Pharmacol.* **1973**, 23, 709.

[11] Yokoyama, H., et al.:*Yakugaku Zasshi* **1982**, 102, 1191.

[12] Nagao, K., et al.:*Shoyakugaku Zasshi* **1986**, 40, 375.

[13] Kubo, M., et al.:*Shoyakugaku Zasshi* **1986**, 40, 367; Takahashi, K., et al.:*Kagakuryoho Kenkyusho Iho* **1960**, 14, 24.

[T. Kimura]

157.　　　　　*Arctium lappa* L.　　(Compositae)

Niu–bang (C), Ngau–bong (H), Gobo (J), U–eong (K)

Fruit　(CP)

Local Drug Name: Niu–bang–zi (C), Ngau–bong–gee (H), Go–bo–shi, Aku–jitsu (J), U–bang–ja (K).

Processing: 1) Eliminate foreign matter, wash and dry. Break into pieces before use (C, K).

　　　　　　2) Stir–fry until inflated and slightly scented. Break into pieces before use (C).

Method of Administration: Oral (decoction: C, H, J, K).

Folk Medicinal Uses:

　　　　　1) Cough and expectoration in influenza or upper respiratory infection (C, H, J,).

　　　　　2) Measles (C, H, K).

　　　　　3) Rubella (C, H).

　　　　　4) Sore throat (C, J, K).

　　　　　5) Mumps (C, H).

　　　　　6) Erysipelas, abscess, carbuncles and sores (C, H, J, K).

Contraindications:

　　　　　1) Insufficiency of the spleen–yang (C).

　　　　　2) Diarrhea (C).

Root, Stem, Leaf

Local Drug Name: Go–bo (J).

Processing: Fresh juice (J).

Method of Administration: Topical (J).

Folk Medicinal Uses:

　　　　　1) Insect bite (J).

Scientific Researches

Chemistry

　1) Lignans: arctiin, arctigenin, lappaol A–F, H [1,2].

　2) Acetylenes: lappaphen A, B, (*S*)–12,13–epoxy–2,4,6,8,10–tridecapentaynne, 1–tridecen–3,5,7,9,11–
　　　　　pentayne, arctinal, arctic acid–b,[3–6].

　3) Triterpenes: α–amyrin, β–amyrin, lupeol, 4–taraxasterol [7].

　4) Essential oil: aplotaxene, dihydroaplotaxene, cyperene, 1–pentadecene, 1–heptadecene,β–elemene,
　　　　　caryophyllene, α–guaiene, clovene, phenylacetaldehyde, benzaldehyde, decanal,
　　　　　6,2–alky–3–methoxypyrazines, 2–methoxy–3–methylpyrazine, 2–methylpropionic acid,
　　　　　3–octenoic acid, costic acid, dehydrocostus lactone, dehydrodihydrocostus lactone [8].

　5) Others: ubiquinone, inulin [9, 10].

Pharmacology

　1) Antibiosis (water extract) [1].

　2) Anticancer effect (arctigenin) [1].

3) Hypoglycemic effect [1].
4) Paralysis effect [1].
5) Ameliorating and protective effect on toxicities caused by chemicals and food colors (dietary fibre) [11, 14].
6) Adsorptive effect of heavy metals [15].

Literatures:

[1] "*Zhongyao Zhi*", Vol. 2, **1979**, 252.
[2] "*Zhongyao Dacidian*", **1977**, 430.
[3] Washino, T. et al.:*Agric. Biol. Chem.* **1987**, 51(6), 1475.
[4] Washino, T. et al.:*ibid.* **1986**, 50(2), 263.
[5] Washino, T. et al.:*Nippon Nogei Kagaku Kaishi* **1986**, 60(5), 377.
[6] Takasugi, M. et al.:*Phytochem.* **1987**, 26(11), 2957.
[7] Iochkova, I. et al.:*Dokl. Bolg. Akad. Nauk*, **1989**, 42(10), 43.
[8] Washino, T. et al.:*Nippon Nogei Kagaku Kaishi* **1985**, 59(4), 389.
[9] Kamei, M. et al.:*Int. J. Vitam. Nutr. Res.* **1986**, 56(1), 57.
[10] Chalcarz, W. et al.:*Herba Pol.* **1984**, 30(2), 109.
[11] Kimura, T. et al.:*J. Nutr.* **1980**, 110(3), 513.
[12] Jsujita, J. et al.:*Nutr. Rep. Int.* **1979**, 20(5), 625.
[13] Ebihara, K,. et al.:*Nippon Nogei Kagaku Kaishi* **1982**, 56(3), 195.
[14] Takeda, H. et al.:*Biosci. Biotechnol. Biochem.* **1992**, 56(4), 551.
[15] Suemitsu, R. et al.:*Sci. Eng. Rev. Doshisha Univ.* **1990**, 31(3), 235.

[J.X. Guo]

158. *Artemisia annua* L. (Compositae)

Huang–hua–hao (C), Kusoninjin (J), Gae–ddong–ssuk (K)

Aerial Part (CP)
Local Drug Name: Qing–hao (C), Ching–ho (H), Hwang–hwa–ho (K).
Processing: Dry in the shade (C).
Method of Adminiatration: Oral (decoction: C).
Folk Medicinal Uses:

      1) Fever caused by summer–heat (C, H, J).
      2) Afternoon fever in deficiency of yin (C, J).
      3) Malaria with chills and fever (C, H).
      4) Jaundice (C, H, J).

Scientific Researches:
Chemistry
1) Volatile oils: artemisia ketone, isoartemisia ketone, 1–camphor,β –artemisia alcohol acetate, cuminal, cadinene, etc. [1].
2) Sesquiterpenes: arteannuin B [2], arteannuin (= artemisinin, qinghaosu) [3], arteannuin A, hydro–arteannuin [4], arteannuin C [5], artemisilactone [6], artemisitene [7], epideoxyarteannuin B [8], artemisic acid [9], artemisininic acid [10], epoxyarteannuinic acid [11], 11R–(–)–dihydroarteannuic acid [12], artemisinine I, III [13], artemisinine IV, V [14].
3) Flavonoids: 3,6,7,3"–tetra–*O*–methyl–5,3'–dihydroxy flavone [15], 3,3',5–trihydroxy–4',6,7–trimethoxy–flavone, artemetin [16], auratimide acetate, 5–hydroxy–3,6,7,3,4"–pentamethoxyflavone, 5–hydroxy–3,6,7,4'–tetramethoxyflavone [17], casticin, chrysosphenetin, artemetin [18], quercetagetin–3–methyl ether, 2',4',5–trihydroxy–5',6,7–trimethoxyflavone, 3',5,7,8–tetra–hydroxy– 3,4–dimethoxyflavone [19], 5,4'–dihydroxy–3,6,7,3'–tetramethoxy–flavone [20],

164

6–methoxy–heampferol–3–glycoside [21].

4) Coumarins: scopoletin, coumarin [16], esculetin [22], 7,8–dimethoxycoumarin (daphnetin dimethyl ether), 7,8–methylenedioxy–coumarin (daphnetin methylene ether), 7–methoxycoumarin (herniarin) [23].

5) Others: campesterol, stigmasterol, β–sitosterol [23], lipopolysaccharides [24], annuadiepoxide [25], α–myrcene hydroperoxide (3–hydroxy–2–methyl–6–methylene–1,7–octadiene),β–myrcene hydroperoxide (2–hydroxy–2–methyl–6–methylene–3,7–octadiene) [26].

Pharmacology

1) Antimalarial effect (arteannuin, = artemisinin, qinghaosu) [3, 27].

2) Antischistosomal effect (arteannuin) [28].

3) Immunoregulatory effect (arteannuin) [29].

4) Antirheumatism effect (lipopolysarides) [24].

5) Antibacterial effect (artemisic acid, artemisinol, artemisic acid Me ether) [30].

Literatures:

[1] Takemoto, T. et al.:*Yakugaku Zasshi*, **1962**, 82, 1323.

[2] Stefanovic, M.: *Glas. Hem. Drus. Beograd* **1977**, 42(3), 227.

[3] Liu, J. M. et al.:*Huaxue Xuebao*, **1979**, 37(2), 129.

[4] Tian, Y. et al.:*Zhongcaoyao*, **1982**, 13(6), 9.

[5] Misra, L.:*Phytochem.* **1986**, 25(12), 2892.

[6] Zhu, D. Y. et al.:*Huaxue Xuebao*, **1984**, 42(9), 937.

[7] Acton, N. et al.:*Planta Med.*, **1985**, 5, 441.

[8] Roth, R. J. et al.:*ibid*, **1987**, 53(6), 576.

[9] Deng, A. D. et al.:*Kaxue Tongbao* **1981**, 26(19), 1209.

[10] Tu, Y. Y. et al.:*Zhongyao Tongbao* **1981**, 6(20), 31.

[11] Wu, Z. H.: *Huaxue Xuebao*, **1984**, 42(6), 596.

[12] Huang, J. J. et al.:*ibid.*, **1987**, 5(6), 609.

[13] Tu, Y. Y. et al.:*Yaoxue Xuebao* **1981**, 16(5), 366.

[14] Tu, Y. Y. et al.:*Planta Med.* **1982**, 44(3), 143.

[15] Jeremic, D.: *Glas.Hem. Drus. Beograd* **1979**, 44(9–10), 615.

[16] Liu, H. M. et al.:*Yaoxue Tongbao* **1980**, 15(10), 39.

[17] Tu, Y. Y. et al.:*Zhongcaoyao* **1985**, 16(5), 200.

[18] Baeva, R. T. et al.:*Khim. Prir. Soedin.* **1988**, 2, 289.

[19] Shilib, Y. et al.:*Phytochem.* **1989**, 28(5), 1509.

[20] Bhardwaj, D. K. et al.:*Proc. Indian Katl. Sci. Acad.(A)*, **1985**, 51(4), 741.

[21] Marco, J.A. et al.:*Pharmazie* **1990**, 45(5), 382.

[22] Aleslerova, A. N. et al.:*Izu. Akad. Nauk. Az. SSR, Ser. Biol. Nauk,***1985**, (2), 25.

[23] Hiroko, S. et al.:*Phytochem.* **1979**, 18(10), 1761.

[24] Soma, G.:*Jpn. Kokai Tokyo Koho JP*04 49 241 (92 49, 241)(cl. A 61 K35178).

[25] Manns, D. et al.:*J. Nat. Prod.* **1992**, 55(1), 29.

[26] Ruecker, G. et al.:*ibid.* **1987**, 50(2), 287.

[27] "Qinghao" Collaborative Research Group:*Yaoxue Tongbao* **1979**, (2), 49.

[28] Chen, D. J. et al.:*Zhonghua Yixue Zazhi* **1980**, 60(7), 422.

[29] Qian, R. S. et al.:*Zhongyi Zazhi* **1981**, 22(6), 63.

[30] Zhu, D. Y. et al.:*Zhongcaoyao* **1982**, 13(2), 6.

[J.X. Guo]

159. *Artemisia princeps* **Pamp.** (Compositae)
(= *A. indica* Willd. var. *maximowiczii* Hara)

Huang–hua–ai (C), Yomogi (J), Ta–rae–ssuk (K)

Leaf
Local Drug Name: Ai–ye (C), Gai–yo (J), Ae–yeop (K).
Processing: Dry under the sun (C, K).
Method of Adminiatration: Oral (moxibustion or fuming and washing (C, K).
Folk Medicinal Uses:

> 1) Dysfunctional uterine bleeding (C,K).
> 2) Threatened abortion (C).
> 3) Cutaneous pruritus (C).
> 4) Bleeding (J).
> 5) Stomach ache (J, K).
> 6) Low back pain (J).
> 7) Traumatic injary (J).
> 8) Epistaxis (K).
> 9) Dirrhea (K).

Side Effects: Toxication: Highly exciting central nervous system.

Scientific Researches:
Chemistry
  1) Coumarins: herniazin, dimethylescletin, scopoletin, isofraxidin [1].
  2) Polysacchaides: AAF–IIb–2 and IIb–3 [2].
Pharmacology
  1) Anti–complementary [2].

Literatures:
[1] Matsueda, S. et al.: *Sci. Rep. Hirosaki Univ.* **1980**, 27(1), 17.
[2] Yamada, H. et al.: *Planta Med.* **1985**, 2, 121.

[J.X. Guo]

160. *Aster tataricus* **L.** (Compositae)

Zi–wan (C), Gee–yuan (H), Shion (J), Gae–mi–chwi (K)

Root (CP)
Local Drug Name: Zi–wan (C), Gee–yuan (H), Shi–on (J), Ja–weon (K).
Processing: 1) Soften briefly, cut into thick slices, and dry (C, H, J, K).
              2) Dilute the refined honey with a quantity of water at first, then add it to the slices and mix
                 well in a closed vessel untill they are infused thoroughly. Roast them in a closed pot
                 with gentle heat untill no more sticky to fingers (C).
Method of Administration: Oral (decoction: C, H, J, K).
Folk Medicinal Uses:

> 1) Sputum (J, K).
> 2) Cough (J, K).
> 3) Expectorant (H, K).
> 4) Antitussive (H, K).
> 5) Hemoptysis in consumptive diseases (C).
> 6) Asthma (K).

7) Acute or chronic cough and asthma with copious expectoration (C).
Contraindications: In high fever, constipation.

Scientific Researches:
Chemistry
1) Triterpenes: shionone [1,2], friedelin, epifriedelinol [4].
2) Monoterpenes: shionoside A, B [5].
3) Triterpene saponins: aster saponin A, B, C, D [6], aster saponin E, F [7], aster saponin Ha, Hb, Hc, Hd, foetidissimoside [8], hederagenin mono-glucoside [3].
4) Flavonoids: quercetin [1].
Pharmacology
1) Antitussive activity.
2) Antimicrobial activity.
3) Anticancer activity (epifriedelanol).

Literatures:
[1] Nakaoki, T.: *Yakugaku Zasshi* **1929,** 49, 1169.
[2] Idem: *ibid.* **1932,** 52, 499.
[3] Koyama, T. et al.: *Kumamoto Pharm. Bull.* **1955,** 2, 66.
[4] Takahashi, T. et al.: *Yakugaku Zasshi* **1959,** 79, 1281.
[5] Nagao, T. et al.: *Chem. Pharm. Bull.* **1988,** 36(2), 571.
[6] Nagao, T. et al.: *Chem. Pharm. Bull.* **1989,** 37(8), 1977.
[7] Nagao, T. et al.: *Chem. Pharm. Bull.* **1990,** 38(3), 783.
[8] Tanaka, R. et al.: *Chem. Pharm. Bull.* **1990,** 38(5), 1153.

[C.K. Sung]

161.   *Atractylodes lancea* **DC.** (Compositae)

Mao-cang-zhu, Nan-cang-zhu (C), Chong-soet (H), Hosobaokera (J).

Related plant: *Atractylodes chinensis* Koidz. (=*A. lancea* DC. var. *chinensis* Kitamura):
Bei-cang-zhu (C), Shinaokera (J)

Rhizome   (CP, JP)
Local Drug Name: Cang-zhu (C), Chong-soet (H), So-jutsu (J), Chang-chul (K).
Processing: 1) Dry under the sun. 2) Stir-fry with bran until their outer surface turned deep yellow (C).
Method of Administration: Oral (decoction: C, H, J).
Folk Medicinal Uses:
1) Dyspepsia (C, H, J).
2) Edema (C, H, J).
3) Gastrointestinal disorder (C, H, J).
4) Diarrhea (C, H).
5) Rheumatic arthralgia (C), rheumatalgia (H).
6) Common cold (C, H, J).
7) Night blindness (C).
8) Malarial disease (H).
9) Phlegm (H).

Scientific Researches:
Chemistry
1) Sesquiterpenoids: hinesol, β-eudesmol, (-)-α-bisabolol, β-selinene, atractylon,

5α,10β–selina–4(14),7(11)–dien–8–one [1].

2) Sesquiterpene glycosides: atractyloside A, B, C, D, E, F, G, H, I [2].

3) Polyacetylenes: atractylodin, atractylodinol, acetylatractylodinol [1].

Pharmacology

1) Increasing excretion of Na, K and Cl ions, nevertheless not observed increasing urination (decoction) [3, 9].

2) Depressing functions of yellow body (water extract) [4].

3) Blood sugar lowering (ethanol extract) [5].

4) Antihistaminic (ethanol extract) [6].

5) Prevention against gastric ulcer. Inhibition of gastric secretion (50 % methanol extr.) [7].

6) Choleretic (ethyl acetate extr., atractylodin) [8].

7) Sedative, extention of sleep, antispasmodic and intestine movement stimulation (benzene extr., a mixture of β–eudesmol and hinesol) [9].

8) Against hepatitis (β–eudesmol, hinesol) [10].

9) Others [11].

Literatures:

[1] Yosioka, I., Kimura, T.: *Chem. Pharm. Bull.* **1969**, 17, 856; *Yakugaku Zasshi* **1976**, 96, 1229; Nishikawa, Y., et al.: *Shoyakugaku Zasshi* **1976**, 30, 132; *Yakugaku Zasshi* **1976**, 96, 1322.

[2] Yahara, S., et al.: *Chem. Pharm. Bull.* **1989**, 37, 2995.

[3] Haginiwa, T., et al.: *Shoyakugaku Zasshi* **1963**, 17, 6; Lu, X. H.: *Yaoxue Xuebao* **1966**, 13, 454.

[4] Usuki, S., et al.: *Wakan Iyakugaku Zasshi* **1987**, 4, 264.

[5] Koda, A., et al.: *Nippon Yakurigaku Zasshi* **1971**, 67, 223; Nogami, M., et al.: *Chem. Pharm. Bull.* **1986**, 34, 3854.

[6] Itokawa, H., et al.: *Shoyakugaku Zasshi* **1983**, 37, 223.

[7] Kubo, M., et al.: *Yakugaku Zasshi* **1983**, 103, 442; Nogami, M., et al.: *ibid.* **1985**, 105, 973 978.

[8] Yamahara, J., et al.: *Shoyakugaku Zasshi* **1983**, 37, 17.

[9] Yamahara, J., et al.: *Yakugaku Zasshi* **1977**, 97, 873.

[10] Kiso, Y., et al.: *J. Nat. Prod.* **1983**, 46, 651.

[11] Kimura, M., et al.: *Phytother. Res.* **1987**, 1, 107; Yamahara, J., et al.: *Chem. Pharm. Bull.* **1990**, 38, 2033; Matsuda, H. et al.: *Yakugaku Zasshi* **1987**, 107, 429.

[T. Kimura]

162.　　　*Atractylodes macrocephara* **Koidz.** (= *A. ovata* DC.) (Compositae)

Bai–zhu (C), Bak–soet (H), Obana–okera (J)

Related plants:　*Atractylodes japonica* Koidz. ex Kitamura: Okera (J), Sap–ju (K).

Rhizome (CP, JP, KP)

Local Drug Name: Bai–zhu (C), Bak–soet (H), Byaku–jutsu (J), Baek–chul (K).

Processing:　1) Dry under the sun.

2) Stir–fry with yellow sand (Terra Flava Vsta) until the surface ashen, and shift out the sand (C).

3) Stir–fry with bran and honey until turned burnt yellow and smelled burnt aroma, and shift out the bran (C).

Method of Administration: Oral (decoction: C, H, J, K).

Folk Medicinal Uses:

1) Gastrointestinal disorder (C, J, K).

2) Gastric neurosis (J, K).

3) Edema (C, H, J, K).

4) Rheumatalgia, arthritis (H, J, K).

5) Weakness (J, K).

6) Hypofunction of the spleen with anorexia (C, H).

7) Diarrhea (C, K).

8) Dizziness and palpitation due to retension of phlegm and fluid (C).

9) Phlegm (H).

10) Oliguria (H).

11) Headache (H).

12) Neuralgia (K).

13) Mastitis (K).

Scientific Researches:

Chemistry

1) Sesquiterpenoids: atractylon, 3β-hydroxyatractylon, 3β-acetoxyatractylon, $5\alpha,10\beta$-selina-4(14),7(11)-dien-8-one, atractylenolide I, II, III [1]. γ-Cadinene, γ-patchoulene [5].

2) Aldehydes: acetaldehyde, 2-furaldehyde [2].

3) Polyacetylenes: diacetyl-atractylodiol, (4E,6E,12E)-tetradecatriene-8,10-diyne-1,3-diol diacetate, (6E,12E)-tetradecadiene-8,10-diyne-1,3-diol diacetate [3].
(4E,6E,12E)-1-acetoxy-3-senecioyloxytetradeca-4,6,12-trien-8,10-diyn-14-ol [6],
(4E,6E,12E)-1-acetoxy-3-isovaleryloxytetradeca-4,6,12-triene-8,10-diyne-14-ol [7].

4) Sugars: atractan A, B, C [4].

5) Phenolic compounds: butenolide A [5], scopoletin [6].

Pharmacology

1) Weak diuretic activity (decoction, water extract, ethanol extract) [8].

2) Inhibition of stress ulcer (50 % methanol extract) [9].

3) Inhibition of acetic acid stimulation on blood capillary permeability (eudesma-4(14),7(11)-diene-8-one, atractylenolide I) [10].

4) Inhibition of adjubant arthritis (water extract) [11].

5) Protection activity for carbon tetrachloride hepatitis and choleretic activity (ethyl acetate extract) [12].

6) Stimulaton of bowel movement was observed, nevertheless central nervous system depressing, anti-inflammatory and diuretic effects were not observed (benzene extract) [13].

7) Antitumor effect (water extract) [14].

8) Inhibition of experimental hepatitis (atractylon) [12, 15].

9) Blood sugar lowering (atractan A, B, C) [16].

10) Reticulo-endothelial phagocytic system stimulation (inulin) [17].

Literatures:

[1] Hikino, H., et al.:*Chem. Pharm. Bull.* **1962**, 10, 640; **1964**, 12, 755; Nishikawa, Y., et al.: *Shoyakugaku Zasshi* **1975**, 29, 139; *Yakugaku Zasshi* **1976**, 96, 1089; **1977**, 97, 515; Takahashi, S.: *Shoyakugaku Zasshi* **1961**, 15, 255; **1965**, 19, 49; Nishikawa, Y., et al.:*ibid.* **1975**, 29, 139: **1976**, 30, 132; *Yakugaku Zasshi* **1977**, 97, 515; Yosioka, I., et al.:*ibid.* **1976**, 96, 1229.

[2] Takahashi, S., et al.:*Yakugaku Zasshi* **1959**, 79, 541.

[3] Yosioka, I., et al.:*Chem. Pharm. Bull.* **1974**, 22, 1943; Kano, Y., et al.:*Chem. Pharm. Bull.* **1989**, 37, 193.

[4] Konno, C., et al.:*Planta Med.* **1985**, 51, 102.

[5] Chen, Y., et al.:*Anal. Chem.* **1987**, 59, 744.

[6] Chen, Z. L.:*Planta Med.* **1987**, 53, 493.

[7] Kano, Y., et al.:*Chem. Pharm. Bull.* **1990**, 38, 1082.

[8] Haginiwa, T., et al.:*Shoyakugaku Zasshi* **1963**, 17, 16; Tsurumi, S., et al.:*Gifu Ikadaigaku Kiyo* **1963**, 11, 129, 138.

[9] Kubo, M., et al.:*Yakugaku Zasshi* **1983**, 103, 442.

[10] Endo, K. et al.:*Chem. Pharm. Bull.* **1979**, 27, 2954.

[11] Cho, S., et al.:*Shoyakugaku Zasshi* **1982**, 36, 78.

[12] Yamahara, J., et al.:*Shoyakugaku Zasshi* **1983**, 37, 17.

[13] Yamahara, J., et al.:*Yakugaku Zasshi* **1977,** 97, 873.

[14] Jo, K., et al.:*Wakan Iyakugaku Zasshi* **1986,** 3, 31; More, H., et al.:*Japan. J. Pharmacol.* **1988,** 48, 37; **1989,** 49, 423.

[15] Kiso, Y., et al.:*J. Nat. Prod.* **1983,** 46, 651; *Planta Med.* **1985,** 51, 97.

[16] Konno, C., et al.:*Planta Med.* **1985,** 51, 102.

[17] Matsuda, H., et al.:*Yakugaku Zasshi* **1987,** 107, 429.

[T. Kimura]

163.   *Dandranthema morifolium* **(Ramat.) Tzvel.**   (Compositae)
(= *Chrysanthemum morifolium*Ramat.)

Ju (C), Guk–fa (H), Kiku (J), Guk–hwa (K)

Inflorescence (CP)

Local Drug Name: Ju–hua (C), Guk–fa (H), Kiku–ka (J), Guk–hwa (K).

Processing: Dry in the shade, bake or dry under the sun after fuming and steaming (C, J, K).

Method of Administration: Oral (decoction: C, J, K).

Folk Medicinal Uses:

　　　　1) Eye disease (C, H, K).

　　　　2) Dizziness (C, H, K).

　　　　3) Headache (H, J, K).

　　　　4) Fever (H, K).

　　　　5) Gastropathy (K).

　　　　6) Weakness (K).

　　　　7) Bee sting (K).

　　　　8) Dysuria (K).

　　　　9) Conjunctivitis (H).

　　　　10) "Wind–heat" type common cold.

　　　　11) Common cold (J).

　　　　12) Pyodermas (H).

Leaf

Local Drug Name: Guk–yeop (K).

Processing: Dry under the sun (K).

Method of Administration: Oral (decoction: K).

Folk Medicinal Uses: 1) Dandruff (K).

Scientific Researches:

Chemistry

　1) Sesquiterpenes: chlorochrymorin [1], chrysandiol [2, 3], chrysantemin A, B [4].

　2) Flavonoids: acaciin (luteolin–7–O–β–D–glucopyranoside) [5], apigenin 7–O–β–D–gluco–pyranoside [6], acacetin 7–O–glucoside, diosmetin–7–O–glucoside [9], luteolin, apigenin.

　3) Anthocyanins: cyanidin 3–O–(6–O–malonyl–β–D–glucopyranoside) [7, 11].

　4) Catechol derivtives: 3,4–dihydroxyacetophenone, 3,4–dihydroxyphenylacetone [11].

　5) Essential oils: aromadendrene, 1,8–cineole, β–selinene, β–chamigrene, α–bergamotene, thymol, eugenol [12].

　6) Triterpenes [13].

　7) Protein: phytotropin [8].

Pharmacology

　1) Gonadotropin–like action (phytotropin) [8].

Literatures:

[1] Osawa, T. et al.: *Tetrahedron Lett.* **1973**, 5135.

[2] Osawa, T. et al.: *Agric. Biol. Chem.* **1974**, 38, 685.

[3] Osawa, T. et al.: *Tetrahedron Lett.* **1974**, 1569.

[4] Romo, J. et al.: *Phytochemistry* **1970**, 9, 1615.

[5] Hwu, K. K. et al.: *Taiwan Ke Hsueh* **1964**, 18, 102.

[6] Arisawa, M. et al.: *Shoyakugaku Zasshi* **1969**, 23, 49.

[7] Kawase, K. et al.: *Plant Cell Physiol.* **1970**, 11(2), 349.

[8] Shomer–Ilan, A. et al.: *Aust. J. Biol. Sci.* **1973**, 26(1), 105.

[9] Asen, S. et al.: *Phytochemistry* **1975**, 14(5–6), 1443.

[10] Chang, C.-F. et al.: *Agric. Biol. Chem.* **1975**, 39(2), 573.

[11] Saito, N. et al.: *Phytochemistry* **1988**, 27(9), 2963.

[12] Ito, T. et al.: *Iwate Daigaku Nogakubu Hokoku* 20(1), 35.

[13] Yahara, S. et al.: *Shoyakugaku Zasshi* **1990**, 44(4), 335.

[C.K. Sung]

164. *Cirsium japonicum* **DC.** (Compositae)

Ji (C), Die–gait (H), Noazami (J)

Related plants: *Cirsium japonicum* var. *ussuriense*: Eong-geong-kwi (K).

Herb (CP)

Local Drug Name: Da–ji–cao (C), Die–gait (H), Dae–gye(K).

Processing: 1) Cut into sections and dry (C, H, K). 2) Stir–fry until the outer surface becomes charred–black (C).

Method of Administration: Oral (decoction: C, H, K); topical (paste of pounded fresh herb: C).

Folk Medicinal Uses:

1) Hematuria (C, H).

2) Abnormal uterine bleeding (C, H).

3) Cough (K).

4) Headache (K).

5) Lassitude (K).

6) Anemia (K).

7) Menoxenia (K).

8) Mammary cancer (K).

9) Swelling (K).

10) Pneumonia (K).

11) Gonorrhoea (K).

12) Hemorrhoid (K).

13) Epistaxis (C).

14) Spitting of blood (C).

15) Hematochezia (C).

16) Traumatic bleeding (C).

17) Carbuncles and sores (C).

18) Hematemesis (H).

19) Hemoptysis (H).

20) Epistaxis (H).

21) Hepatitis (H).

22) Nephritis (H).

23) Mastitis (H).

24) Contusion (H).
25) Furunculosis (H).
26) Hypertension (H).

Root (CP)
Local Drug Name: Da–ji–gen (C), Tai–kei (J), Dae–gye (K).
Processing: Dry under the sun (J, K).
Method of Administration: Oral (decoction: J, K); topical (fresh juice: J).
Folk Medicinal Uses:
1) Edema (J).
2) Neuralgia (J).
3) Nocturia (J).
4) Insect bite (J).
5) Scalds (J).
6) Eczema (J).
7) Hematemesis (K).
8) Abdominal pain (K).
9) Hematuria (C).
10) Abnormal uterine bleeding (C, H).
11) Epistaxis (C).
12) Spitting of blood (C).
13) Hematochezia (C).
14) Traumatic bleeding (C).
15) Carbuncles and sores (C).

Scientific Researches:
Chemistry
1) Hydrocarbons: aplotaxene, dihydro–, tetrahydro–, hexahydro–aplotaxene, 1–pentadecene, cyperene, caryophyllene, thujopsene, α–himachalene [1].
Pharmacology
1) Hypotensive activity.
2) Antibacterial activity.

Literature:
[1] Yano, K. et al.: *Phytochemistry* **1977**, 16(2), 263.

[C.K. Sung]

165.   *Eclipta prostrata* **L.**   (Compositae)
(= *E. alba* (L.) Hassk., *E. erecta* L.)

Mo–han–lian (C), Hon–lin–cho (H), Takasaburo (J), Han–ryun–cho (K)

Whole plant (CP)
Local Drug Name: Mo–han–lian (C), Hon–lin–cho (H), Reicho (J), Muk–han–ryun (K).
Processing: Eliminate foreign matter, wash briefly, cut into sections, dry under the sun.
Method of Administration: Oral or topical (decoction: C, H, J, K).
Folk Medicinal Uses:
1) Hematemesis, epistaxis, hematuria, melena (C, H, J, K).
2) Uterine bleeding (C, H, J).
3) Chronic hepatitis (C, H).
4) Enteritis, dysentery (C, H, K).

5) Infantile malnutrition (C, H).

6) Tinnitus, premature greying of hair (C, H).

7) Neurasthenia (C, H).

8) Tinea pedia (C, H, J).

9) Eczema (C, H, J).

10) Ulcer, wound bleeding (C, H, J).

11) Looseness of teeth (C).

12) Dizziness (C).

13) Aching and weakness of the loins and knees (C).

14) Traumatic bleeding (C).

15) Leukorrhea (K).

Scientific Researches:

Chemistry

1) Ecliptine, wedelolactone, demethylwedelolactone, demethylwedelolactone–7–O–glucoside [1–2].

2) α–Terthienyl, 2–formyl– α–terthienyl, thiophene acetylenes, diisovalerate, α–terthienylmethanol, 5–(3–buten–1–ynyl)–2,2'–bithieny [7].

3) Ecliptal [6].

Pharmacology

1) Against snake–bite [3,4]; wedelolactone, sitosterol and stigmasterol were able to neutralize three lethal doses of rattle–snake venom. Aqueous extracts of the plant inhibited the release of creatine kinase from isolated rat muscle exposed to the crude venom [5].

2) Antihepatoxic effects [8].

3) Antiinflammatory effects (through inhibition on 5–lipoxygenase) [9].

Literatures:

[1] Bhargava, K.K. et al.:*Indian J. Chem.* **1970**, 8, 664–5.

[2] Bhargava, K.K. et al.:*Indian J. Chem.* **1972**, 10, 810–1.

[3] Mors, W.B.:*Mem. Inst. Oswaldo Cruz (Brazil)* **1991**, 86 Suppl 2, 193.

[4] Martz W.:*Toxicon* **1992**, 30, 1131–42.

[5] Mors, W.B.:*Toxicon* **1989**, 27, 1003–9.

[6] Das, B. et al.:*Indian J. Chem.* **1991**, 30B, 1052–3.

[7] Krishnaswamy, N.R. et al.:*Tetrahedron Lett.* **1966**, 35, 4227–30.

[8] Wagner, H. et al.*Planta Med.* **1986**, (5), 370–4.

[9] Wagner, H. et al.*Planta Med.* **1986**, (5), 374–7.

[10] Bhargava, K.K. et al.:*J. Res. Indian Med.* **1974**, 9(1), 9–15.

[P.P.H. But]

166.   *Inula helenium* **L.**   (Compositae)

Tu–mu–xiang (C), Muk–heung (H), Oguruma (J), Mok–hyang (K)

Related plant: *Inula racemosa* Hook.f.: Zong–zhuang–tu(qing)–mu–xiang (C).

Root (CP)

Local Drug Name: Tu–mu–xiang (C), Muk–heung (H), Do–mok–ko (J), To–mok–hyang (K).

Processing: Eliminate foreign matter, wash clean, cut into slices, dry under the sun.

Method of Administration: Oral (decoction: C, H, J, K).

Folk Medicinal Uses:

1) Chest distention and pain (C, H, J).

2) Vomiting (C, H, J).

3) Diarrhea, dysentery (C, H, J).
4) Malarial disease (C).
5) Bronchitis, whooping cough (C, J, K).
6) Threatened abortion (C).

Scientific Researches:
Chemistry
  1) Sesquiterpenes: alantolactone, helenine, isoalantolactone, dihydroisoalantolactone, alantic acid, alantol, dammaradienyl acetate, alantopicrin, inunolide [1, 2].
Pharmacology
  1) Antibacterial effect.
  2) Clonorchicidal effect [2–5].

Literatures:

[1] Ozeki, S. et al.: *Proc. Imp. Acad. (Tokyo)* **1936**, 12, 233–4.
[2] Go, T.: *Japan J. Med. Sci. IV. Pharmacol.* **1941**, 13, 75–93.
[3] Kim, C.S. et al.: *J. Taegu Med. Soc.* **1962**, 3, 176–80.
[4] Rhee, J.K. et al.: *Am. J. Chin. Med.* **1981**, 9, 277–84.
[5] Rhee, J.K. et al.: *Am. J. Chin. Med.* **1985**, 13, 119–25.

[P.P.H. But]

167.　　　　*Senecio scandens* Buch.–Ham. (= *S. chinensis* DC.)　(Compositae)

Qian–li–guang (C), Chin–lay–gwong (H)
Herb
Local Drug Name: Qian–li–guang (C), Chin–lay–gwong (H), Sen–ri–ko (J).
Processing: Dry under the sun or use in fresh (C).
Method of Adminiatration: Oral (decoction: C, H).
Folk Medicinal Uses:
  1) Upper respiratory tract infection, tonsillitis (C, H, J).
  2) Acute enteritis, acute bacillary dysentery (C, H, J).
  3) Acute appendicitis (C, H).
  4) Acute and subacute conjunctivitis (C, J).
  5) Eczematosis, dermatitis (C, H).
  6) Hemorrhoid (H).
  7) Erysipelas (H).
  8) Tonsillitis (J).
Side Effects: Nausea, anorexia, hypersensitive epispasis (C). Hepatotoxicity (H).

Scientific Researches:
Chemistry
  1) Flavonoids: flavoxanthin, chrysanthemaxanthin [1].
  2) Alkaloids: senecionine, seneciphylline [2].
  3) Phenolic acids: p–hydroxy–phenylacetic acid, vanillic acid, salicylic acid, pyromucic acid [3].
  4) Hydroquinone [3].
Pharmacology
  1) Bacteriostasis (hydroquinone, p–hydroxy–phenylacetic acid) [3].
  2) Antileptospiral effect [4].
  3) Antitrichomonal effect [4].
  4) Antitussive effect (vanillic acid) [5].
  5) Antitumour effect (senecionine) [6].

174

Literatures:

[1] Valadon, L. R. G. et al.:*Phytochem.* **1976**, 6, 983.

[2] Batza, Y. et al.:*Curr. Sci.* **1977**, 46(5), 141.

[3] Wang, X. F. et al.:*Yaoxue Xuebao* **1980,** 15(8), 503.

[4] Wang, Y.S. et al.: *'Zhongyao Yaoli Yu Yingyong'* **1983,** 115.

[5] Kupchan, S. M. et al.:*J. Pharm. Sci.* **1967**, 56(4), 541.

[6] Culvenor, C. C. J.:*ibid.* **1968**, 57(7), 1112.

[J.X. Guo]

168.   *Siegesbeckia pubescens* **Makino**   (Compositae)
               (= *S. orientalis* L. var. *pubescens* Makino)

Xian–geng–xi–xian (C), Hay–gim–cho (H), Menamomi (J), Teol–jin–deuk–chal (K)

Related plant: *Siegesbeckia orientalis* L.: Xi–xian (C); *S. glabrescens* Makino: Mao–geng–xi–xian (C).

Aerial part

Local Drug Name: Xi–xian–cao (C), Hay–gim–cho (H), Ki–ren–so (J), Heui–cheom (K).

Processing: Dry under the sun (C. K).

Method of Adminiatration: Oral (decoction: C, H, K).

Folk Medicinal Uses:

            1) Rheumatic arthritis (C, H, J).

            2) Hypertension (C, K, H, J).

            3) Malaria (C, H).

            4) Hemiplegia (H).

            5) Hepatitis (H).

            6) Neurasthenia (H).

            7) Common cold (J).

            8) Apoplexy (K).

Scientific Researches:

Chemistry

    1) Diterpenes: darutoside [1], pimar–8(14)–ene–6β–15,16,18–tetraol, (–)–16,17–dihydroxy–16β–kauran–
          19–oic acid, (–)–17–hydroxy–16β–kauran–19–oic acid [2], kirenol [3], siegesbeckioside,
          siegesbeckiol, siegesbeckic acid [4].

    2) Alkaloids [5].

Pharmacology

    1) Anti–inflammatory effect ((–)–16,17–dihydroxy–16β–kauran–19–oic acid, (–)–17–hydroxy–16β–
          kauran–19–oic acid [2]).

    2) Antihypertensive effect [6] ((–)–16,17–dihydroxy–16β–kauran–19–oic acid) [2].

Literatures:

[1] Kim, J. H. et al.:*Phytochem.* **1979**, 18(5), 894.

[2] Han, K.D. et al.:*Terpenoids, Proc. Symp.,* **1974**, 17.

[3] Takao, M. et al.: *Tetrahed. Lett.* **1973**, (50), 4991.

[4] Xiong, J. et al.:*Phytochem.* **1992**, 31(33), 917.

[5] Woo, L.K. et al.:*Soul Taehakkyo Saengyak Yonguso Opjukjip,* **1978**, 17, 17.

[6] Xue, W.: *Zhonghua Neike Zazhi,* **1960**(2), 115.

[J.X. Guo]

169.   *Taraxacum mongolicum* **Hand.–Mazz.**   (Compositae)

Pu–gong–ying (C), Po–kung–ying (H), Moko–tanpopo (J)

Related plant: *Taraxacum officinale* Weber: Pu–gong–ying (C), Po–kung–ying (H), Sei–yo–tanpopo (J),
Seo–yang–min–deul–re (K).

Whole plant (CP)
Local Drug Name: Pu–gong–ying (C), Po–kung–ying (H), Ho–ko–ei (J), Po–gong–yeong (K).
Processing: Eliminate foreign matter, wash, dry under the sun.
Method of Administration: Oral (decoction: C, H, J), topical (juice: C, H, J, K).
Folk Medicinal Uses:
        1) Upper respiratory tract infection, acute tonsillitis (C, H, J).
        2) Conjunctivitis (C, H).
        3) Epidemic parotitis, acute mastitis (C, H, J).
        4) Gastritis, enteritis, dysentery (C, H, J, K).
        5) Hepatitis, cholecystitis (C, H).
        6) Acute appendicitis (C, H).
        7) Urinary tract infection (C, H, J).
        8) Pelvic inflammatory disease (C, H).
        9) Boils, pyodermas, snake bites (C, H).
        10) Lymphoma (K).
Side Effects: Pallor and shivering in some cases receiving intravenous injections; nausea, dizziness,
sweating or even urticaria in cases receiving tincture of the herb.

Scientific Researches:
Chemistry
  1) Taraxinic acid 1'–O–β–glucopyranoside [3].
  2) Taraxasterol, choline, inulin, pectin, taraxol, taraxerol.
  3) Neosanthin, flavosanthin, chrysanthemaxanthin [6, 7].
  4) Fatty acids [14, 15].
  5) Tetrahydroridentin [18].
Pharmacology
  1) Antibacterial effects.
  2) Hypoglycemic effects [1, 11].
  3) Antiviral effects [8].
  4) Stimulatory effects on phagocytosis in mouse reticuloendotherial system (inulin) [9].
  5) Antineoplastic effects [10].
  6) Endothelium–dependent vasorelaxant effects [12].

Literatures:
[1] Akhtar, M.S. et al.:*J. Pak. Med. Assoc.* **1985**, 35, 207–10.
[2] Hausen, B.M. et al.:*Derm. Beruf. Umwelt.* **1978**, 26, 198.
[3] Hausen, B.M.:*Derm. Beruf. Umwelt.* **1982**, 30, 51–3.
[4] Racz–Kotilla, E. et al.:*Planta Med.* **1974**, 26, 212–7.
[5] Rutherford, P.P. et al.: Biochem. J.**1972**, 126, 569–73.
[6] Nitsche, H. et al.:*Phytochem.* **1972**, 11. 3383.
[7] Bergeron, J.M. et al.:*Can. J. Zool.* **1980**, 58, 1575–81.
[8] Zhang, M.S.: *Chinese J. Integrated Trad. West. Med.***1990**, 10, 39–41.
[9] Matsuda, H. et al.:*Yakugaku Zasshi* **1987**, 107, 429–34.
[10] Baba, K. et al.:*Yakugaku Zasshi* **1981**, 101, 538–43.
[11] Swanston–Flatt, S.K. et al.:*Diabetes Res.* **1989**, 10, 69–73.
[12] You, C.L. et al.:*Niigata Igakkai Zasshi***1992**, 106, 513–7.

[13] Besora, C.: *Circ. Farm.* **1974**, 32, 641–3.

[14] Takanashi, M. et al.: *Yakagaku* **1973**, 22, 269–71.

[15] Mitsuhashi et al.: *Tokyo Gakugei Daigaku Kiyo, Dai–4–Bu* **1978**, 30, 91–5.

[16] Pickett, J.A. et al.: *J. Chem. Ecol.* **1980**, 6, 435–44.

[17] Samokhvalova, G.V. et al.: *Vestn. Mosk. Univ., Ser. 16: Biol.* **1981**, (1), 24–7.

[18] Hänsel, R. et al.: *Phytochem.* **1980**, 19, 857–61.

[P.P.H. But]

170. *Tussilago farfara* L. (Compositae)

Kuan–dong (C), Foon–dung–fa (H), Fukitanpopo (J), Gwan–dong (K)

Bud (CP)

Local Drug Name: Kuan–dong–hua (C), Foon–dung–fa (H), Kan–to–ka (J), Gwan–dong–hwa (K).

Processing: 1) Eliminate foreign matter and residual pedicels (C). 2) Stir–fry with honey (C).

Method of Adminiatration: Oral (decoction: C, H, J).

Folk Medicinal Uses:

     1) Acute or chronic cough with dyspnea and copious expectoration (C, H, J).

     2) Hemoptysis in consumptive diseases (C, H).

Side Effects: Digestive tract reaction, vexation, insomnia (C). Hepatotoxicity (H).

Scientific Researches:

Chemistry

  1) Alkaloids: senkirkine [1], tussilagine [2], senecionine [3].

  2) Sesquiterpenes: tussilagin [4] (= tussilagone [5], farfaratin [6], L–653, 469 [7], 14–acetoxy–7β–[3'–ethyl–crotonoloxy]–notonipetranone), 14–acetoxy–7β–[3'–ethyl crotonoloxy]–1α–[2'–methylbutylryl–oxy]–notonipetranone, 7β–[3'–ethylcrotonoloxy]–1α–[2'–methyl–butylryloxy]–3,14–dehydro–Z–notonipetranone.

  3) Volatile oil: (5Z)–1,5–undecadiene, (5Z)–tridecadiene, (5Z,8Z)–1,5,8–heptadecatriene, etc. [8].

  4) Organic acids: fezudic acid, p–hydroxybenzoic acid, caffeic acid, caffeoyltartaric acid [9].

  5) Flavonoids: quercetin, kaempferol, quercetin 3–arabinoside, kaempferol 3–arabinoside, quercetin 4'– glucoside, kaempferol 3–glucoside [9].

  6) Others: faradiol, arnidiol.

Pharmacology

  1) Antitussive, expectorant, and antiasthmatic effects (decoction)[10].

  2) Respitation–excitatory effect (alc. and ether ext., tussilagin) [10, 11].

  3) Effect of increasing blood pressure (tussilagin) [11].

  4) Inhibitory effect on gastrointestinal tract smooth muscle, excitatory effect on uterine smooth muscle.

  5) Inhibitory effect on both platelet activating factor (PAF) and Ca^{2+} entry blocker binding to membrane vesicles (tussilagin) [4, 7].

  6) Antibacterial effect [12].

  7) Antiphlogistic, immunoslenoulating and cytoprotective effect [13].

Litratures:

[1] Luethy, J. et al.: *Mitt. Geb. Lebensmittelunters. Hyg,* **1980**, 71(1), 73.

[2] Roeder,E. et al.: *Planta Med.,* **1981**, 43(1), 99.

[3] Rosberger, D.F. et al.: *Mitt. Geb. Lebensmittelunters.Hyg,* **1981**, 72(4), 432.

[4] Han, G.Q. et al.: *Beijing Yike Daxue Xuebao,* **1987**, 19(1), 33.

[5] Ying, B.P. et al.: *Huaxue Xuebao,* **1987**, 45(5), 450.

[6] Wang, C.D. et al.: *Yaoxue Xuebao,* **1989**, 24(12), 913.

[7] Hwang, S.B. et al.: *Eur. J. Pharmacol,* **1987**, 14(2), 269.

[8] Suzuki, N. et al.: *Yakugaku Zasshi,* **1992**, 112(8), 571.
[9] Didry, N. et al.: *Ann. Pharm. Fr.,* **1980**, 38(3), 237.
[10] Wang, Y.S. et al.: *"Zhongyao Yaoli Yu Yingyong",* **1983,** 1132.
[11] Li, Y.P. et al.: *Zhongguo Yaoli Xuebao,* **1986**, 7(4), 333.
[12] Didry, N. et al.: *Ann. Pharm. Fr.,* **1982**, 40(1), 75.
[13] Wickman, L. et al.: *Eur. Pat.* Appl. EP 213, 099.

[J.X. Guo]

171. *Xanthium sibiricum* Patrin. (Compositae)

Cang–er (C), Chong–yee (H), Do–ggo–ma–ri (K)

Related Plant: *Xanthium strumarium* L.: Onamomi (J).

Fruit (CP)
Local Drug Name: Cang–er–zi (C), Chong–yee–gee (H), So–ji–shi (J), Chang–i–ja (K).
Processing: Stir–frying (C). Dry under the sun (J).
Method of Adminiatration: Oral (decoction: C, H, J, K).
Folk Medicinal Uses:
        1) Headache caused by "wind–cold" (C, H, J, K).
        2) Sinusitis with nasal discharge (C, H, J).
        3) Urticaria with itching (C, H, J, K).
        4) Arthritis with limited motion of the joint (C, H, K).
        5) Uterine bleeding (H).
        6) Deep abscesses (H).
        7) Leprosy, eczema (H).
        8) Gout (K).
        9) Dermatopathy (K).
Side Effects: Toxic (fresh fruit, atractyloside).

Scientific Researches:
Chemistry
    1) Glycosides: xanthostrumarin [1], atractyloside [2], carboxyatractyloside [3].
    2) Steroids: β–sitosterol, stigmasterol [4].
    3) Others: xanthanol, isoxanthanol, hydroquinone [5].
Pharmacology
    1) Hypoglycemic effect (A2 [6], carboxyatractyloside [3]).
    2) Antitussive effect [2].
    3) Inhibitory effect on heart [7].
    4) Antibacterial effect [7].

Literatures:
[1] Wehemer, C.: *"Die Pflanzenstoffe",* Vol. 2, **1931**, 1223.
[2] Wang, S.X. et al.: *Zhongcaoyao,* **1983,** 14(12), 1.
[3] Tumer, C.E. et al.: *US Patent,* 33,922,263, **1975**.
[4] Nishioka, I. et al.: *Chem. Pharm. Bull.,* **1965**, 13, 379.
[5] Kuzel, N.R. et al.: *J. Amer. Pharm. Ass. (Sci. Ed.),* **1950**, 36(4), 202.
[6] Shong, Z.Y. et al.: *Yaoxue Xuebao,* **1962**, 9(11), 678.
[7] Wang, Y.S. et al.: *"Zhongyao Yaoli Yu Yingyong",* **1983**, 509.

[J.X. Guo]

172.   *Alisma orientale* (Sam.) **Juzepczuk**   (Alismataceae)
            (= *A. plantago – aquatica* L. subsp. *orientale* Sam.)

Zexie (C), Jark–sair (H), Jil–gyung–i–taek–sa (K).

Related Plant: *Alismata plantago – aquatica* L.: Sajiomodaka (J).

Corm (Rhizome)   (CP, JP, KP)
  Local Drug Name: Ze–xie (C), Jark–sair (H), Taku–sha (J), Taek–sa (K).
  Processing: Air dry.
  Method of Administration: Oral (decoction: C, H, J, K).
  Folk Medicinal Uses:
                  1) Edema (C, H, J, K).
                  2) Dyspepsia (C, J).
                  3) Gonorrhoea (K).
                  4) Vomiting (H).
                  5) Dysentery (H).
                  6) Beriberi (H).
                  7) Dysuria (H, J).
                  8) Hematuria (H).
                  9) Diarrhea with diminished discharge of urine (C).
                  10) Vertigo due to retention of fluid (C).
                  11) Acute urinary infection with difficult painful urination (C).
                  12) Hyperlipemia (C).

Scientific Researches:
  Chemistry
    1) Triterpenoids: alisol A, alisol A monoacetate, alisol B, alisol B monoacetate [1, 2].
    2) Sesquiterpenes [2].
    3) Polysaccharides [3].
  Pharmacology
    1) Diuretic (water extract) [4].
    2) Against fatty liver (choline, lecithin, alisol A monoacetate) [5].
    3) Sodium excretion increasing in urea [6].
    4) Inhibition of artery contraction (alisol) [7].
    5) Blood circulation (alisol) [8].

Literatures:
[1] Murata, T., et al.: *Chem. Pharm. Bull.* **1970,** 18, 1347, 1354, 1362, 1369; Fujioka, S., et al. *Takeda Kenkyusho Nenpo* **1975,** 34, 351.
[2] Oshima, Y., et al.: *Phytochemistry* **1983,** 22, 183.
[3] Tomoda, et al. : *Chem. Pharm. Bull.* **1984,** 32, 2845; **1987,** 35, 3918.
[4] Tsurumi, S., et al.: *Gifu Ikadaigaku Kiyo* **1963,** 11, 129; Haginiwa, T., et al.: *Shoyakugaku Zasshi* **1963,** 17, 6; Tanaka, S., et al.: *Yakugaku Zasshi* **1984,** 104, 601; Hsü. C. T.: *Acta Sch. Med. Gifu* **1957,** 5, 485.
[5] Kobayashi, T.: *Yakugaku Zasshi,* **1960,** 80, 1456, 1460, 1465, 1612, 1617; Imai, Y., et al. *Japan. J. Pharmacol.* **1970,** 20, 222; Imai, Y., et al.: *Takeda Kenkyusho Hokoku,* **1970,** 29, 462; Tamura, S., et al.: *ibid.* 467.
[6] Hikino, H. et al.: *Shoyakugaku Zasshi,* **1982,** 36, 150.
[7] Yamahara, J., et al.: *Chem. Pharm. Bull.* **1986,** 34, 4422; Matsuda, H., et al.: *Life Sci.* **1987,** 41, 1845; Matsuda, H., et al.: *Japan. J. Pharmacol,* **1988,** 46, 331.
[8] Yamahara, J., et al.: *Phytother. Res.* **1989,** 3, 57, 72.

[T. Kimura]

173.   *Allium chinense* **G. Don** (= *A. bakeri* Regel)   (Liliaceae)

Hua–xie–bai (C), Kiu (H), Rakkyo (J), San–bu–chu (K)

Related Plant: *Allium macrostemon* Bunge: Xiao–gen–suan (C).

Bulb
Local Drug Name: Xie–bai (C), Kiu–tou (H), Gai–haku (J), Hae–baek (K).
Method of Administration: Oral (decoction: C, J), topical (Juice: C).
Folk Medicinal Uses:

        1) Colds (C).
        2) Burns (C).
        3) Traumatic injury (C).
        4) Cough and sputum (C).
        5) Diarrhea (C).
        6) Boils (C).
        7) Leukorrea (C).
        8) Stenocardia (C).
        9) Cardiac infanction (J).
        10) Cerebral embolism (J).
        11) Hypertension (J).

Scientific Researches:
Chemistry
  1) N–(p-$trans$-Coumaroyl)–tyramine, N–(p-cis-coumaroyl)–tyramine, lunularic acid, p–coumaric
        acid [1].
Pharmacology
  1) Antibacterial effects (leaf extracts).
  2) Inhibitory effects on prostaglandin and thromboxane synthetases [1].
  3) Inhibitory effects on platelet aggregation [1, 2].

Literatures:
[1] Goda, Y. et al.: *Chem. Pharm. Bull.* **1987**, 35, 2668–74.
[2] Morimitsu, Y. et al.: *J. Agric. Food. Chem.* **1992**, 40, 368–72.

                                            [P.P.H. But]

174.   *Allium sativum* **L.**   (Liliaceae)

Da–suan (C), Die–soon (H), Ninniku, Seiyoninniku (J), Ma–neul (K).

Bulb
Local Drug Name: Da–suan (C), Die–soon (H), Tai–san (J), Dae–san (K).
Method of Administration: Oral (decoction or raw: C, H, J, K).
Folk Medicinal Uses:

        1) Indigestion (C, J, K).
        2) Epigastric pain (C, H, J, K).
        3) Whooping cough (C, K).
        4) Edema (C, J).
        5) Diarrhea (C, H, J).
        6) Malarial diseases (C).
        7) Pyrodermas (C).

8) Tinea (C).

9) Snake and insect bite (C, K).

Contraindications: Yin–deficiency with fire–excess, eye diseases, oral diseases.

Side Effects: Contact dermatitis [6, 54, 61].

Scientific Researches:

Chemistry

1) Allicin, alliin, S–allylcysteine.

2) S–Allylcysteine sulphoxide, a sulphur–containing amino acid [4].

3) Ajoene [9].

4) Mannose–binding lecitins [15].

5) Scordinin A_1 [16, 17].

6) Polysaccharide [31].

7) γ–Glutamyl peptides: γ–L–glutamyl–S–(trans–1–propenyl)–L–cysteine, γ–L–glutamyl–S–allyl–
        L–cysteine, γ–L–glutamyl–S–allylthio–L–cysteine [80].

Pharmacology

1) Antibacterial effects [1, 26, 30, 34, 35, 36, 51, 52, 56, 64, 71].

2) Antifungal effects [25, 28, 32, 37, 43, 44, 48, 66, 69].

3) Antiprotozoan effects [62].

4) Antitumor effects [40, 60, 63, 70, 72].

5) Cytotoxic effects [2].

6) Protective effects against isoproterenol–induced heart, liver and pancreas damage [3], and against
        collagen and arachidonic acid toxicity [13].

7) Antidiabetic effects in alloxan diabetic rats [4].

8) Inhibitory effects on cytochrome P–450 reductases [5].

9) Anticlastogenic effects [7].

10) Cardioprotective effects [8, 67, 68].

11) Anti–platelet aggregation effects [9, 65].

12) Palliate hepatopulmonary syndrome [10].

13) Hypocholesterolaemic effects [11, 29, 39, 41].

14) Virucidal effects [12].

15) Depressant effects on automaticity and tension development in the heart [13].

16) Preventive effects against hepatocarcinogenesis (diallyl disulphide), stimulatory effects on hepato–
        carcinogenesis (diallyl sulphide) [14].

17) Anticoagulant effects on blood [20, 21].

18) Anticandidal effects [24].

19) Anthelmintic effects [27].

20) Hypotensive effects [33, 59].

21) Increase weight of seminal vescicle [42].

22) Anti–atherosclerotic effects [49].

23) Detoxification effects [45, 47].

24) Antimutagenic effects [46].

25) Hepatoprotective effects [57].

26) Immunoprotective effects [58].

27) Antiallergic effects [73].

28) Antioxidant effects [75].

29) Antiproliferative effects on neuroblastoma cells S–allylcysteine) [76].

30) Inhibitory effects on hepatocarcinogenesis induced by diethylnitrosamine [78].

Literatures:

[1] Didry, N. et al.: *Pharmazie* **1987**, 42, 687–8.

[2] Shah, A.H. et al.: *Fitoterapia* **1989**, 60, 171–3.

[3] Ciplea, A.G. et al.: *Arzneimittelforchung* **1988**, 38, 1583–92.

[4] Sheela, C.G. et al.:*Indian J. Exp. Biol.* **1992**, 30, 523–6.

[5] Oelkers, B. et al.:*Arzneimittelforschung* **1992**, 42, 136–9.

[6] Lembo, G. et al.:*Contact Dermatitis* **1991**, 25, 330–1.

[7] Das, T. et al.:*Environ. Mol. Mutagen* **1993**, 21, 383–8.

[8] Isensee, H. et al.: Arzneimittelforschung **1993**, 43, 94–8.

[9] Tatarintsev, A.V. et al.:*Vestn. Ross. Akad. Med. Nauk.* **1992**, (11–12), 6–10.

[10] Caldwell, S.H. et al.:*J. Clin. Gastroenterol.* **1992**, 15, 248–50.

[11] Rotzsch, W. et al.:*Arzneimittelforschung* **1992**, 42, 1223–7.

[12] Weber, N.D. et al.:*Planta Med.* **1992**, 58, 417–23.

[13] Alnaqeeb, M.A. et al.:*Prostaglandins, Leukotrienes Essent. Fatty Acids* **1992**, 46, 301–6.

[14] Takahashi, S. et al.:*Carcinogenesis* **1992**, 13, 1513–8.

[15] Kaku, H. et al.:*Carbohydr. Res.* **1992**, 229, 347–53.

[16] Kominato, K.:*Chem. Pharm. Bull.* **1969**, 17, 2193–7.

[17] Kominato, K.:*Chem. Pharm. Bull.* **1969**, 17: 2198–208.

[18] Abdo, M.S. et al.:*Jpn. J. Pharmacol.* **1969**, 19, 1–4.

[19] Fujiwara, M. et al.:*Nature* **1967**, 216, 83–4.

[20] Song, C.S. et al.:*Yonsei Med. J.* **1963**, 4, 21–6.

[21] Song, C.S. et al.:*Yonsei Med. J.* **1963**, 4, 17–20.

[22] Augusti, K.T. et al.:*Indian J. Exp. Biol.* **1973**, 11, 239–41.

[23] Tynecka, Z. et al.:*Acta Microbiol. Pol. [B]* **1973**, 5, 51–62.

[24] Barone, F.E. et al.:*Mycologia* **1977**, 69, 793–825.

[25] Tynecka, Z. et al.:*Ann. Univ. Mariae Curie Sklodowska [Med]* **1975**, 30, 5–13.

[26] Uchida, Y. et al.:*Jpn. J. Antibiot.* **1975**, 28. 638–42.

[27] Raj, R.K.:*Indian J. Physiol. Pharmacol.* **1975**, 19(1),

[28] Fromtling, R.A. et al.:*Mycologia* **1978**, 70, 397–405.

[29] Augusti, K.T.:*Indian J. Exp. Biol.* **1977**, 15, 489–90.

[30] Sharma, V.D. et al.:*Indian J. Exp. Biol.* **1977**, 15, 466–8.

[31] Das, N.N. et al.:*Carbohydr. Res.* **1977**, 56, 337–49.

[32] Prasad, G. et al.:*Br. Vet. J.* **1980**, 136, 448–51.

[33] Malik, Z.A. et al.:*J. Pak. Med. Assoc.* **1981**, 31, 12–3.

[34] Paszewski, A. et al.:*Ann. Univ. Mariae Curie Sklodowska [Med]* **1978**, 33, 415–22.

[35] Dankert, et al.:*Zentralbl. Bakteriol.* **1979**, 245, 229–39.

[36] Kumar, A. et al.:*Indian J. Med. Res.* **1982**, 76 Suppl, 66–70.

[37] Caporaso, N. et al.:*Antimicrob. Agents Chemother.* **1983**, 23, 700–2.

[38] Dixit, V.P. et al.:*Indian J. Exp. Biol.* **1982**, 20, 534–536.

[39] Kamanna, V.S. et al.:*Lipids* **1982**, 17, 483–8.

[40] Rao, A.R. et al.:*Indian J. Exp. Biol.* **1990**, 28, 405–8.

[41] Dausch, J.G. et al.:*Prev. Med.* **1990**, 19, 346–61.

[42] al–Bekairi, A.M. et al.:*J. Ethnopharmacol.* **1990**, 29, 117–25.

[43] Davis, L.E. et al.:*Antimicrob. Agents Chemother.* **1990**, 34, 651–3.

[44] Ghannoum, M.A.:*J. Appl. Bacteriol.* **1990**, 68, 163–9.

[45] Unnikrishnan, M.C. et al.:*Nutr. Cancer* **1990**, 13, 201–7.

[46] Zhang, Y.S. et al.:*Mutat. Res.* **1989**, 227, 215–9.

[47] Cha, C.W.:*J. Korean Med. Sci.* **1987**, 2, 213–24.

[48] Louria, D.B. et al.:*J. Med. Vet. Mycol.* **1989**, 27, 253–6.

[49] Lata, S. et al.:*J. Postgrad. Med.* **1991**, 37, 132–5.

[50] Fehri, B. et al.:*J. Pharm. Belg.* **1991**, 46, 363–74.

[51] Elnima, E.I.:*Pharmazie* **1983**, 38, 747–8.

[52] Adetumbi, M.A. et al.:*Med. Hypotheses* **1983**, 12, 227–37.

[53] Rodriguez, S.M. et al.:*Rev. Med. Panama* **1983**, 8, 206–11.

[54] Papageorgiou, C. et al.:*Arch. Dermatol. Res.* **1983**, 275, 229–34.

[55] Delaha, E.C. et al.:*Antimicrob. Agents Chemother.* **1985**, 27, 485–6.

[56] Tongia, S.K.:*Indian J. Physiol. Pharmacol.* **1984**, 28, 250–2.

[57] Hikino, H. et al.:*Planta Medica* **1986**, 163–8.

[58] Lau, B.H. et al.:*J. Urol.* **1986**, 136, 701–5.

[59] Ribeiro, R. de A. et al.:*J. Ethnopharmacol.* **1986**, 15, 261–9.

[60] Aboul–Enein, A.M.:*Nahrung* **1986**, 30, 161–9.

[61] Fernandez, de Corres L. et al.:*Allergol. Immunopathol.* **1985**, 13, 291–9.

[62] Mirelman, D. et al.:*J. Infect. Dis.* **1987**, 156, 243–4.

[63] Wargovich, M.J.:*Carcinogenesis* **1987**, 8, 487–9.

[64] Marsh, C.L. et al.: *J. Urol.* **1987**, 137, 359–62.

[65] Mohammad, S.F. et al.:*Thromb. Res.* **1986**, 44, 793–806.

[66] Adetumbi, M. et al.:*Antimicrob. Agents Chemother.* **1986**, 30, 499–501.

[67] Kendler, B.S.:*Prev. Med.* **1987**, 16, 670–85.

[68] Ernst, E.: *Pharmatherapeutica* **1987**, 5, 83–9.

[69] Ghannoum, M.A.:*J. Gen. Microbiol.* **1988**, 134, 2917–24.

[70] Wargovich, M.J. et al.:*Cancer Res.* **1988**, 48, 6872–5.

[71] Gimenez, M.A. et al.:*Rev. Argent Microbiol.* **1988**, 20, 17–24.

[72] Brady, J.F. et al.:*Cancer Res.* **1988**, 48, 5937–40.

[73] Tanaka, Y. et al.:*Osaka–furitsu Koshu Eisei Kenkyusho Kenkyu Hokoku, Shokuhin Eisei Hen***1991**, 22, 7–13.

[74] Morimitsu, Y. et al.:*J. Agric. Food Chem.* **1992**, 40, 368–72.

[75] Yang, G.C. et al.:*J. Food Drug Anal. (Taiwan)* **1993**, 1, 357–64.

[76] Welch, C. et al.: *Cancer Lett. (Shannon, Irel.)* **1992**, 63, 211–9.

[77] Didry, N. et al.:*Pharm. Acta Helv.* **1992**, 67, 148–51.

[78] Lee, Y.S. et al.:*Environ. Mutagens Carcinog.* **1991**, 11, 21–8.

[79] Pino, J.A.:*J. Sci. Food Agric.* **1992**, 59, 131–3.

[80] Muetsch–Eckner, M. et al.:*Phytochem.* **1992**, 31, 2389–91.

[P.P.H. But]

175.   *Allium tuberosum* Rottler   (Liliaceae)

Jiu–cai (C), Gou–choi (H), Nira (J), Bu–chu (K)

Leaf

Local Drug Name: Jiu–cai (C), Gou–choi (H), Kyu–haku (J), Gu–chae (K).

Processing: Use in fresh.

Method of Administration: Oral or topical (juice or as food: C, H, J, K).

Folk Medicinal Uses:

         1) Chest discomfort (C, H).

         2) Hiccup (C, H).

         3) Nausea (C).

         4) Hematuria, hematemesis, epistaxis (C).

         5) Diarrhea (C, J, K).

         6) Prolapse of rectum (C).

         7) Traumatic injury (C).

         8) Insect bite (C, K).

         9) Hemorrhoid (C).

         10) Tonic (K).

         11) Tinea pedis (K).

Contraindications: Eye diseases.

Seed (CP)

Local Drug Name: Jiu–zi (C), Gou–choi–gee (H), Kyu–shi (J), Gu–ja (K).

Processing: Eliminate foreign matter and dry, or stir–fry the clean seeds with salt–water and then dry.

Method of Administration: Oral (decoction: C, H, K).

Folk Medicinal Uses:

      1) Spermatorrhea (C, H, J).

      2) Frequent urination (C, J).

      3) Lumbago (C).

      4) Leukorrhea (C, H).

      5) Diarrhea (J).

      5) Toothache (K).

Contraindications: Yin–deficiency with fire–excess.

Root

Local Drug Name: Jiu–gen (C), Gu–geun (K).

Method of Administration: Oral or topical (decoction or juice: C).

Folk Medicinal Uses:

      1) Leukorrhea (C).

      2) Chest distention (C).

      3) Traumatic injury (C).

      4) Tinea (C).

      5) Hematuria (C).

      6) Epistaxis (C).

Scientific Researches:

Chemistry

1) Dimethyl disulphide, diallyl sulphide, methylallyl disulphide, dimethyl trisulphide, diallydisulphide, methylallyl trisulphide, dimethyl tetrasulphide, linalool [1].

2) Hexadecanoic acid, 1,3–dithiane, 2–methyl–1,3–oxathiane, di–2–propenyl–trisulphide, 2,4–di-methyl–thiophene [2].

3) Cysteine synthase [3].

4) Thilanes: trans– and cis–3,5–diethyl–1,2,4–trithiolane, trans– and cis–3–methyl–5–ethyl–1,2,4-–trithiolane [5].

Pharmacology

1) Antibacterial effects.

Literatures:

[1] Kameoka, H. et al.: *Nippon Nogei Kagaku Kaishi* **1974**, 48, 385–8.

[2] Yi, Y.H. et al.: *Zhongguo Yaoxue Zazhi* **1991**, 26, 648–9.

[3] Ikegami, F. et al.: *Phytochem.* **1992**, 32, 31–4.

[4] Mackenzie, I.A. et al.: *Phytochem.* **1977**, 16, 763–4.

[5] Kameoka, H. et al.: *Tennen Yuki Kagobutsu Toronkai Koen Yoshishu, 21st.* **1978**, 199–205.

[P.P.H. But]

176.   *Anemarrhena asphodeloides* **Bunge**   (Liliaceae)

Zhi–mu (C), Gee–mo (H), Hanasuge (J), Ji–mo (K).

Rhizome (CP, JP, KP)

Local Drug Name: Zhi–mu (C), Gee–mo (H), Chi–mo (J), Ji–mo (K).

Processing: 1) Dry under the sun, and remove hairs and scraps.

          2) Stir–fry with salt water until dryness (C).

Method of Administration: Oral (decoction: C, H, J, K).
Folk Medicinal Uses:
1) Fever (C, J, K). Febrile diseases (C, H).
2) Diabetes (C, H, J, K).
3) Dire thirst (C, K).
4) Heat in the lung with dry cough (C).
5) Constipation (C, H).
6) Cough (C, H, K).
7) Oliguria (H, J).

Scientific Research:
Chemistry
1) Saponins: asphonin [1], sarsasapogenin, timosaponin A–I, A–II, A–III, A–IV, B–I, B–II [2] .
2) Phenolic compounds: *cis*–hinokiresinol [3].
3) Polysaccharides: anemaran A, B, C, D [4].
4) Xanthones: mangiferin (= chimonin) [5].
Pharmacology
1) Blood sugar lowering (water extract, anemaran A, B, C, D) [6,7,8].
2) Blood ketones lowering in mouce with diabetes (water extract) [7].
3) Inhibition fo stress ulcer (water extract) [9].
4) Antipyretic (decoction) [10].
5) Platelet coagulation inhibiting (timosaponin A–III, markogenin glycoside) [11].
6) Hemolytic (timosaponia A–III) [11].
7) Inhibition of cyclic AMP phosphodiesterase (*cis*–hinokiresinol) [12].
8) Sadative (*cis*–hinokiresinol) [12].

Literatures:
[1] Kodama, J.:*Manshu Igakkai Zasshi* **1934**, 21, 211.
[2] Takeda, K. et al.:*Yakugaku Zasshi* **1953**, 73, 29; **1954**, 74, 1371; Kawasaki, T. et al.:*ibid.* **1963**, 83, 892; *Chem. Pharm. Bull.* **1963**, 11, 1221.
[3] Saito, T. et al.:*Ann. Meeting, Jap. Soc. Pharmacognosy, abstr* **1975**.
[4] Hikino, H. et al.:*Planta Med.* **1985**, 100.
[5] Morita, N. et al.:*Yakugaku Zasshi* **1965**, 85, 374.
[6] Bin, H. :*Nippon Yakubutsugaku Zasshi* **1930**, 11, 22; Koda, A. et al.:*Nippon Yakurigaku Zasshi,* **1971**, 67, 223.
[7] Kimura, M.:*Nippon Rinsho* **1967**, 25, 2841.
[8] Takahashi, M. et al.:*Planta Med.* **1985**, 51, 100.
[9] Yamazaki, M. et al.:*Shoyakugaku Zasshi* **1981**, 35, 96.
[10] Noguchi, M.:*Shoyakugaku Zasshi* **1967**, 21, 17.
[11] Niwa, A. et al.:*Yakugaku Zasshi* **1988**, 108, 555.
[12] Nikaido, T. et al. :*Planta Med.* **1981**, 43, 18.

[T. Kimura]

177. *Fritillaria thunbergii* **Miq.** (Liliaceae)

Zhe–bei–mu (C), Jzit–bui–mo (H), Amigasayuri (J), Jung–guk–pae–mo (K)

Bulb (CP)
Local Drug Name: Zhe–bei–mu (C), Jit–bui–mo (H), Bai–mo (J), Pae–mo (K).
Processing: Cut into thick slices and dry, or pound to pieces (C).
Eliminate skins, keep a few days with slaked lime and dry under the sun (J).

Method of Adminidstration: Oral (decoction or power: C, H, J).
Folk Medicinal Uses:

　　　　1) Cough caused by wind–heat, dryness–heat or phlegm–heat (C, H, J, K).
　　　　2) Lung abscess (C, H, J, K).
　　　　3) Mastitis (C, J).
　　　　4) Scrofula (C, H).
　　　　5) Depression (C).
　　　　6) Hematemesis (C, H).
　　　　7) Epistaxis (C, H).

Scientific Researches:

Chemistry
　1) Alkaloids: peimine (verticine), peiminine (verticinine), isopeiminine, peimisine, peimiphine, peimidine, peimitidine, baimonidine, isobaimonidine, verticine *N*–oxide, verticinine *N*–oxide, verticinine *N*–oxide, fritillarizine [1–5], zhebeinine [6].
　2) Alkaloidal glycosides: peiminoside [7].
　3) Steroids: propeimin.
Pharmacology
　1) Antitussive effect (peimine, peiminine) [8].
　2) Atropine–like effect (alkaloids) [9].
　3) Antihypertensive effect (peimine, peiminoside) [10].

Literatures:

[1] Xu, D. M. et al.:*Zhongcaoyao*, **1991,** 22, 132.
[2] Kaneko, K. et al.:*Chem. Pham. Bull.*, **1980,** 28, 1345, 3711.
[3] Kaneko, K. et al.:*Tetrahedron Lett.*, **1979,** 35, 3737.
[4] Kitajima, J. et al.:*Phytochem.*, **1982,** 21, 187.
[5] Kitajima, J. et al.:*Heterocycles*, **1981,** 15, 791.
[6] Zhang, J. X. et al.:*Yaoxue Xuebao*, **1991,** 26, 231.
[7] Marimate, H. et al.:*Chem. Pharm. Bull.*, **1960,** 8, 302.
[8] Nanjing College of Pharmacy: *"Zhongcaoyao Xue"*, Vol. 3, **1980,** 1301.
[9] Zhang, C. S. et al.: *Chinese Med. J.*, **1949,** 35, 353.
[10] Kikuchi, K. et al.:*Nippon Yakurigaku Zasshi*, **1961,** 61, 493.

　　　　　　　　　　　　　　　　　　　　　　　　　　　　　　　[J.X. Guo]

178.　　　　　　　*Lilium brownii* F.E. Brown var. *vivridulum* Baker　　(Liliaceae)

Bai–he (C), Bak–hup (H)

Related Plants:　*Lilium auratum* Lindl: Yamayuri (J);*L. lancifolium* Thunb.: Juan–dan (C), Oniyuri (J), Cham–na–ri (K);*L. pumilum* DC.: Xi–ye–bai–he (C).

Bulb

Local Drug Name: Bai–he (C), Bak–hup (H), Byaku–go (J), Baek–hap (K).
Processing:　　　1) Wash clean, heat with boiling water briefly and dry (C, J, K).
　　　　　　　　　2) Stir–fry with honey to no longer stick (C).
Method of Administration: Oral (decoction: C, H, J, K); topical (Powder: C, H).
Folk Medicinal Uses:

　　　　1) Deficiency of yin with chronic cough and bloody sputum (C, H, J).
　　　　2) Fidgetness, palpitation, insomnia, dream–disturbed sleep and absent–mindedness (C, H).
　　　　3) Pulmary tuberculosis (H).

4) Bronchitis (H).
5) Hemoptysis (H).
6) Hematemesis (H).
7) Weakness (J).
8) Mastitis (K).
9) Furuncle (K).

Scientific Researches:
Chemistry
  1) Alkaloids: colchicine, etc. [1]
  2) Starch, protein, fat [1].
Pharmacology
  1) Antitussive, antiasthmatic effects [2].
  2) Hemostyptic effect [2].

Literatures:
[1] Nanjing College of Pharmacy: "*Zhongcaoyao Xue*", Vol. 3, **1980**, 1309.
[2] "*Zhongyao Zhi*", Vol. 2, **1982**, 348.

[J.X. Guo]

179.   *Ophiopogon chekiangensis* **K.Kimura et H. Migo**   (Liliaceae)

Mai–dong (C), Mak–moon–dung (H), Sekko–ryunohige (J), So–yeop–maek–mun–dong (K)

Related plants: *Ophiopogon japonicus* Ker Maek–Gawl.: Janohige (J).
          Liriope platyphylla Wang et Tang (= *L. muscari* L. H. Bailey): Yaburan (J), Maek–
          mun–dong (K).

Tuberous root (CP, JP, KP)
  Local Drug Name: Mai–dong (C), Mak–moon–dung (H), Baku–mon–do (J), Maek–mun–dong (K).
  Processing: Dry under the sun.
  Method of Administration: Oral (decoction: C, H, J, K).
  Folk Medicinal Uses:
          1) Phlegm (J, K).
          2) Bronchitis (J, K).
          3) Bronchial asthma (J, K).
          4) Cough (H, J, K), dry cough, phthisical cough (C).
          5) Hemoptysis (H).
          6) Diabetes caused by internal heat (C, H).
          7) Febrile diseases (H). Diphtheria (C).
          8) Constipation (C, H).
          9) Thirst due to impairment of body fluid (C).
          10) Fidgetness and insomnia (C).

Scientific Researches:
Chemistry
  1) Saponins: ophiopogonin A, B, C, D [1].
  2) Monoterpenoids: borneol derivative [2].
  3) Oligosaccharides [3].
  4) Homoisoflavonoids [4].
Pharmacology

187

1) Blood sugar lowering (decoction) [5].

2) Antiinflammatory (methanol extract) [6].

3) Antiallergic (ophiopogonin D) [7].

Literatures :

[1] Kato, H., et al.:*Yakugaku Zasshi* **1968**, 88, 710; Shoji, J., et al.:*Chem. Pharm. Bull.* **1972**, 20, 1729; **1973**, 21, 308; **1977**, 25, 3049; Watanabe, Y., et al.:*Chem. Pharm. Bull.* **1983**, 31, 3486; **1984**, 32, 3994.

[2] Kaneda, N., et al.:*Yakugaku Zasshi* **1983**, 103, 1133.

[3] Tomoda, S., et al.:*Shoyakugaku Zasshi* **1966**, 20, 12; *Chem. Pharm. Bull.* **1968**, 16, 113; **1973**, 25, 659.

[4] Tada, A., et al. :*Chem. Pharm. Bull.* **1980**, 28, 1477, 2039, 2487; Zhu, Y. X., et al.: *Phytochemistry* **1987**, 26, 2873 ; *J. Chromatogr.* **1988**, 437, 265; *Yaowu Fenxi Zazhi* **1988**, 8, 343.

[5] Koda, A., et al.:*Nippon Yakurigaku Zasshi* **1971**, 67, 223.

[6] Shibata, M., et al.:*Hoshi Yakkadaigaku Kiyo* **1971**, 13, 66.

[7] Mita, A., et al. :*Biomedicine* **1979**, 31, 223.

[T. Kimura]

180. *Polygonatum odoratum* (Mill.) Druce var. *pluriflorum* (Miq.) Ohwi
(Liliaceae)

Yu–zhu (C), Yuk–juk (H), Amadokoro (J), Dung–gul–re (K)

Rhizome (CP)

Local Drug Name: Yu–zhu (C), Yuk–juk (H), I–zui (J), Ok–juk (K).

Processing: Soften throughly, cut into thick slices or sections and dry (C). Steam and sun–dry (H), dry under the sun (J, K).

Method of Administration: Oral (decoction: C, H, J, K).

Folk Medicinal Uses:

1) Reconvalescence after sickness (H, J, K).

2) Febrile diseases (H, K).

3) Weakness (J, K).

4) Frequent urination (C, H).

5) Gastritis (J).

6) Gastric ulcer (J).

7) Spermatorrhea (J).

8) Bruise, sprain (J).

9) Impairment of yin of the lung and the stomach with dry cough, dryness of the throat and thirst(C)

10) Diabetes caused by internal heat (C).

11) Cough (H).

12) Lumbago (H).

Scientific Researches:

Chemistry

1) Flavonoids: polygonatiin, cosmosiin, vitexin 2"–glucoside, saponarin [1].

Literature:

[1] Morita, N. et al.:*Yakugaku Zasshi* **1976,** 96(10), 1180.

[C.K. Sung]

181.   *Smilax china* **L.**   (Liliaceae; Smilacaceae)

Ba–qia (C), Gum–gong–teng (H), Sarutori–ibara (J), Cheong–mi–rae–deong–gul (K)

Rhizome
Local Drug Name: Ba–qia (C), Gum–gong–teng (H), Bak–katsu (J), Bal–gye (K).
Processing: Cut and dry under the sun (J, K).
Method of Administration: Oral (decoction) (C, H, J, K).
Folk Medicinal Uses:
1) Syphilis (J, K).
2) Burn (C, H).
3) Cancer (C, H).
4) Chronic aperient (K).
5) Appendicitis (K).
6) Cough (K).
7) Perspiration (K).
8) Diabetes (H, K).
9) Taenia (K).
10) Pyoderma (H).
11) Abscess, pain (J).
12) Edema (J).
13) Rheumatic arthralgia (C).
14) Injury from fall or beat (C).
15) Dysentery (C, H).
16) Phlegm (C).
17) Acute lymphadenitis (C).
18) Boils (C).
19) Gastroenteritis (C).
20) Rhematic arthritis (H).
21) Traumatic injury (H).
22) Enteritis (H).
23) Chyluria (H).
24) Psoriasis (H).

Scientific Researches:
Chemistry
1) Saponins: smilax saponin.
2) Ketones: 16–hentriacontanone[1].
3) Carotenoids: β–carotene, neo–β–carotene, cryptoxanthin, lutein, lutein epoxide [2].
4) Amino acids: 4–methylene–, 4–methyl– and 4–hydroxy–4–methyl–glutamic acid, arginine,
     N–α–acylarginine, acidic N–α–acylarginine deriv [3, 4].

Literatures:
[1] Isono, H. et al.: *Yakugaku Zasshi* **1974,** 94(3), 404.
[2] Kudritskaya, S. E. et al.: *Khim. Prir. Soedin,* **1987**(5), 759.
[3] Kasai, T. et al.: *Agric. Biol. Chem.* **1984,** 48(9), 2271.
[4] Kasai, T. et al.: *Phytochem.* **1983,** 22(1), 147.

[C.K. Sung]

182.   *Stemona japonica* **Miq.**   (Stemonaceae)

Man–sheng–bai–bu (C), Bak–bo (H), Tsurubyakubu (J)

Related plants: *Stemona sessiliflora* (Miq.) Miq.: Zhi–li–bai–bu (C), Tachibyakubu (J);
                   S. tuberosa Lour.: Dui–ye–bai–bu (C), Tamabyakubu (J).

Root tuber (CP)
Local Drug Name: Bai–bu (C), Bak–bo (H), Byaku–bu (J).
Processing: (1) Eliminate foreign matter, wash clean, soften thoroughly, cut into thick slices, dry
            (2) Stir–fry with honey until not sticky to touch (C).
Method of Administration: Oral (decoction: C, H, J); Topical (decoction or alcoholic extract: C).
Folk Medicinal Uses:
            1) Pulmonary tuberculosis (C, H, J).
            2) Cough, whooping cough (C, H, J).
            3) Senile asthma (C).
            4) Ascariasis (C, J).
            5) Tinea (C).
            6) Eczema (C).

Scientific Researches:
Chemistry
    1) Alkaloids: didehydroprotostemonine, isoprotostemonine, isostemonidine, neostemonine, paipunine,
            protostemonine, sinostemonine, stemodiol, stemonidine, stemonine, tuberostemonine
            [1,2,4,8].
Pharmacology
    1) Antibacterial effects [5].
    2) Insecticidal effects [6, 7].
    3) Tuberostemonine acts as an open–channel blocker at the crayfish neuromuscular junction [1].
    4) Anthelmintic effects [3].
    5) LD_{50} of paipunine = 38,95 ± 2.09 mg/kg i.v. in mice, LD_{50} of sinostemonine 757 ± 53.5 mg/kg i.v.
            in mice [8].

Literatures:
[1] Shinozaki, H. et al: *Brain Res.* **1985**, 334, 33–40.
[2] Ye, Y. et al.: *Chin. Chem. Lett.* **1992**, 3(7), 511–4.
[3] Terada, M. et al.: *Nippon Yakurigaku Zasshi* **1982**, 79, 93–103.
[4] Cong, X.D. et al.: *Yaoxue Xuebao* **1992**, 27, 556–60.
[5] Wang, Y. et al.: *Zhiwu Xuebao* **1954**, 3, 121–131.
[6] Wang, L.S.: *Chin. Med. J.* **1938**, 54, 151–8.
[7] Chao, C.S.: *Chin. Med. J.* **1941**, 60, 517–28.
[8] Lee, H.M. et al.: *J. Amer. Pharmaceut. Ass.* **1940**, 29, 391–4.

[P.P.H. But]

183.   *Curculigo orchioides* **Gaertn.**   (Hypoxidaceae)

Xian–mao (C), Sin–mao (H), Kinbaizasa (J)

Rhizome (CP)
Local Drug Name: Xian–mao (C), Sin–mao (H), Sen–bo (J).
Processing: Eliminate foreign matter, wash clean, cut into sections, dry.
Method of Administration: Oral (decoction: C, H, J).

Folk Medicinal Uses:
1) Lumbago (C, H, J).
2) Impotence (C, H).
3) Menopausal (C, H).
4) Spermatorrhea (C, H).
5) Hypertension (C, H).
6) Chronic nephritis (C, H).
7) Scrofula (C).
8) Rheumatism (J).
9) Limpness of the limbs (C).
10) Knees joints (C).
Contraindications: Yin–deficiency with fire–excess.

Scientific Researches:
Chemistry
1) Sponins: curculigosaponins A, B, C, D, E, F [12], G, H, I, J [2], K, L, and M, curculigenins A, B and C [12, 13].
2) Curculigol [6], 25–dihydroxy–33–methylpentatricantan–one [5].
3) Corchioside A, hentriacontanol, sitosterol, stigmasterol, cycloartenol, sucrose [7].
4) Curculigoside [8,11], orcinol glucoside [11].
5) Glycosides: curculigoside B, curculigines B and C [3].
6) 5,7–dimethoxy myricetin 3–O–α–L–xylopyranosyl 4–O–β–D–glucopyranoside [1].
7) N–Acetyl–N–hydroxy–2–carbamic acid methyl ester, 3–acetyl–5–carbomethoxy–2H–3,4,5,6–tetrahydro–1,2,3,5,6–oxatetrazine,N,N,N',N'–tetramethylsuccinamide [9].
8) Curculigine A [10], 31–methyl–3–oxo–20–ursen–28–oic acid [14].
Pharmacology
1) Immunopotentiating effects [2, 4].
2) Adaptive effects, enhancing tolerance towards high temperature and hypoxia [4].
3) Sedative, anticonvulsant and androgen–like effects [4].
4) Phagocytic effects (curculigoside) [8].

Literatures:
[1] Tiwari, R.D. et al.:*Planta Med.* **1976**, 29, 291–4.
[2] Xu, J.P. et al.:*Planta Med.* **1992**, 58, 208–10.
[3] Xu, J.P. et al.:*Yaoxue Xuebao* **1992**, 27, 353–7.
[4] Chen, Q.S.: *Chung Kuo Chung Yueh Tsa Chih* **1989**, 14, 618–20, 640.
[5] Mehta, B.K. et al.:*Indian J. Chem.* **1990**, 25B, 493–4.
[6] Misra, T.N. et al.:*Phytochem.* **1990**, 29, 929–31.
[7] Garg, S.N. et al.:*Phytochem.* **1989**, 28, 1771–2.
[8] Kubo, M. et al.:*Planta Med.* **1983**, 47. 52–5.
[9] Porwal, M. et al.:*Indian J. Chem.* **1988**, 27B, 856–7.
[10] Xu, J.P. et al.:*Zhongcaoyao* **1987**, 18, 194–5, 222.
[11] Xu, J.P. et al.:*Zhongcaoyao* **1986**, 17, 248–9, 278.
[12] Xu, J.P. et al.:*Phytochem.* **1992**, 31, 233–6.
[13] Xu, J.P. et al.:*Phytochem.* **1992**, 31, 2469–71.
[14] Mehta, B.K. et al.:*Indian J. Chem.* **1991**, 30B, 989–90.

[P.P.H. But]

184.   *Dioscorea opposita* Thunb. (= *D. batatas* Decne.)   (Dioscoreaceae)

Shu–yu (C), Why–saan (H), Nagaimo (J), Ma (K).

Related plant: *Dioscorea japonica* Thunb.; Yamanoimo (J).

Tuber   (CP, JP, KP)
Local Drug Name: Shan–yao (C), Why–saan (H), San–yaku (J), San–yak (K).
Processing: 1) Eliminate foreign matter, soak and soften thoroughly, cut into thick slices and dry (C).
               2) Stir–fry the slices with bran to yellowish (C).
Method of Administration: Oral (decoction: C, H, J, K).
 Folk Medicinal Uses:
               1) Weakness (C, H, J, K).
               2) Dyspepsia (C, J, K).
               3) Furuncle (K).
               4) Diarrhea (C, H, J, K).
               5) Seminal emission, excessive leukorrhea, frerquency of urination or diabetes due to
                  defficiency condition of the kidney (C).

Scientific Researches:
 Chemistry
   1) Glycoprotein [1].
   2) Polysaccharides: dioscoran A∼F [2], dioscoreamucilage B [3].
 Pharmacology
   1) Blood sugar lowering (dioscoran A∼F, dioscoreamucilage B) [2,3]

Literatures:
[1] Tomoda, M., et al.: *Chem. Pharm. Bull.* **1981**, 29, 3256; Kiho, T., et al.: *ibid.* **1985**, 33, 270.
[2] Hikino, H., et al.: *Planta Med.* **1986**, 52, 168.
[3] Tomoda, M. et al.: *Planta Med.* **1987**, 53, 8.

[T. Kimura]

185.   *Dioscorea bulbifera* L.   (Dioscoreaceae)

Huang–du (C), Wong–yuek–gee (H), Nigakashu–u (J), Dung–geun–ma (K)

Tuber
Local Drug Name: Huang–yao–zi (C), Wong–yuek–gee (H), O–yaku–shi (J), Hwang–yak–ja (K).
Processing: Wash clean, cut into slices, dry under the sun.
Method of Administration: Oral or topical (decoction: C, H, J).
Folk Medicinal Uses:
               1) Goiter (C, H).
               2) Tuberculosis lymphadenitis (C, H).
               3) Gastrointestinal cancer (C, H).
               4) Hematemesis, hemoptysis, uterine bleeding (C, H, J).
               5) Boils (C, H, J).
               6) Thyroid tumor (C).
               7) Cough, asthma (C).
               8) Soar throat (J).
Side Effects: Burning sensation of mouth and tongue, vomiting, abdominal pain, coma.

Bulbil
Local Drug Name: Huang–du–ling–yu–zi (C), O–doku–rei–yo–shi (J), Hwang–dok–ryung–yeo–ja (K).
Method of Administration: Oral (decoction: C).
Folk Medicinal Uses:
    1) Whooping cough (C).
    2) Cough (C).
    3) Headache (C).
    4) Gastrointestinal cancer (C).
Side Effects: Hepatotoxic, renotoxic [1].

Scientific Researches:
Chemistry
    1) Diosgenin, diosbulbins.
    2) 4–hydroxy–[2–*trans*–3'7'–dimethyl–octa–2',6'–dienyl]–6–methoxyacetopheone, 4,6–dihydroxy–2–
        O–(4'hydroxybutyl)acetopheone [5].
    3) Demethylbatatasin IV, dihydroresveratrol in bulbils infected with *Botryodiplodia theobromae*[6].
Pharmacology
    1) Anorexient effect [4].
    2) Antifungal effect by demethylbatatasin IV and dihydroresveratrol [6].

Literatures:
[1] Song, C. S.:*Zhongyao Tongbao* **1983**, 8, 34–6.
[2] Martin, F. W. et al.:*J. Agric. Food Chem.* **1974**, 22, 335–7.
[3] Telek, L. et al.:*J. Agric. Food Chem.* **1974**, 22, 332–4.
[4] Jindal, M. N. et al.:*Indian J. Med. Res.* **1969**, 57, 1075–80.
[5] Gupta, D. et al.:*Phytochem.* **1989**, 28, 947–9.
[6] Adesanya, S. A. et al.:*Phytochem.* **1989**, 28, 773–4.

[P.P.H. But]

186.   *Belamcanda chinensis* (L.) DC.   (Iridaceae)

She–gan (C), Sair–gon (H), Hiogi (J), Beom–bu–chae (K)

Rhizome (CP)
Local Drug Name: She–gan (C), Sair–gon (H), Ya–gan (J), Sa–gan (K).
Processing: Cut into thin slices, and dry.
Method of Administration: Oral (decoction: C, H, J, K).
Folk Medicinal Uses:
    1) Wheezing (C, H).
    2) Cough (C, H, J).
    3) Sore throat (C, H, K).
    4) Rice–field dermatitis (C, H).
    5) Pharyngitis (H, J, K).
    6) Tonsillitis (H, J, K).
Contraindications: Pregnancy.

Scientific Researches:
Chemistry
    1) Belamcandin, iridin, irigenin, tectorigenin, tectoridin, dimethyltectorigenin, muningin,
        5,3'–dihydroxy–4'5'–dimethoxy–6,7–methylenedioxyisoflavone, methyl irisolidone,
        irisflorentin, iristectorigenins A and B [1, 7, 8, 9].

2) Mangiferin [3].

3) (+)-(6 *R*,10*S*,11*S*,14*S*,26*R*)-26-hydroxy-15-methylidenespiroirid-16-enal, iso-iridogermanal, belamcandal, deacetyl belamcandal, 16- *O*-acetyl iso-iridogermanal [4].

4) Belamcandols A and B [5].

Pharmacology

1) Antibacterial effects.

2) Anti-inflammatory effects [2].

3) Promote saliva secretion.

4) Belamcandal stimulates throat mucous membrane [4].

5) Inhibitory effects of belamcandol A on 5-lipoxygenase [5].

6) Allergy inhibitory effects (tectorigenin) [6].

Literatures:

[1] Wu, Y. X. et al.: *Yaoxue Xuebao* **1992**, 27, 64-8.

[2] Hu, X. L.: *Chung Yao Tung Pao* **1982**, 7, 29-30.

[3] Bate-Smith, E. C. et al.: *Nature* **1963**, 198, 1307-8.

[4] Abe, F. et al.: *Phytochem.* **1991**, 30, 3379-82.

[5] Fukuyama, Y. et al.: *Chem. Pharm. Bull.* **1991**, 39, 1877-9.

[6] Tsuchiya, H. et al.: *Jpn. Kokai Tokkyo Koho JP* 63 30,417 [88 30,417]. **1988**.

[7] Lee, S. O. et al.: *Saengyak Hakhoechi* **1989**, 20, 219-22.

[8] Yamaki, M. et al.: *Planta Med.* **1990**, 56, 335.

[9] Eu, G. H. et al.: *Saengyak Hakhoechi* **1991**, 22, 13-7.

[P.P.H. But]

187.   *Crocus sativus* **L.**   (Iridaceae)

Fan-hong-hua (C), Fan-hung-fa (H), Safuran (J), Sa-peu-ran (K).

Stigma   (CP, JP, KP)

Local Drug Name: Xi-hong-hua (C), Fan-hung-fa (H), Safuran (J), Sa-peu-ran (K).

Processing: Air dry (C, J).

Method of Administration: Oral (decoction: C, H, J, K).

Folk Medicinal Uses:

1) Women's diseases (J, K).

2) Hypertension (J).

3) Feeling of cold (J).

4) Intestinal catarrh (K).

5) Amenorrhea (H).

6) Hemoptysis (H).

7) Traumatic injury (H).

8) Eruption in infectious diseases (C).

9) Emotional dejection, mania (C).

Scientific Researches:

Chemistry

1) Carotenoids and the degradation products: protocrocin, crocin, crocetin, picrocrocin, safranal [1].

Pharmacology

1) Uterotonic (ethanol extract, ether extract) [2].

2) Inhibition of blood and platelet coagulation (powder) [3].

3) Vasodilation aorta and coronary artery (powder) [4].

4) Inhibition of experimental arterosclerosis (crocetin) [5].

194

Literatures:

[1] Kimura, Y., et al.:*Yakugaku Zasshi* **1953**, 73, 25.

[2] Zhang, P. D., et al:*Yaoxue Xuebao* **1964**, 11, 94.

[3] Nishio, T. et al.:*Shoyakugaku Zasshi* **1987**, 41, 271.

[4] Yu, M. et al.:*Wakan Iyaku Gakkaishi***1987**, 4, 352; Nishimoto, T.:*Ibid.* **1988**, 5, 266.

[5] Gainer, J. L. et al.:*Experientia* **1975**, 31, 548; Pool, J. D. et al.:*Adv. Exp. Med. Biol.* **1976**, 67, 205; Kuwano, S.: *Gendai Toyo Igaku***1983**, 4, 57.

[T. Kimura]

188.   *Iris lactea* **Pall. var.** *chinensis* **Koidz**   (Iridaceae)
                 (= *I. lactea* Pallas; *I. pallasii* var. *chinensis* Frisch)

Ma–lin (C), Nejiayame (J), Ta–rae–but–ggot (K)

Seed

Local Drug Name: Ma–lin–zi (C), Ba–rin–shi (J), Ma–rin–ja (K).

Processing: Eliminate foreign matter, break into pieces after stir–frying or fry with vinegar (C). Dry under the sun (J).

Method of Adminiatration: Oral (decoction: C); topical (powder: C).

Folk Medicinal Uses:

     1) Spitting blood, apostaxis, dysfunctional uterine bleeding (C, J).

     2) Acute infectious icterohepatitis, bone tuberculosis (C).

     3) Hernia (C).

     4) Carbuncle, traumatic bleeding(C, J).

     5) Menorrhagia (J).

     6) Leukorrhea (J).

     7) Sore throat (J).

     8) Epistaxis (J).

     9) Insect or snake bite (J).

     10) Acne (J)

Flower

Local Drug Name: Ma–lin (C), Ba–rin–ka (J), Ma–rin–hwa (K).

Processing: Dry in the shade (C, J).

Method of Adminiatration: Oral (decoction: C, J).

Folk Medicinal Uses:

     1) Spitting blood, hemoptysis, apostaxis, sore throat (C, J).

     2) Oliguria, urinary infection (C).

     3) Carbuncles and boils, traumatic bleeding (C, J).

Root

Local Drug Name: Ma–lin (C), Ba–rin–kon (J), Ma–rin–geun (K).

Processing: Wash clean, cut into sections, dry under the sun (C).

Method of Adminiatration: Oral (decoction: C).

Folk Medicinal Uses:

     1) Acute pharyngitis, infectious hepatitis.

     2) Hemorrhoid.

     3) Toothache.

Scientific Researches :(Seed)

Chemistry

  1) Quinones: pallasone A (inisquinone) [1], pallasone B, C [2].

2) Tritepenes: betulin, lupene–3–one [3].
3) Steroids: β–sitosterol [3].
4) Fatty acid: linolenic acid [4].
Pharmacology
1) Antinidatory effect [5].
2) Antitumor effect (pallasone A) [6].
3) Radiation–resistant effect (pallasone A) [7].
4) Promoting immunologic function (pallasone A) [8].

Literatures:

[1] Wu, S.J. et al.:*Huaxue Xuebao,* **1980,** 38(2), 156.
[2] Wu, S.J. et al.:*ibid,* **1981,** 39(8), 767.
[3] Wu, S.J. et al.:*Zhongcaoyao,* **1984,** 15(4), 1.
[4] Zhang, J.Y. et al.:*ibid,* **1983,** 14(3), 7.
[5] "*Quanguo Zhongcaoyao Huibian*", Vol. 1, **1975,** 85.
[6] Li, D.H. et al.:*Zhongguo Yaoli Xuebao,* **1981,** 2(2), 131.
[7] Wang, S.X. er al.:*Tianjin Yixue,* **1981,** (5), 300.
[8] Li, W.M. et al.:*Yaoxue Tongbao,* **1981,** 16(9), 19.

[J.X. Guo]

189.   *Juncus effusus* L.,   (Juncaceae)
                  J. effusus L. var. *decipiens* Buch.

Deng–xin–cao (C), Dung–sum–cho (H), Igusa (J), Gol–pul (K)

Stem pith (CP) or **whole plant**
Local Drug Name: Deng–xin–cao (C), Dung–sum–cho (H), To–shin–so (J),
            Deung–sim–cho (K).
Processing: Remove pith from stem, cut into sections or fold and tie in bundles.
Method of Administration: Oral (decoction: C, H, J, K).
Folk Medicinal Uses:
          1) Edema (C, H, J, K).
          2) Jaundice (C, H).
          3) Sore throat (C).
          4) Hemorrhoid (C).
          5) Urethritis (C, J).
          6) Hemorrhinia (C).
          7) Fidgetness and insomnia with oliguria (C).
          8) Buccal or tongue ulcer (C).
          9) Toothache (K).

Root
Local Drug Name: Deng–xin–cao-gen (C).
Method of Administration: Oral (decoction: C).
Folk Medicinal Uses:
          1) Jaundice (C).
          2) Mastitis (C).

Scientific Researches:
Chemistry
    1) Undecan–2–one, tridecan–2–one, *p*–methylone–4–en–3–one, α–ionone, β–ionone, 1,2–dihydro–1,5,8–

trimethylnaphthalene, β–bisabolene, *p*–cresol, 6,10,14–trimethyl–pentadecan–2–one, dihydroactinodiolide, cyperone.

2) Luteolin, luteolin–7–glucoside, mono–p–coumaroyl glyceride [1, 2, 5].

3) Phenanthrenes: effusol, dehydroeffusal, dehydroeffusol, dehydrojuncusol, juncunol, juncunone, juncusol, micrandol B and others [2–4].

4) α–Tocopherol [6].

Pharmacology

1) Antitumor and cytotoxic effects [3, 4].

2) Antioxidant and antimicrobial effects [6].

Literatures:

[1] Arisawa, M. et al.:*Shoyogaku Zasshi* **1969**, 23, 49–52.
[2] Shima, K. et al.:*Phytochem.* **1991**, 30, 3149–51.
[3] Della Greca, M. et al.:*Tetrahedron Lett.* **1992**, 33, 5257.
[4] Della Greca, M. et al.:*Tetrahedron* **1993**, 16, 3425–32.
[5] Stabursvik, A.:*Acta Chem. Scand.* **1968**, 22, 2371–3.
[6] Oyaizu, M. et al.:*Yukagaku* **1991**, 40, 511–5.

[P.P.H. But]

190.   *Lophatherum gracile* **Brongn.**   (Gramineae)

Dan–zhu–ye (C), Dam–juk–yip (H), Sasakusa (J), Jo–rit–dae–pul (K)

Whole plant (CP)

Local Drug Name: Dan–zhu–ye (C), Dam–juk–yip (H), Tan–chiku–yo (J), Dam–juk–yeop (K).

Processing: Eliminate foreign matter, cut into sections and dry.

Method of Administration: Oral (decoction: C, H, J).

Folk Medicinal Uses:

      1) Febrile diseases (C, H, J).

      2) Pharyngitis, stomatitis (C, H, J).

      3) Buccal sore, swollen gums (C, H).

      4) Hematuria, oliguria, urinary tract infection (C, H, J).

Contraindications: Pregnancy.

Rhizome and root–tuber

Local Drug Name: Sui–gu–zi (C).

Method of Administration: Oral (decoction: C).

Folk Medicinal Uses:

      1) Febrile disease (C).

      2) Oliguria (C).

Contraindications: Pregnancy.

Scientific Researches:

Chemistry

1) Arundoin, cylindrin, taraxerol, friedelin [1].

Pharmacology

1) Antipyretic effect.

2) Diuretic effect.

3) LD_{50} of methanol–water extract of stem and root are both >1 g/kg i.p. in mice [2].

Literatures:
[1] Ohmoto, T. et al. *Phytochem.* **1970**, 9: 2137–48.
[2] Nakanishi, K. et al. *Chem. Pharm. Bull.* **1965**, 13, 882–90.

[P.P.H. But]

191.   *Oryza sativa* **L.**   (Gramineae)

Dao (C), Do (H), Ine (J), Byeo (K)

Kernel
Local Drug Name: Jing–mi (C), Migh (H), Ko–bei (J), Kyung–mi (K).
Method of Administration: Oral (decoction or cooked rice: C, H, J, K).
Folk Medicinal Uses:
>   1) Dysentery (C, H, J).
>   2) Thirst (C, H, J).
>   3) Fever due to heat stroke (C, H).
>   4) Stomacache (J).
>   5) Erysipelas (K).
>   6) Acute gastritis (J).

Side Effects: rice albumin proteins causes allergy in some persons [7].

Leaf and stem
Local Drug Name: Dao–cao (C), To–so (J), Do–cho (K).
Method of Administration: Oral (decoction: C, J, K).
Folk Medicinal Uses:
>   1) Hiccup (C, J).
>   2) Nausea (C, J).
>   3) Indigestion (C, J).
>   4) Dysentery (C).
>   5) Diabetes (C).
>   6) Jaundice (C).
>   7) Hemorrhoid (C).
>   8) Burns (C).
>   9) Urticaria (K).

Sprout (CP)
Local Drug Name: Dao–ya (C), Guk–nga (H), Koku–ga (J), Gok–a (K).
Processing: (1) Eliminate foreign matter and dry. (2) Stir–fry until dark yellow.
Method of Administration: Oral (decoction: C, H, J, K).
Folk Medicinal Uses:
>   1) Indigestion (C, H, J, K).
>   2) Dysentery (C, H).
>   3) Anroexia (C).

Scientific Researches:
Chemistry
>   1) Oryzacystatin I and oryzacystatin II, both lack disulfide bonds [2].
>   2) Oryzarans A, B, C, D from root [3].
>   3) Polysaccharides: oryzabrans A, B, C, and D from bran [4].
>   4) Momilactones A and B [5].
>   5) 2–Acetyl–1–pyrroline [6].

Pharmacology
1) Boiled and cooled supernatants of rice–water decreased cholera toxin–induced net water secretion or reversed it to net absorption in rats [1].
2) Hypoglycemic effects (oryzarans [3] and oryzabrans [4]).

Literatures:
[1] Rolston, D.D. et al.:*Trans. R. Soc. Trop. Med. Hyg.* **1990**, 84, 156–9.
[2] Abe, K. et al.:*Biomed. Biochim. Acta* **1991**, 50, 637–41.
[3] Hikino, H. et al.:*Planta Med.* **1986**, (6), 490–2.
[4] Hikino, H. et al.:*Planta Med.* **1988**, 54, 1–3.
[5] *J. Chem. Soc. Perkins I* **1977**, 250
[6] Lin, C.F. et al.:*J. Food Sci.* **1990**, 55, 1466–67,1469.
[7] Matsuda, T. et al.:*Agr. Biol. Chem.* **1991**, 55, 509–13.

[P.P.H. But]

192.　　　　　　　　*Phragmites communis* (L.) Trin.　　　　(Gramineae)

Lu–wei (C), Lo–wai (H), Yoshi (J), Gal–dae (K)

Rhizome　(CP)
Local Drug Name: Lu–gen (C), Lo–gun (H), Ro–kon (J), No–geun (K).
Processing: Wash clean, cut into section, dry under the sun (C).
Method of Administration: Oral (decoction: C, H, J, K).
Folk Medicinal Uses:
1) Feverish disease (C, H).
2) Nausea, vomiting (C, J, K).
3) Hiccup (C, J).
4) Pulmonary tuberculosis (C).
5) Constipation (C, J).
6) Sore throat (C).
7) Spermatorrhea (C).
8) Food intoxication (J).
9) Jaundice (J).
10) Peritonitis (K).

Leaf
Local Drug Name: Lu–ye (C), No–yeop (K).
Method of Administration: Oral (decoction: C).
Folk Medicinal Uses:
1) Vomiting (C).
2) Diarrhea (C).
3) Hematemesis (C).
4) Hemorrhinia (C).

Flower
Local Drug Name: Lu–hua (C), No–hwa (K).
Method of Administration: Oral (decoction: C, K).
Folk Medicinal Uses:
1) Vomiting (C).
2) Diarrhea (C).
3) Hemorrhagia (C, K).

4) Hemorrhinia (C).

Scientific Researches:
Chemistry
　1) Coixol, *p*–hydroxybenzaldehyde, vanilic acid, ferulic acid, *p*–coumaric acid [1], tocopherols,
　　　　　polyphenols (caffeic acid, gentisic acid) [2].
　2) Polysaccharide composed of arabinose, xylose and glycose (10:19:94) [3].
　3) Wax [4].
Pharmacology
　1) Inhibitory effects on cyclic adenosine 3',5'-monophosphate phosphodiesterase [1].
　2) Antibacterial effects [2].
　3) Immunomodulatory effects (polysaccharide) [3].

Literatures:
[1] Nikaido, T. et al.:*Chem. Pharm. Bull.* **1984**, 32, 578–84.
[2] Tsitsa–Tzardi, E. et al.:*Ann. Pharm. Fr.* **1990**, 48, 185–91.
[3] Fang, J.N. et al.:*Phytochem.* **1990**, 29, 3019–21.
[4] Kashnoula, T.B. et al.:*J. Agric. Water Resour. Res.***1988**, 7, 49.

[P.P.H. But]

193.　　　　　　　　　　*Trachycarpus wagnerianus* Becc.　　　　　(Palmae)

Zong–lu (C), Chung–lui (H), Toshuro (J), Wae–jong–ryeo–na–mu (K)

Related plant:　　*Trachycarpus fortunei*H. Wendl.: Shuro (J).

Petiole (CP)
　Local Drug Name: Zong–lu (C), Chung–lui–pay (H), Shu–ro (J), Jong–ryeo–pi (K).
　Processing: Ashed.
　Method of Administration: Oral or topical (decoction: C, H, J).
　Folk Medicinal Uses:
　　　　　　　1) Hematemesis (C, H).
　　　　　　　2) Hemorrhinia (C, H, J).
　　　　　　　3) Dysentery (C).
　　　　　　　4) Leukorrhea (C, H).
　　　　　　　5) Traumatic injury (C, J).
　　　　　　　6) Tinea (C).
　　　　　　　7) Uterine bleeding (C).

Fruit
　Local Drug Name: Zong–lu–zi (C), Chung–lui–gee (H), Shu–ro–jitsu (J), Jong–ryeo–ja (K).
　Processing: Eliminate foreign matter, dry under the sun.
　Method of Administration: Oral (decoction: C, H, J).
　Folk Medicinal Uses:
　　　　　　　1) Dysentery (C, J).
　　　　　　　2) Hypertension (C, J).
　　　　　　　3) Leukorrhea (C, H, J).
　　　　　　　4) Spermatorrhea (C).
　　　　　　　5) Cerebral apoplexy (J).

Flower

Local Drug Name: Zong–lu–hua (C), Shu–ro–ka (J), Jone–ryeo–hwa (K).
Method of Administration: Oral (decoction: C, J).
Folk Medicinal Uses:

        1) Dysentery (C).
        2) Hypertension (C, J).
        3) Leukorrhea (C).
        4) Scrofula (C).

Root

Local Drug Name: Zong–lu–gen (C), Shu–ro–kon (J), Jong–ryeo–geun (K).
Processing: Eliminate foreign matter, dry under the sun.
Method of Administration: Oral (decoction: C, J).
Folk Medicinal Uses:

        1) Leukorrea (C).
        2) Scrofula (C).
        3) Hematemesis (C, J).
        4) Traumatic injury (C).
        5) Edema (C).
        6) Hemorrhagia (C, J).

Scientific Researches:

Chemistry
  1) Tannins, leucoanthocyanins [1], fatty acids [2], sialic acids [3], amino acids [4].
  2) Glycosides [5]: glucoluteolin, luteolin–7–O–rutinoside (= scolymoside), dioscin, methyl proto–dioscin, diosgenin 3–O–α–L–rhamnopyranosyl–(1→4)–α–L–rhamnopyranosyl–(1→4)–[α–L–rhamnopyranosyl–(1→2)]–β–D–gluycopyranoside (tentatively named Pb when originally identified in *Paris polyphylla* [6]) and methyl proto–Pb.
Pharmacology
  1) Molluscidal effects [5].

Literatures:

[1] Mizuno, T. et al.: *Nippon Nogei Kagaku Kaishi* **1967**, 41, 512–20.
[2] Litchfield, C.: *Chem. Phys. Lipids* **1970**, 4, 96–103.
[3] Ferrara, L.: *Boll. Soc. Ital. Biol. Sper.* **1975**, 51, 696–8.
[4] Murakoshi, I.: *Shoyakugaku Zasshi* **1984**, 38, 355–8.
[5] Hirai, Y. et al.: *Chem. Pharm. Bull.* **1984**, 32, 295–30.
[6] Nohara, T. et al.: *Chem. Pharm. Bull.* **1973**, 21, 1240–7.

[P.P.H. But]

194.   *Acorus gramineus* **Soland**   (Araliaceae)

Shi–chang–pu (C), Sak–cheong–po (H), Sekisho (J), Seok–chang–po (K)

Rhizome

Local Drug Name: Shi–chang–pu (C), Sak–cheong–po (H), Seki–sho (J), Seok–chang–po (K).
Processing: Dry under the sun (C, H, J, K).
Method of Administration: Oral (decoction: C, H, J, K); bathing (J, K).
Folk Medicinal Uses:

        1) Epilepsy (C, H, J).
        2) Stomach ache (J, K).

3) Rheumatalgia, arthritis (C, H).
4) Traumatic injury (C, H).
5) Gastralgia, abdominal pain (C, H).
6) Amnesia (J).
7) Rheumatism (J).
8) Gynecologic backache (J).
9) Hysteria (J, K).
10) Neurasthenia (K).
11) Delirium (H).
12) Deafness (H).
13) Tinnitus (H).
14) Lumbago (H).
15) Productive cough (H).
16) Gastritis (C).
17) Pleuro–abdominal distension (C).
18) Intestinal colic (C).
19) Chronic tracheitis (C).
20) Carbuncle (C).
21) Sarcoptidosis and tinea (C).

Scientific Researches:
Chemistry
 1) Essential oils: α–asarone, β–asarone, 1–allyl–2,4,5–trimethoxybenzene [1].
 2) Lignans: bisasaricin [2].
Pharmacology
 1) Spasmolytic activity (α–asarone, β–asarone, 1–allyl–2,4,5–trimethoxybenzene) [1].
 2) Hypolipemic activity (bisasaricin) [2].
 3) Induction of structural chromosomal aberrations (β–asarone) [3, 4].

Literatures:
[1] Liu, G. Q. et al.:*Yaoxue Xuebao* **1983,** 4, 95.
[2] Yuan, Y. H. et al.:*Zhongcaoyao* **1982,** 13, 387.
[3] Goggelmann, W. et al.:*Mutat. Res.* **1983,** 121, 191.
[4] Abel, G.:*Planta Med.* **1987,** 251–3.

[C.K. Sung]

195.　　　　　　　　　　　*Pinellia ternata* **Breitenbach**　　　　　　　(Araceae)

Ban–xia (C), Boon–har (H), Karasubishaku (J), Ban–ha (K).

Corm (Tuber) (CP, JP, KP)
Local Drug Name: Ban–xia (C), Boon–har (H), Han–ge (J), Ban–ha (K).
 Processing:　　1) Dry under the sun. 2) Processed with alum. Soak in 8% alum solution until the center is
　　　　　　　　　　devoid of a dry core.
　　　　　　　3) Processed with ginger. Soak in water until the center is devoid of dry core. Add alum and the
　　　　　　　　　　decoction of ginger and boil thoroghly.
　　　　　　　4) Processed with Glycyrrhizae Radix. Soak in water as same above. Remove the water, add
　　　　　　　　　　Glycyrrhiza–lime solution, stir 1–2 times a day with maintain pH 12 until the drug has a
　　　　　　　　　　slight numbing taste and the color becomes yellow. Then, wash and dry (C).
Method of Administration: 1) Oral (decoction: C, H, J, K); topical (rubbed into juice or ground into
　　　　　　　　　　powder and applied after mixing with liquor: C).

Folk Medicinal Uses:
>   1) Vomiting, vomiting of pregnancy (C, H, J, K).
>   2) Pharyngitis (C, J).
>   3) Damp and phlegm (C, H, H, K).
>   4) Headache (C, H).
>   5) Furunculosis (H).
>   6) Eyebrow soot (K).
>   7) Boils, sores and lymphadenitis (externally).
>   8) Cough and asthma with phlegm (C).
>   9) Dizziness and palpitation due to retention of phlegm and fluid (C).
>   10) Vertigo caused by wind–phlegm (C).

Side Effects: Inflammation when used orally unprocessed drug.

Scientific Researches:

Chemistry
>   1) Steroids: β–sitosterol, β–sitosteryl–D–glucoside [1].
>   2) Alkaloids: (–)–ephedrine [2].
>   3) Polysaccharides: araban [3].
>   4) Phenolic compounds: 3,4–diglycosilic benzaldehyde [4].

Pharmacology
>   1) Depression of vomiting (decoction, polysaccharides) [5, 10].
>   2) Saliva secretion (decoction) [6].
>   3) Inhibition of stress ulcer (water extract) [7].
>   4) Increasing serum corticosterone density (water extract) [8].
>   5) Anti–inflammatory (water extract) [9].
>   6) Decreasing secretion of gastric juice and stimulation of bowel movement (50% methanol extract) [10].

Literatures:
[1] Murakami, T., et al.:*Yakugaku Zasshi* **1965,** 85, 832, 845; Ozeki, S.:*Yakugaku Zasshi* **1961,** 81, 1706, **1962,** 82, 766.
[2] Oshio, H., et al.:*Chem. Pharm. Bull.* **1978,** 26, 2096.
[3] Maki, T., et al.:*J. Agr. Food Chem.* **1985,** 33, 1024; *Planta Med.* **1987,** 53, 410.
[4] Suzuki, M.:*Arzneim. –Forsch.* **1969,** 19, 1307.
[5] Suzuki, T.: *Tohoku J. Exptl. Med.* **1931,** 17, 219; Takabe, N.: *Gifu Ikadaigaku Kiyo* **1958,** 6, 243; Maki, T., et al.:*Planta Med.* **1987,** 53, 410.
[6] Takabe, N.: *Gifu Ikadaigaku Kiyo* **1959,** 7, 1279.
[7] Yamazaki, M., et al.:*Shoyakugaku Zasshi* **1981,** 35, 96.
[8] Maeda, T., et al.:*Wakan Iyakugaku Zasshi* **1986,** 3, 450.
[9] Sengoku, T., et al.:*Wakan Iyakugaku Zasshi* **1988,** 5, 470.
[10] Kasahara, Y., et al.:*Shoyakugaku Zasshi* **1983,** 37, 73.

[T. Kimura]

196.   *Typha latifolia* L.   (Typhaceae)

Kuan–ye–xiang–pu (C), Po–wong (H), Gama (J), Keun–bu–deul (K)

Related plants: *Typha angustata* Bory et Chaub.: Zhang–bao–xiang–pu (C), Himegama (J);
                   T. orientalis Presl.: Dong–fong–xiang–pu (C), Kogama (J).

Pollen grain
   Local Drug Name: Pu–huang (C), Po–wong (H), Ho–o (J), Po–hwang (K).
   Processing: Dry under the sun (C, H, J, K).

Method of Administration: Oral (decoction: C, H, J, K); topical (C).

Folk Medicinal Uses:

      1) Contusion (H, J, K).

      2) Hematuria (C, H).

      3) Epistaxis (C, H).

      4) Leukorrhea (C, H).

      5) Scrofula (C, H).

      6) Traumatic injury (H, J).

      7) Edema (K).

      8) Acute gastritis by milk (K).

      9) Aphtha (K).

      10) Mastitis (K).

      11) Melena (J).

      12) Hematemesis (C, J).

      13) Hematochezia and haematuria due to heat in blood (C).

      14) Anemia and abdominalgia due to stagnation of blood (C).

      15) Puerperal abdominalgia caused by stasis (C).

      16) Dysfunctional uterine bleeding (C).

      17) Traumatic bleeding (C).

      18) Lochia (C).

Contraindications: Pregnancy (C).

Scientific Researches:

Chemistry

  1) Flavonoids: isorhamnetin–3–O–glucoside, isorhamnetin 3–O–neohesperidoside, isorhamnetin 3–rutinoside 7–rhamnoside, 3,3'–di–O–methylquercetin 4'–O–glucoside [1–3], naringenin, isorhamnetin, quercetin, kaempferol–3–O–neohesperidoside [9].

  2) Carotenoid like compd.: blumenol A [2].

  3) Sterols: typhasterol [4], (20S)–4–methyl–24–methylene–cholest–7–en–3–ol, β–sitosterol, (20 S)24–methylene–lophenol, stigmas–4–ene–3,6–dione [6–8].

  4) Triterpenes: α–, β–amyrin [7].

Pharmacology

  1) Using as hemostatics, diuretics, uterine contrctants, tuberculostatics (isorhamnetin) [1].

  2) Antihemorrhagic action (flavonoid glucoside) [5].

  3) Plant growth promoting action (typhasterol) [4].

Literature:

[1] Kosuge, T. et al.:*Jpn. Kokai Tokkyo Koho* JP 01,213,294, 28 Aug. **1989**.

[2] Della, G. M. et al.:*J. Nat. Prod.* **1990,** 53(4), 972.

[3] Woo, W. S. et al.:*Phytochem.* **1983,** 22(12), 2882.

[4] Schneider, J. et al.:*Tetrahedron Lett.* **1983**(36), 3859.

[5] Ishida, H. et al.:*Chem. Pharm. Bull.* **1988,** 36(11), 4414.

[6] Della G. M. et al.:*Phytochem.* **1990,** 29(6), 1797.

[7] Hooper, S. et al.:*J. Ethnopharmacol.* **1984,** 10(2), 181.

[8] Aliotta, G. et al.:*J. Chem. Ecol.* **1990,** 16(9), 2637.

[9] Liao, M. et al.:*Zhiwu Xuebao* **1989,** 31(12), 939.

[C.K. Sung]

197.   *Alpinia zerumbet* **(Pers.) Burtt et Smith**   (Zingiberaceae)
                           (= *A. speciosa* K. Schm.)

Yan–shan–jiang (C), Die–cho–kou (H), Getto (J)

Seed
Local Drug Name: Da–cao–kou (C), Die–cho–kou (H), Shiro–de–izu–shuku–sha (J).
Method of Administration: Oral (decoction: C, H, J).
Folk Medicinal Uses:
                1) Stomachache (C, H, J).
                2) Abdominal distention (C, H).
                3) Excessive sputum (C, H).
                4) Indigestion, vomiting (C, H, J).
                5) Diarrhea (C, H, J).

Scientific Researches:
Chemistry
  1) Cardamonin, alpinetin [8], 5,6–dehydrokawain, dihydro–5,6–dehydrokawain [7].
Pharmacology
  1) Anti–platelet aggregation effects (dehydrokawains) [1].
  2) Intra–peritoneal administration of the hydroalcoholic extract at 100 to 1400 mg/kg or oral
                administration of the extract at 2500–18000 mg/kg produced in mice: writhing, psychomotor
                excitation, hypokinesis and pruritus [2].
  3) LD_{50} of the hydroalcoholic extract is 0.760± 0.126 g/kg i.p. and 10.0± 2.5 g/kg p.o. Subacute toxicity
                made by injecting daily for 30 days the LD_{10} in rats caused an increase in transaminases
                and lactate dehydrogenase, whereas other parameters such as blood glucose, urea and
                creatinine were normal. No change in liver, spleen, gut, lung and heart was found [2].
  4) Slight diuretic effects [3].
  5) Hypotensive effects [3].
  6) Protective effects against gastric and duedenal lesions [7].
  7) Anti–ulcer effects [8].

Literatures:
[1] Teng, C.M. et al.: *Chin. J. Physiol.* **1990**, 33, 41–8.
[2] Mendonca, V.L. et al.: *Mem. Inst. Oswaldo Cruz (Brazil)* **1991**, 86 (Suppl 2), 93–7.
[3] Laranja, S.M. et al.: *Mem. Inst. Oswaldo Cruz (Brazil)* **1991**, 86 (Suppl 2), 237–40.
[4] Kimura, Y. et al.: *Yakugaku Zasshi* **1966**, 86, 1184–6.
[5] Fujita, H. et al.: *Yakugaku Zasshi* **1973**, 93, 1635–8.
[6] Hsu, S.Y.: *Taiwan I Hsueh Hui Tsa Chih* **1987**, 86, 58–64.
[7] Hsu, S.Y.: *Chung–hua Yao Hsueh Tsa Chih* **1988**, 40, 41–8.
[8] Krishna, B.M. et al.: *Phytochem.* **1973**, 12, 238.
[9] Wang, Y.T. et al.: *Taiwan I Hsueh Hui Tsa Chih* **1972**, 71, 256–9.

[P.P.H. But]

198.   *Bletilla striata* **(Thunb.) Reichb. f.**   (Orchidaceae)

Bai–ji (C), Bak–kup (H), Shiran (J), Ja–ran (K)

Rhizome (CP)
Local Drug Name: Bai–ji (C), Bak–kup (H), Byak–kyu (J), Baek–geup (K).
Proceesing: Wash clean, soften thoroughly, cut into thin slices, and dry under the sun (C).

Method of Administration: Oral or topical (powder: C, H).
Folk Medicinal Uses:
        1) Hemoptysis in pulmonary tuberculosis, hematemesis in peptic ulcer, trumatic bleeding (C, H, J).
        2) Boils and sores (C, H, J).
        3) Rhagadia of limbs (C, H, J).
        4) Tinea (H).
Contraindications: Incompatible with Radix Aconiti and allied drugs (C).

Scientific Researches:
Chemistry
  1) Stilbenoids: 2,4,7,-trimethoxyphenanethrene, 2,4,7,-tri-methoxy-9,10-dihydropenanthrene, 2,3,4,7- tetramethoxyphenanthrene, 3,5-dimethoxy bibenzyl, 3,3',5-trimethoxybibenzyl [1].
  2) Biphenanthrenes: blestriarens A, B, C, batatasin III, 3'-O-methylbatatasin [2].
  3) Anthroquinones: physcion [1].
  4) Polysaccharides [3].
Pharmacology
  1) Styptic effect [4].
  2) Antibacterial effect [4, 5].
  3) Antitumor effect [6].
  4) Liver-protective effect [7].

Literature:
[1] Yamaki, M. et al.: *Phytochem.*, **1991,** 30(8), 2759.
[2] Yamaki, M. et al.: *ibid*, **1987,** 28(12), 2503.
[3] Tomoda, M. et al.: *Chem. Pharm. Bull.,* **1973**, 31, 2607.
[4] Ma, X.: *Zhonghua Yixue Zazhi,* **1964**, 50, 246.
[5] Wang, Y. et al.: *Zhiwu Xuebao,* **1953,** (2), 312.
[6] Dept. of Chinese Traditionnal and Herbal Drugs, et al.: *Wuhan Yixueyuan Xuebao,* **1978,** (2), 115.
[7] Wu, Z.B. et al.: *ibid*, **1978,** (2), 121.

[J.X. Guo]

199.   *Dendrobium nobile* Lindl.   (Orchidaceae)

Jin-chai-shi-hu (C), Shek-huk (H), Koki-sekkoku (J), Go-gwi-seok-gok (K)

Stem (CP)
  Local Drug Name: Shi-hu (C), Shek-huk (H), Sek-koku (J), Seok-gok (K).
  Processing: Remove roots, wash clean, cut into sections, and dry (C).
  Method of Administration: Oral (decoction: C, H).
  Folk Medicinal Uses:
        1) Feverish disease (C, H, J).
        2) Yin-deficiency (C, H).
        3) Blurry eye (C, H).
        4) Loss of appetite with nausea (C, J).
        5) Night sweating (K).
        6) Lumbago (J).

Scientific Researches:
Chemistry
  1) Alkaloids: Dendrobine [1], dendramine [2, 7], nobilonine [3], dendroxine [4], dendrine, 6-hydroxy-

206

dendroxine, 6–oxydendroxine [5], 4–hydroxydendroxine, nobilomethylene [6].
2) Essential oil: manool [10].
Pharmacology
1) Strychnine–like effects on nervous system (dendrobine) [9].

Literatures:

[1] Onaka, T. et al.:*Chem. Pharm. Bull.* **1964**, 12, 506.
[2] Inubushi, Y. et al.:*Chem. Pharm. Bull.* **1964**, 12, 1175.
[3] Onaka, T. et al.:*Chem. Pharm. Bull.* **1965**, 13, 745.
[4] Okamoto, T. et al.:*Chem. Pharm. Bull.* **1966**, 14, 672.
[5] Okamoto, T. et al.:*Chem. Pharm. Bull.* **1966**, 14, 676.
[6] Okamoto, T. et al.:*Chem. Pharm. Bull.* **1972**, 20, 418.
[7] Inubushi, Y. et al.:*Chem. Pharm. Bull.* **1966**, 14, 668.
[8] Hedman, K. et al.:*Acta Chem. Scand.* **1972**, 26, 3177.
[9] Kudo, Y. et al.:*Br. J. Pharmacol.* **1983**, 78, 709.
[10] Li, M. F. et al.:*Youji Huaxue* **1991**, 11, 219.

[P.P.H. But]

200.   *Gastrodia elata* **Blume**   (Orchidaceae)

Tian–ma (C), Tin–ma (H), Oninoyagara (J), Cheon–ma (K)

Rhizome (CP)
Local Drug Name: Tian–ma (C), Tin–ma (H), Ten–ma (J), Cheon–ma (K).
Processing: Wash clean, steam to soften, cut into slices, and dry (C, J, K).
Method of Adminiatration: Oral (decoction: C, H, J, K).
Folk Medicinal Uses:
    1) Headache, dizziness and numbness of the limbs (C, H, J, K).
    2) Infantile convulsion (C, H, K).
    3) Epilepsy (C, H).
    4) Tetanus (C, H).
    5) Hemiplegia (H).
    6) Neurasthenia (K).
    7) Hemeralopia (K).

Scientific Researches:
Chemistry
1) Phenolic compounds: vanillin [1], gastrodin, *p*–hydroxy–benzyl alcohol [2, 3], *p*–hydroxy–aldehyde
    [3], 4,4'–dihydroxy–diphenylmethane, 4,4'–dihydroxydibenzyl ether, 4–ethoxymethlphenyl
    4'–hydroxybenzyl ether, 3,4–dihydroxybenzaldehyde,*p*–hydroxybenzyl ethyl ether, parishin
    [4], gastrodioside, 4–(4'–hydroxybenzyloxy)benzyl methyl ether, bis–(4–hydroxy–benzyl)–
    ether [5].
2) Organic acids: citric acid, palmitic acid [2], succinic acid [3].
3) Steroids: β–sitosterol, daucosterol [2].
4) Carbohydrates: sucrose [1, 2], polysaccharide [6].
5) Protein: GAFP [7].
Pharmacology
1) Sedative effect (vanillin, gastrodin) [8].
2) Anticonvulsive effect [9, 10].
3) Anti–inflammatory effect [11].
4) Antiepileptic, hypnotic, analgesic effects [12].

5) Antifungal effect (protein) [7].

Literatures:

[1] Liu, X.K. et al.: *Shanghai Diyi Yixueyuan Xuebao,* **1958,** (1), 57.
[2] Fang, X.Z. et al.:*Huaxue Xuebao,* **1979**, 37(3), 175.
[3] Zhou, J. et al.:*ibid,* **1979**, 37(3), 183.
[4] Zhou, J. et al.:*Kexue Tongbao.,* **1981**, 26(18), 1118.
[5] Taguchi, H. et al.:*Chem.Pharm. Bull.* **1981**, 29(1), 55.
[6] Hu, M.Q. et al.: *Tiedao Yixue* **1988**, 16(4), 203.
[7] Hu, Z. et al.:*Yuannan Zhiwu Yanjiu* **1988**, 10(4), 373.
[8] Deng, S.X. et al.:*ibid,* **1979**, 1(2), 66.
[9] Shen, D.X. et al.:*Huaxue Xuebao* **1979**, 37(3), 183.
[10] Jiang, Z.Y. et al.:*Shengli Xuebao* **1961**, 24, 187.
[11] Wang, L.S. et al.:*Zhongcaoyao* **1989**, 20(5), 19.
[12] Lu, G.W. et al.:*ibid*, **1985**, 18(9), 424.

[J.X. Guo]

PLANT NAME INDEX (in Plant No.)

210

中文索引　　（繁体字、简体字、日字）(in Plant No.)

213

MEDICINAL USE INDEX (in Plant No.)

217

febrile 15, 99, 126, 148, 176, 179, 180, 190
fever 9, 11, 13, 14, 15, 21, 28, 30, 31, 37, 42, 44,
 46, 63, 65, 66, 77, 100, 109, 115, 121, 124,
 128, 140, 142, 143, 147, 152, 158, 163, 176,
 191, 192, 198
fever, epidemic 14, 61, 143, 146
fidget 31, 178, 179, 189
filariasis 134
fluid 52, 179, 195
food poisoning 30, 31, 38, 77, 140, 192
fracture 10, 40, 152
freckle 96
frequent urination 7, 27, 103, 175, 180, 184
frigidity 108
frost-bite 7, 11, 28, 56, 63, 69, 100
furuncle 19, 22, 40, 53, 66, 71, 85, 127, 131, 155,
 164, 178, 184, 195

G
galactosemia 94
gallstone 88, 91
gastralgia 96, 98, 194
gastrectasis 152
gastric canser 2, 34, 68, 149, 185
gastric disease 19, 80
gastric ulcer 10, 36, 64, 69, 180
gastritis 51, 65, 78, 85, 92, 105, 107, 108, 136,
 147, 149, 151, 163, 169, 180, 191, 194, 196
gastroatony 85, 108
gastroenteritis 32, 36, 40, 48, 93, 134, 137, 181
gastrointestinal pain 127
gastrointestinal neurosis 108, 162
gastrointestinal disorder 18, 19, 26, 28, 58, 60, 64,
 66, 69, 73, 75, 77, 88, 161, 162
gastropathy 163
gastroptosis 73
gingivitis 20, 68
glaucoma 60
goitre, goiter 17, 141, 185
gonalgia 113
gonorrh(o)ea 33, 56, 68, 105, 151, 164, 172
gout 171
gynecologic back-ache 194

H
hair loss 8
hair, premature greying 16, 123, 148, 150, 165
hang-over 89
harsh throat 49
headache 21, 25, 28, 30, 42, 43, 45, 60, 63, 65, 67,
 93, 106, 111, 115, 119, 128, 131, 135, 136,
 138, 139, 141, 142, 162, 163, 164, 171, 185,
 195, 200
heart disorder 2
heart exitability 19
heart failure 108
heat 177, 191
heat in the blood 18, 126, 143, 196
heat in the liver 67
heat in the lung 38, 143, 146, 176
hematemesis 8, 10, 23, 24, 44, 48, 51, 56, 126,
 142, 143, 148, 164, 165, 175, 177, 178, 185,
 192, 193, 196, 198
hematochezia 48, 67, 81, 133, 142, 164, 196
hematoma 53, 85, 138
hematorrhea 23
hematuria 18, 22, 23, 24, 46, 48, 67, 103, 126,

 129, 131, 138, 146, 150, 151, 164, 165, 172,
 175, 190, 196
hemeralopia 60, 135, 146, 161, 200
hemiplegia 29, 110, 114, 128, 168, 200
hemoptysis 8, 18, 24, 41, 46, 48, 56, 126, 137,
 146, 160, 164, 170, 178, 179, 185, 187, 188,
 198
hemorrhage 6, 8, 13, 32, 36, 56, 67, 137, 192, 193
hemorrhage, duodenal 18
hemorrhage, intestinal 67, 93
hemorrhage, uterine 10, 24, 54, 67, 81, 99, 101,
 108, 143, 159, 164, 185
hemorrhinia 23, 24, 51, 67, 129, 146, 189, 192,
 193
hemorrhoid 10, 13, 14, 15, 20, 23, 24, 30, 41, 53,
 56, 65, 67, 93, 95, 97, 98, 99, 100, 106, 107,
 131, 146, 164, 167, 175, 188, 189, 191
hemostyptic 56
hepatitis 3, 12, 20, 47, 51, 60, 62, 64, 71, 72, 98,
 115, 124, 127, 132, 134, 137, 141, 151, 164,
 165, 168, 169, 188
hepatopathy 97
hepatosplenomegaly 61, 71
heptidis 2
hernia 32, 51, 75, 78, 83, 117, 188
hiccup 5, 51, 89, 175, 191, 192
hoarseness of voice 156
hookworms 62, 83
hydrocele 117
hydrothorax 70
hyperacidity 31, 36, 150
hypercholesterolemia 16
hyperlipemia 16, 172
hyperplasia of breast 141
hypertension 8, 12, 18, 23, 28, 41, 46, 58, 59, 60,
 65, 67, 75, 128, 133, 141, 143, 146, 164,
 168, 173, 183, 187, 193
hypoacidity 152
hypochondria 33, 83
hypofunction 129, 162
hypogalactia 59, 96, 154
hypogastric pain 138
hypotonia 50, 108, 110
hysteria 91, 108, 110, 111, 194

I
icteric hepatitis 98, 127, 188
impaired eyesight 123
impairment of yin 148, 180
impetigo 11, 83
impotence 103, 105, 108, 129, 183
indigestion 3, 17, 56, 78, 174, 191, 197
infantile asthma 150
infantile convulsion 128, 145, 200
infantile epilepsy 5, 29
infantile maldigestion 102
infantile malnutrition 165
inflammation 14, 37, 39, 43, 98, 121, 126, 134,
 143, 151
influenza 6, 12, 40, 61, 63, 157
injury due to fall 152, 181
insect bite 14, 33, 72, 98, 139, 157, 163, 164, 174,
 175, 188
insecticide 82
insomnia 3, 8, 16, 27, 50, 57, 62, 63, 84, 90, 95,
 104, 108, 178, 179, 189
intercostal neuralgia 98

218

swelling, throat 18
syphilis 56, 181
systremma 49, 50

T

taeniasis 48, 87, 98, 101, 130, 181
tenderness 73
tenesmus 73
tetanus 119, 200
thirst 10, 65, 78, 89, 94, 97, 100, 108, 118, 176,
179, 180, 191
thorn sticking 87
threatened abortion 13, 143, 159, 166
throat ache 14, 49, 180
throat, swelling 18
thrombotic angiitis 86
thyroid tumor 185
tinea capitis 39, 83
tinea pedis 19, 66, 76, 82, 93, 99, 101, 111, 125,
142, 153, 165, 174, 175, 182, 186, 193, 194,
198
tinnitus 103, 123, 129, 148, 165, 194
tongue ulcer 189
tonic 175
tonsillitis 14, 21, 30, 48, 62, 66, 68, 82, 86, 101,
132, 137, 147, 167, 169, 186
toothache 10, 11, 20, 25, 31, 42, 47, 75, 76, 79,
99, 111, 139, 145, 175, 188, 189
toxicity reduction 64
tracheitis 8, 47, 113, 147, 194
trachoma 151
traumatic injury 10, 13, 18, 20, 21, 22, 23, 28, 39,
40, 43, 44, 45, 48, 53, 54, 56, 57, 59, 61, 71,
76, 78, 79, 83, 85, 104, 105, 109, 114, 127,
128, 134, 135, 137, 139, 145, 148, 159, 173,
175, 181, 187, 188, 193, 194, 196, 198
trichomoniasis 48, 53, 62, 83
tuberculosis 31, 46, 62, 98, 100, 127, 141, 178,
182, 185, 188, 198
tuberculous adenopathy 16
tumor 2, 3, 4, 85
twist 126
tympanitis 38, 56, 71

U

ulcer 10, 13, 30, 36, 42, 64, 76, 77, 96, 165, 189,
198
upper respiratory infection 121, 137, 157, 167, 169
urethral calculus 21, 46, 151
urethritis 4, 17, 38, 134, 189
urinary calculus 21, 46, 151
urinary tract disease 5, 13, 20, 23, 24, 32
urinary tract infection 38, 77, 94, 121, 132, 134,
147, 169, 172, 188, 190
urination, frequent 7, 27, 103, 175, 180, 184
urolithiasis 21, 46, 151
urticaria 11, 16, 24, 78, 83, 119, 147, 171, 191
uterine bleeding 46, 99, 101, 142, 159, 164, 165,
171, 185, 188, 193, 196
uterine hemorrhage 10, 24, 54, 67, 81, 99, 101,
108, 143, 159, 164, 185
uterus cancer 147
uveitis 23

V

valetudinarianism 154
vertigo 75, 123, 142, 172, 195

vexation 63
vitiligo 129
vomiting 15, 49, 50, 51, 62, 74, 89, 93, 108, 117,
136, 143, 166, 172, 192, 195, 197
vomiting of pregnancy 140, 195

W

water eczema 125
weakness 3, 5, 8, 12, 16, 27, 37, 49, 50, 58, 68,
75, 103, 104, 105, 108, 109, 110, 116, 122,
123, 148, 150, 153, 162, 163, 165, 178, 180,
184
wheezing 27, 28, 140, 186
whooping cough 31, 36, 98, 127, 166, 174, 182,
185
wind dampness, pathogenic 36, 49, 59, 61
wind expulsion 113
wind-cold 171
wind-heat 163, 177
wind-phlegm 195
withdrawn nipple 98
women's disease 43, 44, 53, 110, 116, 187

221

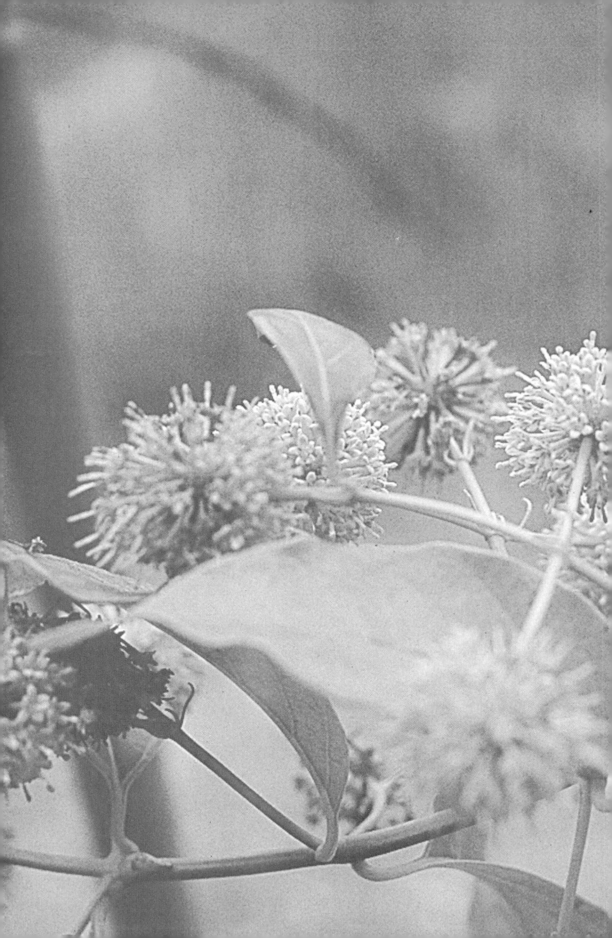